IMMUNOPATHOLOGY

VIIIth INTERNATIONAL SYMPOSIUM, 1980

Academic Press Rapid Manuscript Reproduction

Immunopathology

VIIIth INTERNATIONAL SYMPOSIUM, 1980

Held at San Diego, California
October 27–November 1, 1980

Edited by

FRANK J. DIXON
DEPARTMENT OF IMMUNOPATHOLOGY
RESEARCH INSTITUTE OF SCRIPPS CLINIC
SCRIPPS CLINIC AND RESEARCH FOUNDATION
LA JOLLA, CALIFORNIA

PETER A. MIESCHER
DIVISION D'HÉMATOLOGIE
ET CENTRE DE TRANSFUSION SANGUINE
HÔPITAL CANTONAL
GENEVA, SWITZERLAND

1982

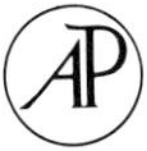

ACADEMIC PRESS

A Subsidiary of Harcourt Brace Jovanovich, Publishers

New York London
Paris San Diego San Francisco São Paulo Sydney Tokyo Toronto

ACADEMIC PRESS, INC.
111 Fifth Avenue, New York, New York 10003

United Kingdom Edition published by
ACADEMIC PRESS, INC. (LONDON) LTD.
24/28 Oval Road, London NW1 7DX

Library of Congress Cataloging in Publication Data
Main entry under title:

Immunopathology : VIII international symposium 1980.

Includes index.
1. Immunopathology--Congresses. I. Dixon, Frank J.
(Frank James), Date. II. Miescher, Peter A.
III. Title. [DNLM: 1. Allergy and immunology--Congresses.
2. Pathology--Congresses. QW 504 I3657 1980]
RC582.15.I48 616.07'9 81-19120
ISBN 0-12-218320-7 AACR2

PRINTED IN THE UNITED STATES OF AMERICA

82 83 84 85 9 8 7 6 5 4 3 2 1

Contents

Cellular Aspects of Murine SLE

Argyrios N. Theofilopoulos and Frank J. Dixon

Retroviral Gene Expression and Murine Systemic Lupus Erythmatosus

Shozo Izui, Ikuo Hara, Vicki E. Kelley, John E. Elder, Patricia J. McConahey, and Frank J. Dixon

Monoclonal Lupus Autoantibodies

Joyce Rauch, Eileen Lafer, Chester Andrzejewski, Jr., Robert S. Schwartz, and B. David Stollar

Alterations of Estrogen Metabolism in SLE

Robert G. Lahita and Henry G. Kunkel

Antibody-Mediated Tubulointerstitial Nephritis

B. Noble, J. R. Brentjens, and G. A. Andres

Human Lymphoplasmacytic Proliferations with Production of Structurally Abnormal Immunoglobulins

Jean-Louis Preud'homme and Maxime Seligmann

Treatment of Autoimmune Diseases with Total Lymphoid Irradiation (TLI)

Samuel Strober, Brian L. Kotzin, and David J. Schurman

Complement Defects, Immunological Health, and Immunological Disease

Peter Lachmann

In Vivo Studies of Fc Receptor Dependent Clearance: Defects in Autoimmune Disease Associated With The HLA B8 DRw3 Haplotype

Michael M. Frank

The Unusual Functional and Structural Versatility of C3 and the Initiation of the Alternative Complement Pathway

Hans J. Müller-Eberhard, Robert D. Schreiber, and Michael K. Pangburn

Complement Receptors—Biological and Biochemical Characterization

Manfred P. Dierich

Biochemistry and Pathophysiologic Effects of the Hageman Factor System

Charles G. Cochrane

Lung Injury Produced by Oxygen Metabolites

Peter A. Ward, Joseph C. Fantone, and Kent Johnson

Contributors

Numbers in parentheses indicate the pages on which the authors' contributions begin.

Guiseppe A. Andres (305), Department of Microbiology, Pathology, and Medicine, State University of New York at Buffalo, Buffalo, New York 14214

Chester Andrzejewski, Jr. (285), Cancer Research Center, Tufts University School of Medicine, Boston, Massachusetts 02152

Deborah P. Beebe (531), Department of Molecular Immunology, Research Institute of Scripps Clinic, La Jolla, California 92037

Dennis J. Beer (77), The Division of Allergy and Immunology and of Experimental Medicine, Department of Medicine, Tufts–New England Medical Center Hospital, Boston, Massachusetts 02111

Barry Bloom (475), Departments of Immunology and Microbiology and of Molecular Pharmacology, Albert Einstein College of Medicine, The Bronx, New York 10461

J. R. Brentjens (305), Department of Microbiology, Pathology, and Medicine, State University of New York at Buffalo, Buffalo, New York 14214

Henry N. Claman (57), Departments of Medicine and of Microbiology and Immunology, University of Colorado School of Medicine, Denver, Colorado 80262

Charles G. Cochrane (443), Department of Immunopathology, Research Institute of Scripps Clinic, La Jolla, California 92037

Neil R. Cooper (531), Department of Molecular Immunology, Research Institute of Scripps Clinic, La Jolla, California 92037

Joseph M. Davie (95), Department of Microbiology and Immunology, Washington University School of Medicine, St. Louis, Missouri 63110

Marc H. De Baets[1] (201), Department of Immunopathology, Research Institute of Scripps Clinic, La Jolla, California 92037, and The Receptor Biology Laboratory, The Salk Institute for Biological Studies, San Diego, California 92112

Manfred P. Dierich (421), Institut für Medizinische Mikrobiologie der Johannes-Guttenberg-Universität, D-6500 Mainz, Federal Republic of Germany

Charles A. Dinarello (77), The Division of Allergy and Immunology and of Experimental Medicine, Department of Medicine, Tufts–New England Medical Center Hospital, Boston, Massachusetts 02111

Frank J. Dixon (225, 263), Department of Immunopathology, Research Institute of Scripps Clinic, La Jolla, California 92037

Thomas S. Edgington (25), Department of Molecular Immunology, Research Institute of Scripps Clinic, La Jolla, California 92037

John E. Elder (263), Department of Immunopathology, Research Institute of Scripps Clinic, La Jolla, California 92037

Daryl S. Fair (25), Department of Molecular Immunology, Research Institute of Scripps Clinic, La Jolla, California 92037

Joseph C. Fantone (459), Department of Pathology, The University of Michigan Medical School, Ann Arbor, Michigan 48109

Carmen Fernandez (129), Department of Immunobiology, Karolinska Institute, Wallenberglaboratory, Stockholm, Sweden

Michael M. Frank (387), Laboratory of Clinical Investigation, National Institute of Allergy and Infectious Diseases, National Institutes of Health, Bethesda, Maryland 20205

Robert S. Fujinami (491), Department of Immunopathology, Research Institute of Scripps Clinic, La Jolla, California 92037

Elizabeth E. Grabau (475), Department of Biology, University of California at San Diego, La Jolla, California 92093

Ikuo Hara[3] (263), Department of Pathology, Montefiore Hospital, Pittsburgh, Pennsylvania 15213

Kyoko Hayakawa (149), Department of Immunology, Faculty of Medicine, University of Tokyo, Tokyo, Japan

Keiichi Hiramatsu (149), Department of Medicine and Microbiology, The Johns Hopkins University, School of Medicine at the Good Samaritan Hospital, Baltimore, Maryland 21239

Mutsuomi Hirashima[2] (111), Department of Medicine and Microbiology, The Johns Hopkins University School of Medicine at the Good Samaritan Hospital, Baltimore, Maryland 21239

John J. Holland (475), Department of Biology, University of California at San Diego, La Jolla, California 92093

Frank Horodyski (475), Department of Biology, University of California at San Diego, La Jolla, California 92093

Peter Isakson (165), Department of Microbiology, Southwestern Medical School, University of Texas Health Science Center, Dallas, Texas 75235

Kimishige Ishizaka[4] (111), Department of Medicine and Microbiology, The Johns Hopkins University, School of Medicine at the Good Samaritan Hospital, Baltimore, Maryland 21239

Shozo Izui[5] (263), Department of Immunopathology, Research Institute of Scripps Clinic, La Jolla, California 92037

Kent Johnson (459), Department of Pathology, The University of Michigan Medical School, Ann Arbor, Michigan 48109

Charlotte Jones (475), Department of Biology, University of California at San Diego, La Jolla, California 92037

David H. Katz (1), The Department of Cellular and Developmental Immunology, Research Institute of Scripps Clinic, La Jolla, California 92037

Vicki E. Kelley[6] (263), Department of Pathology, Montefiore Hospital, Pittsburgh, Pennsylvania 15213

Norman R. Klinman (179), Department of Immunopathology, Research Institute of Scripps Clinic, La Jolla, California 92037

Brian L. Kotzin (345), Division of Immunology, Department of Medicine, Stanford University School of Medicine, Stanford, California 94305

Keith Krolick (165), Department of Microbiology, Southwestern Medical School, University of Texas Health Science Center, Dallas, Texas 75235

Henry G. Kunkel (293), The Rockefeller University, New York, New York 10021

Peter Lachmann (365), MRC Unit on Mechanisms in Tumour Immunity, Cambridge CB2 2QH, England

Eileen Lafer (285), Departments of Biochemistry and Pharmacology, Tufts University School of Medicine, Boston, Massachusetts 02111

Robert G. Lahita (293), The Rockefeller University, New York, New York 10021

Gary A. Levy[7] (25), Department of Molecular Immunology, Research Institute of Scripps Clinic, La Jolla, California 92037

Jon M. Lindstrom (201), The Receptor Biology Laboratory, The Salk Institute for Biological Studies, San Diego, California 92112

Patricia J. McConahey (263), Department of Immunopathology, Research Institute of Scripps Clinic, La Jolla, California 92037

John P. McKearn (95), Department of Microbiology and Immunology, Washington University School of Medicine, St. Louis, Missouri 63110

Stephen D. Miller (57), Departments of Medicine and of Microbiology and Immunology, University of Colorado School of Medicine, Denver, Colorado 80220

Nagahiro Minato (475), Departments of Immunology and Microbiology and of Molecular Pharmacology, Albert Einstein College of Medicine, The Bronx, New York 10461

Göran Möller (129), Department of Immunobiology, Karolinska Institute, Wallenberglaboratory, Stockholm, Sweden

John W. Moorhead (57), Departments of Medicine and of Microbiology and Immunology, University of Colorado School of Medicine, Denver, Colorado 80220

Hans J. Müller–Eberhard (399), Department of Molecular Immunology, Research Institute of Scripps Clinic, La Jolla, California 92037

Moon Nahm (95), Department of Microbiology and Immunology, Washington University School of Medicine, St. Louis, Missouri 63110

Glen R. Nemerow (531), Department of Molecular Immunology, Research Institute of Scripps Clinic, La Jolla, California 92037

B. Noble (305), Department of Microbiology, School of Medicine, State University of New York at Buffalo, Buffalo, New York 14214

Erling Norrby (509), Department of Virology, Karolinska Institute School of Medicine, Stockholm, Sweden

Michael B. A. Oldstone (491), Department of Immunopathology, Research Institute of Scripps Clinic, La Jolla, California 92037

Claes Orvell (509), Department of Virology, Karolinska Institute School of Medicine, Stockholm, Sweden

Michael K. Pangburn (399), Department of Molecular Immunology, Research Institute of Scripps Clinic, La Jolla, California 92037

Jeff W. Paslay[8] (95), Department of Microbiology and Immunology, Washington University School of Medicine, St. Louis, Missouri 63110

Jean-Louis Preud'homme[9] (331), Laboratoire d'Immunochimie et d'Immunopathologie (INSERM U 108), Institut de Recherches sur les Maladies du Sang de l'Université Paris VII, Laboratoire d'Oncologie et d'Immuno-Hématologie due C.N.R.S., Hôpital Saint-Louis, 75475 Paris Cedex 10, France

Ellen Puré (165), Department of Microbiology, Southwestern Medical School, University of Texas Health Science Center, Dallas, Texas 75235

Joyce Rauch[10] (285), Department of Medicine, Tufts University School of Medicine, Boston, Massachusetts 02111

Lola Reid (475), Departments of Immunology and Microbiology and of Molecular Pharmacology, Albert Einstein College of Medicine, The Bronx, New York 10461

Ross E. Rocklin (77), The Division of Allergy and Immunology and of Experimental Medicine, Department of Medicine, Tufts–New England Medical Center Hospital, Boston, Massachusetts 02111

Lanny J. Rosenwasser (77), The Division of Allergy and Immunology and of Experimental Medicine, Department of Medicine, Tufts–New England Medical Center Hospital, Boston, Massachusetts 02111

Robert D. Schreiber (399), Department of Molecular Immunology, Research Institute of Scripps Clinic, La Jolla, California 92037

David J. Schurman (345), Departments of Medicine and Surgery, Stanford University School of Medicine, Stanford, California 94305

Bradford S. Schwartz[11] (25), Department of Molecular Immunology, Research Institute of Scripps Clinic, La Jolla, California 92037

Robert S. Schwartz (285), Department of Medicine, Tufts University School of Medicine, Boston, Msssachusetts 02111

Maxime Seligmann (331), Laboratoire d'Immunochimie et d'Immunopathologie (INSERM U 108), Institut de Recherches sur les Maladies du Sang de l'Université Paris VII, Laboratoire d'Oncologie et d'Immuno-Hématologie du C.N.R.S., Hôpital Saint-Louis, 75475 Paris Cedex 10, France

John H. Slack (95), Department of Microbiology and Immunology, Washington University School of Medicine, St. Louis, Missouri 63110

Katherine Spindler (475), Department of Biology, University of California at San Diego, La Jolla, California 92037

Andrzej A. Stanisz (95), Department of Microbiology and Immunology, Washington University School of Medicine, St. Louis, Missouri 63110

B. David Stollar (285), Departments of Biochemistry and Pharmacology, Tufts University School of Medicine, Boston, Massachusetts 02111

Samuel Strober (345), Division of Immunology, Department of Medicine, Stanford University School of Medicine, Stanford, California 94305

Masaki Suemura[12] (111), Department of Medicine and Microbiology, The Johns Hopkins University, School of Medicine at the Good Samaritan Hospital, Baltimore, Maryland 21239

Gen Suzuki (149), Department of Immunology, Faculty of Medicine, University of Tokyo, Tokyo, Japan

Tomio Tada (149), Department of Immunology, Faculty of Medicine, University of Tokyo, Tokyo, Japan

Masaru Taniguchi (149), Department of Immunology, School of Medicine, Chiba University, Chiba, Japan

Judy M. Teale (179), Department of Immunopathology, Research Institute of Scripps Clinic, La Jolla, California 92037

Argyrios N. Theofilopoulos (225), Department of Immunopathology, Research Institute of Scripps Clinic, La Jolla, California 92037

Jonathan W. Uhr (165), Department of Microbiology, Southwestern Medical School, University of Texas Health Science Center, Dallas, Texas 75235

Ellen S. Vitetta (165), Department of Microbiology, Southwestern Medical School, University of Texas Health Science Center, Dallas, Texas 75235

Peter A. Ward (459), Department of Pathology, The University of Michigan, Medical School, Ann Arbor, Michigan 48109

William O. Weigle (201), Department of Immunopathology, Research Institute of Scripps Clinic, La Jolla, California 92037

Junji Yodoi[13] (111), Department of Medicine and Microbiology, The Johns Hopkins University, School of Medicine at the Good Samaritan Hospital, Baltimore, Maryland 21239

[1]*Present address:* Department of Immunology, Rijksuniversiteit, Limburg Biomedical Center, 6200 MD Maastricht, The Netherlands.

[2]*Present address:* Kumamoto University School of Medicine, Kumamoto 860, Japan.

[3]*Present address:* Okayama University Medical School, Okayama, Japan.

[4]*Present address:* Department of Immunology and Medicine, The Johns Hopkins University School of Medicine at the Good Samaritan Hospital, Baltimore, Maryland 21239.

[5]*Present address:* WHO Immunology Research and Training Center, Geneva 4, Switzerland.

[6]*Present address:* Department of Medicine, Brigham and Women's Hospital, Boston, Massachusetts 02115.

[7]*Present address:* Department of Medicine, University of Toronto, Toronto, Ontario, Canada.

[8]*Present address:* Hypersensitivity Diseases, The Upjohn Company, Kalamazoo, Michigan 49001.

[9]*Present address:* Laboratory of Immunology and Immunopathology, La Milétrie, 86021 Potiers Cedex, France.

[10]*Present address:* Montreal General Hospital Research Institute, Montreal, Quebec H3G 1A4, Canada.

[11]*Present address:* Department of Medicine, University of Wisconsin, Madison, Wisconsin 53792.

[12]*Present address:* Department of Medicine, Osaka University, Osaka, Japan.

[13]*Present address:* Faculty of Medicine, Kyoto University, Sakyo 606, Japan.

Preface

The term "immunopathology" emerged in the late 1950s out of rapid developments in research on the immunological aspects of various disease conditions. At the first International Symposium on Immunopathology held in 1958, R.R.A. Coombs defined the new term as follows: "Immunopathology covers all immune phenomena associated with general pathology, the majority of the reactions of course being physiogenic and beneficial to the host, others being inconsequential or even harmful."

On the occasion of this first symposium, a small group of clinicians and pathologists decided to found an international committee of immunopathology, whose purpose would be, via symposia, to further collaborative efforts among basic scientists, pathologists, microbiologists, and clinicians concerning this new subject. This book sets out the proceedings of the eighth meeting in this series.

Whereas in 1958 the number of immunopathologists was fewer than 100, this field has grown rapidly with the explosive development of basic and applied immunology. However, the problem of rapidly integrating acquired basic knowledge into the overall structure of patient care remains. Because of the fact that there are very few disease states not caused by, complicated by, or accompanied by, immunologic phenomena the impact of immunopathology has been tremendous.

The VIIIth International Symposium reflects this tremendous proliferation. In particular, immunogenetics has become the leading, most rapidly advancing topic over the past 10 years. The most remarkable advances in molecular biology have indeed relied upon the application of genetic methodology to the elucidation of immunological phenomena. Immunogenetics has already had a marked impact on clinical medicine by putting into perspective conditions such as rheumatoid arthritis, systemic lupus erythematosus, multiple sclerosis, and a number of other "autoimmune diseases."

Other topics discussed at the Symposium included: cell-to-cell interactions, regulation of the immune response, and immunological tolerance. Furthermore, some papers dealt with the various pathogenic mechanisms mediated by immunological phenomena in animal models, in particular murine SLE.

As in the past, the main aim of publishing the symposium proceedings is to permit clinicians and pathologists to keep abreast of fascinating developments in basic research relevant to disease-related problems. At the same time, the basic scientist needs to remain in touch with clinical problems. Indeed, scientists engaged in basic biomedical research as well as applied research and clinical medicine are all fighting for a common goal, i.e., prevention of disease and care of the sick. With such an explosive development in immunology at the basic level, this need for exchange of information at all stages has become especially relevant if the patients are to benefit from this progress with minimal delay.

These papers stem from talks originally presented in San Diego, California, October 27 to November 1, 1980, sponsored by the Research Institute of Scripps Clinic. The organizers and speakers greatly appreciate support by Lilly Research Laboratories, a Division of Eli Lilly and Company, that made this seminar possible.

Immunopathology: VIIIth International Symposium, 1980

SELF-RECOGNITION AS THE BASIS OF CELL COMMUNICATION IN REGULATION OF IMMUNE RESPONSES[1]

David H. Katz

The Department of Cellular
and Developmental Immunology,
Scripps Clinic and Research Foundation,
La Jolla, California

I. INTRODUCTION[2]

Since the discovery of immune response (*Ir*) genes by Benacerraf and McDevitt and their colleagues (1), much effort has been directed toward delineating the nature of these genes

[1]*This is publication number 207 from the Department of Cellular and Developmental Immunology and publication number 2302 from the Immunology Departments, Research Institute of Scripps Clinic, La Jolla, California. This work was supported by U.S. Public Health Service Grant AI-13781 and March of Dimes Birth Defects Foundation Grant 1-540.*

[2]*Abbreviations used in this paper: ASC,* Ascaris suum *extract; CFA, complete Freund's adjuvant;* CI, *cell interaction; CTL, cytotoxic T lymphocyte; DNP, 2,4-dinitrophenyl hapten; DTH, delayed-type hypersensitivity; GLT, synthetic random terpolymer of* L-*glutamic acid*^{57}, L-*lysine*^{38}, L-*tyrosine*^{5}*; GLΦ, synthetic random terpolymer of* L-*glutamic acid*^{53}, L-*lysine*^{36}, L-*phenylalanine*^{11}*;* Ir *gene, immune response gene; KLH, keyhole limpet hemocyanin; MHC, major histocompatibility complex; (T,G)-A-L, synthetic branched-chain polymer of (Tyr,Glu)-Ala-*dl-*Lys*.

ISBN 0-12-218320-7

and the mechanism by which they determine the ability of an individual to develop an immune response to a specific antigen. The discovery of major histocompatibility (MHC)-linked genetic control of interactions between T cells and B cells (10, 11, 22) and between T cells and macrophages (27, 28) added additional complexities to these questions, particularly when the cell interaction (*CI*) genes were mapped to the *I* region of the murine *H-2* complex (12, 13).

Even before the final mapping of *CI* genes to the *I* region had been accomplished, experimental evidence was obtained strongly indicating a crucial functional linkage between *CI* and *Ir* genes. The first such evidence was the observation that T cells from (responder × nonresponder) F_1 hybrids primed to the synthetic terpolymer L-glutamic acid, L-lysine, L-tyrosine (GLT) to which responses are governed by *Ir-GLT* genes, were restricted in providing GLT-specific help for 2,4-dinitrophenyl (DNP)-primed B cells only from phenotypic responder parental and F_1 donors in response to DNP-GLT; the same F_1 T-cell population was incapable of helping B cells obtained from nonresponder parental donors (12). Since F_1 T cells can indiscriminately interact effectively with partner B cells from either parent when the carrier antigen employed is not one to which responses are governed by a known *Ir* gene (10, 11), this restricted cooperating phenotype in the DNP-GLT experiment clearly signalled a role for *Ir* genes in determining the partner cell preferences in such cooperative interactions.

As detailed elsewhere (7, 8), for this and other reasons we have concluded that *Ir* and *CI* genes are one and the same. Since expression of *CI* genes determines the self-recognition repertoire of the lymphocytes in a given individual, and since this repertoire is subject to adaptive differentiation during which immunocompetent cells perceive the environmental milieu which they inhabit, thus developing a cooperative phenotype dictated by that environment (6-9, 14, 15, 16), one would predict that if *Ir* and *CI* are identical then the immune response phenotype should exhibit plasticity comparable to that already demonstrated for *CI* gene-determined cooperative phenotypes based on the environment in which stem cells differentiate. Indeed, several reports have appeared indicating that this is so in bone marrow chimeras (2, 4, 5, 23, 24, 32).

Previous studies from our own laboratory (17, 18) have prompted us to speculate (8) about the possible occurrence of anti-*CI* molecule receptor responses as an integral component in processes of adaptive differentiation and, hence, in the appearance of plasticity in the self-recognition repertoire. One of these studies (17) was carried out in the *Ir-GLT* system where it was shown that (responder × nonresponder) F_1 GLT-specific helper cells primed under the influence of a responder parental cell-induced allogeneic effect exhibited good cooperative activity for B cells of nonresponder type, while losing their cooperative activity for B cells of responder parental type. A second line of evidence derived from experiments with lymphocytes from bone marrow chimeras or neonatally tolerant mice (20). Such studies made it obvious that the restricted phenotypes observed with cells primed *in situ* in the chimeric environment were actually pseudorestrictions developing as a consequence of environmental restraint; we speculated that such environmental restraint reflected the development of haplotype-specific anti-*CI* receptor responses that would determine the permissiveness versus nonpermissiveness of the development of respective self-recognizing cell subpopulations in a given environment.

In the present study, we returned to the *Ir-GLT* gene system to probe further the validity of such speculations about anti-*CI* receptor responses as an explanation for adaptive differentiation in general and *Ir* gene expression in particular.

These experiments demonstrate rather conclusively that the plasticity of the immune response phenotype of lymphoid cells of a given origin is not determined by the thymic microenvironment, but rather is strikingly influenced by the non-thymic corporeal environment in which differentiation and exposure to antigen take place. Moreover, it appears that the manner in which elements in the corporeal environment determine the *Ir* phenotype could be explained by anti-*CI* receptor responses.

II. THE RESTRICTED COOPERATING PHENOTYPE OF (RESPONDER × NONRESPONDER) F_1 HELPER T CELLS IS NOT AFFECTED BY TRANSPLANTING PARENTAL THYMUS GRAFTS INTO THYMECTOMIZED $F_1 \rightarrow F_1$ BONE MARROW CHIMERAS

Much speculation has been raised in recent years about the contribution of the thymic microenvironment to the adaptive differentiation of T lymphocytes with regard to their self-specificity restriction phenotypes, in general, and to the expression of *Ir* gene function, in particular. The DNP-GLT system provides an excellent model for exploring the contribution of the thymic microenvironment to *Ir* gene phenotype since conventional (responder × nonresponder) F_1 T cells are restricted in their helper activity for partner B cells of responder type (12). If the thymus is the major determining environment for *Ir* gene phenotype, then one might expect that chimeras constructed by reconstituting thymectomized, lethally irradiated F_1 recipients with F_1 bone marrow cells and parental thymus grafts of nonresponder donor origin might display the nonresponder phenotype characteristic of the parental donors of such thymus grafts. The experiment summarized in Fig. 1 illustrates that this is not the case (21).

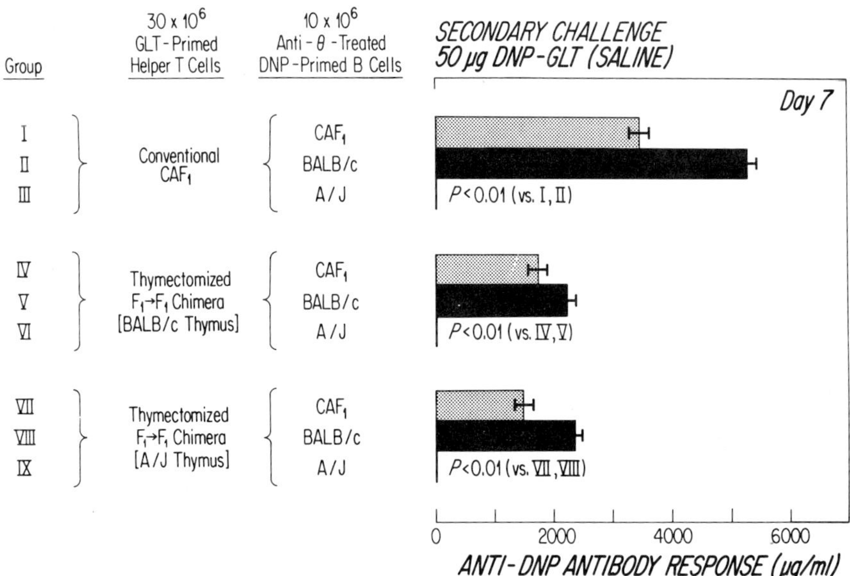

FIGURE 1. The restricted cooperating phenotype of (responder × nonresponder) F_1 helper T cells is not affected by transplanting parental thymus grafts into thymectomized $F_1 \rightarrow F_1$ bone marrow chimeras. Conventional CAF_1 mice and chimeras of the types indicated on the left of the figure were primed with GLT. 30×10^6 spleen cells from such GLT-primed donors were transferred together with 10×10^6 anti-θ-treated DNP-ASC-primed spleen cells from CAF_1, BALB/c or A/J donor mice into 650-rad irradiated CAF_1 recipients. All recipient mice were secondarily challenged with 50 µg of DNP-GLT in saline and bled 7 days later for titration of IgG anti-DNP antibody levels. The data presented on the right of the figure are geometric mean levels and standard errors of serum anti-DNP antibodies in groups of 4 mice each. Relevant *p* values depicting statistically significant differences are indicated beside the corresponding bars.

Groups I-III illustrate the characteristic restricted phenotype of GLT-specific helper T-cell activity of conventional CAF_1 origin which provides excellent helper activity for DNP-primed B cells of responder CAF_1 and BALB/c origins, but not of nonresponder parental A/J origin. Likewise, GLT-specific helper T cells generated in thymectomized $F_1 \rightarrow F_1$

bone marrow chimeras reconstituted with thymus transplants of responder parental BALB/c-type display, as expected, an identical pattern of restricted cooperative activity (groups IV-VI). As shown by groups VII-IX, precisely the same restricted cooperating phenotype is displayed by GLT-specific helper T cells obtained from thymectomized $F_1 \rightarrow F_1$ bone marrow chimeras reconstituted with thymus grafts of nonresponder parental A/J origin.

III. THE CORPOREAL ENVIRONMENT DICTATES THE *Ir* GENE PHENOTYPE IN RESPONSES OF BONE MARROW CHIMERAS TO GLT

It is clear from the preceding results that in the GLT system the cooperating phenotype of (nonresponder × responder) F_1 lymphoid cells differentiating in the environment of F_1 hosts is not influenced to any appreciable extent by the presence of nonresponder parental thymus grafts. In order to explore the influence of the extrathymic corporeal environment on the immune response phenotype, thymic chimeras were constructed by reconstituting lethally irradiated, thymectomized (a) CAF_1, BALB/c, or A/J recipients with CAF_1 bone marrow cells and CAF_1 thymus grafts or (b) CAF_1 recipients with both bone marrow cells and thymus grafts obtained from nonresponder parental A/J donors. These chimeras were then immunized with unconjugated GLT and analyzed for their capacities to develop GLT-specific antibody responses.

As summarized in Table I, $CAF_1 \rightarrow CAF_1$ and $CAF_1 \rightarrow$ BALB/c chimeras, both possessing CAF_1 thymus grafts, developed comparable GLT-specific antibody responses. In striking contrast, chimeras of $CAF_1 \rightarrow$ A/J type possessing thymus grafts of CAF_1 origin failed to produce detectable levels of anti-GLT antibody responses. This failure to respond did not reflect

TABLE I. The Corporeal Environment Dictates the *Ir* Gene Phenotype in Responses of Bone Marrow Chimeras to GLT*

Group	Type of chimera	Antibody responses to: GLT**	KLH***
I	$CAF_1 \rightarrow CAF_1$ [F_1 thymus]	58.7(1.09)	85.7(1.21)
II	$CAF_1 \rightarrow$ BALB/c [F_1 thymus]	57.2(1.16)	Not determined
III	$CAF_1 \rightarrow$ A/J [F_1 thymus]	1.4(1.20)	84.8(1.06)
IV	A/J $\rightarrow CAF_1$ [A/J thymus]	94.7(1.07)	Not determined

*****Radiation bone marrow chimeras were constructed by transferring either CAF_1 bone marrow cells into thymectomized, lethally irradiated (950 rads) CAF_1, BALB/c or A/J recipients (groups I-III) or A/J bone marrow into thymectomized, lethally irradiated CAF_1 recipients (group IV). Recipients were transplanted 2 weeks later with thymuses, of the donor type indicated, under the kidney capsules. All mice were typed for H-2 3 to 4 months after reconstitution and were rested until 9 months after reconstitution before immunization with GLT and/or KLH was performed. Group I consisted of 4 mice and groups II-IV of 3 mice each*

***All mice were immunized ip with 50 μg of GLT in CFA on day 0 and boosted with 50 μg of GLT in saline on day 14. The data presented are mean % binding of ^{125}I-labeled GLT of 1:10 dilutions of individual serum samples from bleedings on day 24 (10 days after boosting). The numbers in parentheses are standard errors.*

****Mice in groups I and III were immunized ip on day 30 (after initiation of GLT immunizations) with 20 μg of KLH in CFA and boosted on day 40 with 10 μg of KLH in saline. The data presented are mean % binding of ^{125}I-labeled KLH of 1:10 dilutions of individual serum samples from bleedings on day 47. The numbers in parentheses are standard errors.*

ineffective thymic reconstitution since such mice were able to develop KLH-specific antibody responses when immunized with unconjugated KLH subsequent to the GLT immunization regimen. On the other hand, chimeras constructed with lymphoid stem cells and thymus grafts of nonresponder A/J parental origin, which had differentiated in the environment of CAF_1 hosts, developed excellent GLT-specific antibody responses (group IV).

IV. GENOTYPIC GLT-RESPONDER BALB/c T CELLS DIFFERENTIATING IN MIXED RESPONDER + NONRESPONDER → F_1 CHIMERIC ENVIRONMENTS PROVIDE GLT-SPECIFIC HELPER ACTIVITY TO F_1, BUT NOT TO EITHER RESPONDER OR NONRESPONDER PARENTAL, B CELLS

In order to ascertain the extent to which lymphoid cells interact with other lymphoid as well as nonlymphoid elements in a chimeric environment, mixed parent chimeras were constructed by reconstituting lethally irradiated CAF_1 recipients with equivalent numbers of responder BALB/c and nonresponder A/J parental bone marrow cells. Six months after reconstitution, these double parent chimeras were primed with GLT in order to generate GLT-specific helper T cells. Spleens were removed from such mice, treated with BALB/c anti-A/J antibodies plus C to remove any cells of parental A/J type or of recipient F_1 type; the remaining "Chim.BALB/c" splenic cells were then tested for cooperative helper activity when cotransferred with DNP-primed B cells of CAF_1, BALB/c, or A/J origin in response to secondary challenge with DNP-GLT. The cooperative phenotype of "Chim.BALB/c" helper T cells was compared with that of GLT-primed helper T cells taken from conventional CAF_1 donors cotransferred with portions of the same populations of DNP-primed cells.

As shown in Fig. 2, GLT-primed conventional CAF_1 helper T cells displayed the normal cooperative phenotype of providing good helper activity for B cells of responder F_1 and parental BALB/c origins, but not for B cells of nonresponder A/J origin. The cooperative phenotype of GLT-primed "Chim.BALB/c" helper T cells provides a striking contrast. Such cells displayed excellent helper activity for DNP-primed partner B cells of CAF_1 type, but failed to engage in effective interactions with either responder BALB/c or nonresponder A/J partner B cells.

The failure of "Chim.BALB/c" T cells to provide GLT-specific helper activity for either BALB/c or A/J partner B cells in response to DNP-GLT is not a reflection of some general abnormality existing in such mixed parental chimeras. Nor are these data a reflection of some unusual properties of the partner B cells employed in this experiment with respect to their ability to interact with mixed parental chimera T cells. Thus, as summarized in Table II, "Chim.BALB/c" helper T cells obtained from the same group of mixed parental → F_1 chimeras, but primed to KLH[3] rather than to GLT, provided adequate helper T cell activity for portions of the same B cells as those used in Fig. 2 in secondary adoptive responses to DNP-KLH. Although such helper activity was comparable with the two parental-type partner B cells (groups II and III), it is noteworthy that significantly higher cooperative responses were obtained between such chimera T cells and CAF_1 B cells (group I). This appears to reflect something particular about the cooperative interactions between "Chim.BALB/c" T cells and F_1 B cells (and not something trivial such as a more hyper-responsive F_1 B cell population) since cooperative responses

[3] *Immunization with KLH was as follows: 20 μg of KLH in CFA ip followed 3 weeks later with 10 μg of KLH in saline; spleen cells taken 10 days after boost.*

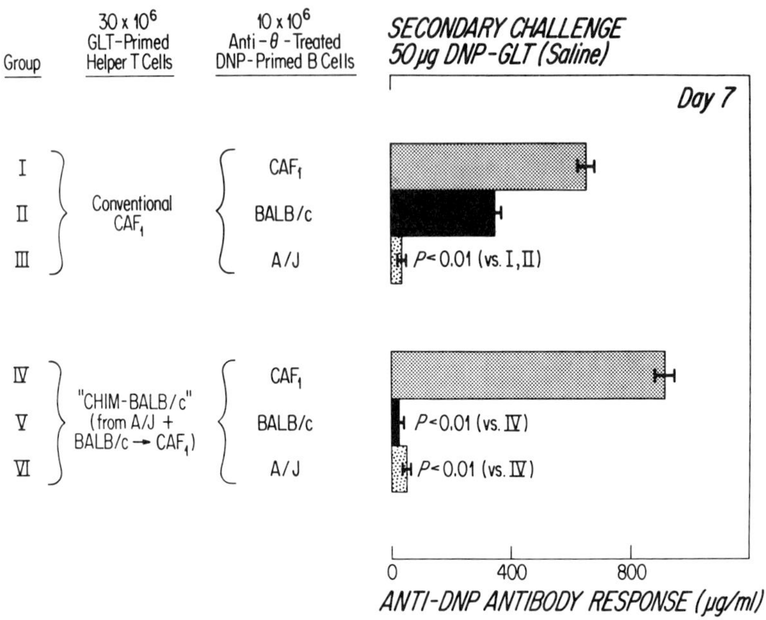

FIGURE 2. Genotypic GLT-responder BALB/c T cells differentiating in mixed responder + nonresponder → F_1 chimeric environments provide GLT-specific helper activity to F_1, but not to either responder or nonresponder parental, B cells. Conventional CAF_1 mice and mixed parental A/J + BALB/c → CAF_1 chimeras were primed to GLT. "Chim.BALB/c" spleen were obtained from such mixed parental → F_1 GLT-primed chimeras by treatment of the spleen cells *in vitro* with BALB/c anti-A/J antibodies + C. 30 × 10^6 GLT-primed conventional CAF_1 and "Chim.BALB/c" spleen cells were transferred together with 10 × 10^6 anti-θ-treated DNP-ASC-primed B cells from CAF_1, BALB/c, or A/J donor mice into 650-rad irradiated CAF_1 recipients. All recipient mice were secondarily challenged with 50 μg of DNP-GLT in saline and bled 7 days later for titration of IgG anti-DNP antibody levels. The data presented on the right of the figure are geometric mean levels and standard errors of serum anti-DNP antibodies in groups of 4 mice each. Relevant *p* values depicting statistically significant differences are indicated beside the corresponding bars.

TABLE II. BALB/c T Cells Differentiating in Mixed Parental → F_1 Chimeric Environments Provide KLH-Specific Helper Activity to Both Parental and F_1 B Cells*

Group	10×10^6 KLH-primed helper T cells	7.5×10^6 DNP B cells	Anti-DNP response (μg/ml - Day 7)
I	"Chim.BALB/c"	CAF_1	7500(1.02)**
II	(from A/J +	BALB/c	2425(1.19)
III	BALB/c → CAF_1)	A/J	1516(1.09)
IV	Conventional CAF_1	CAF_1	2341(1.33)
V		BALB/c	2266(1.26)
VI		A/J	4129(1.36)

Protocol as in Fig. 2 except "Chim.BALB/c" and conventional CAF_1 T cells were primed to KLH and secondary challenge of adoptive recipients was with 20 μg of DNP-KLH in alum. DNP-primed B cells were portions of same populations used in Fig. 2.

**$p < 0.03$ *versus groups II and III.*

between conventional F_1 helper cells and F_1 B cells (group IV) were not significantly different from the cooperative responses between conventional F_1 helper cells and parental BALB/c or A/J B cells (groups V and VI).

V. INTERPRETATIONS

These experiments have demonstrated that the immune response phenotype of a given individual is (a) not dictated by the thymic microenvironment, (b) determined by one or more elements in the extrathymic corporeal environment, and (c) dependent upon as yet undefined interactions between lymphoid stem cells with nonlymphoid corporeal elements and with other cells of lymphoid origin. These conclusions are based on the experiments using thymectomized $F_1 \rightarrow F_1$ chimeras reconstituted with either GLT-responder BALB/c or nonresponder A/J parental thymus grafts (Fig. 1), the caricature of responsiveness to GLT of F_1 → parent and nonresponder parent → F_1 chimeras (Table I), and the unusual cooperating phenotype of responder parental T cells which had differentiated in, and been primed to GLT in, mixed parental → F_1 chimeras (Fig. 2). Some of these observations are in contrast to others reported, whereas others are consistent; the likely explanations for these discrepancies are discussed in detail elsewhere (21).

A. *The Role of Corporeal Elements in Dictating* Ir *Phenotype*

The experiment summarized in Table I appears to offer significant insight into the mechanism(s) by which *Ir* genes determine the immune response phenotype. The most pertinent findings, displayed by groups III and IV, illustrate quite clearly that elements in the corporeal environment determine the *Ir* phenotype of a given individual. This is the only conclusion that one can reach considering that stem cells from phenotypic responder F_1 donors that mature in an environment containing homologous F_1 thymus display the nonresponder phenotype characteristic of the remainder of the corporeal environment provided by the nonresponder parental host. Reciprocally, stem cells from phenotypic nonresponder parental donors differentiate in a corporeal environment provided largely by phenotypic responder F_1 elements, with the exception of the nonresponder parental thymus graft, to display phenotypic responsiveness to GLT. In other words, the *Ir* phenotypes in these circumstances reflect the permissiveness of the phenotypic responder F_1 environment on the one hand and the nonpermissiveness of the phenotypic nonresponder parental environment on the other.

B. *The Nature of the Corporeal Elements Dictating* Ir *Phenotype*

It is impossible to precisely define each (or all) of the elements responsible for dictating *Ir* phenotype. Based on the data from the present study, however, one can hardly escape the conclusion that both nonlymphoid and lymphoid elements participate and, moreover, that these different compartments perceive each other uni- or bidirectionally. Again, this conclusion follows from the data obtained with chimeras in groups III and IV of Table I. In both cases it is clear that nonlymphoid elements of the irradiated host exert a determinative influence on the phenotype of the lymphoid elements reconstituting such individuals that are derived from the donor bone marrow inocula. Thus, it would seem that something(s) within the nonlymphoid compartment is(are) perceived by the lymphoid cells differentiating within such environments and determines permissiveness *versus* nonpermissiveness of the immune response, in this case to GLT. Alternatively, something(s) within the nonlymphoid compartment influences the lymphoid cells within that environment to perceive something(s) about themselves which, in turn, determines permissiveness *versus* nonpermissiveness. Whichever of these alternatives is correct (or both), it is nonetheless clear that interaction(s) between the lymphoid and nonlymphoid compartments is pertinent to, and determinative of, the immune response phenotype of a given individual. Definition of the structure(s) displayed by the nonlymphoid compartment, and even whether MHC genes are related to them, must await further investigation.

It should be noted that no conclusion can be reached about the cellular locus at which the mechanism(s) determining *Ir* phenotype operates. For example, unresponsiveness to GLT displayed by $CAF_1 \rightarrow$ A/J chimeras could reflect a defect at the level of T cells, B cells or macrophages, or any combination thereof, or at one or more of the requisite interactions between such cells. From the data in Fig. 2, it seems clear that nonpermissiveness can at least operate at the level of generation of a relevant subset of GLT-specific helper T cells, but again this could reflect a defect solely at the T cell level or at the level of T-macrophage and/or T-T cell interactions.

C. Responses Against Cell Interaction Molecules Can Determine the Observed Plasticity of the Immune Response Phenotype

As stated at the outset, some of our previous studies (17-20) prompted us to foster the idea that responses against self-specific *CI* molecules may be a central mechanism determining adaptive differentiation of the self-recognition repertoire of a given individual. As postulated elsewhere (8), such anti-*CI* molecule responses could readily explain the mechanism by which *Ir* genes function to determine the *Ir* phenotype; it is only necessary to assume that *Ir* genes encode *CI* molecules. If one considers that *CI* molecules are distinct entities from antigen-specific receptors, then the manner in which *Ir* genes exert such exquisite specificity for antigen in responses over which they display control depends on whether *Ir* genes encode molecules serving as (a) anti-*CI* receptors alone (at least in part), (b) target *CI* molecules themselves, or (c) both anti-*CI* receptors and target *CI* molecules. These three possibilities and the role of responses against self-specific *CI* molecules in determining *Ir* phenotype are explained in detail elsewhere (8); space constraints prohibit full reiteration of these ideas here.

The present experiments are consistent with this notion, and indeed, are difficult to explain by any other mechanism. Thus, it is clear from these findings, as well as from our earlier studies in the *Ir-GLT* system (17) and from the work of others discussed above (2, 5, 23), that expression of *Ir* phenotype is not a reflection of whether or not a given *I* region gene or genes has been deleted from the genome of an individual. Nor, for that matter, is there any structural evidence to indicate whether or not *Ir* phenotype is associated with the expression of the relevant *Ir* gene product(s). Data pertinent to this point in the present study arise from the results obtained with GLT-primed responder BALB/c T cells which had differentiated in the same environment with nonresponder A/J parental cells (Fig. 2). Such cells displayed a cooperating phenotype restricted for DNP-primed partner cells derived from conventional F_1 donors. The fact that differentiation and priming to GLT occurred in an environment where nonresponder parental lymphoid cells were also present obviously determined this unusual cooperating phenotype. We can think of no mechanism by which the presence of the cohabitating nonresponder A/J cells could have regulated expression of the relevant *I* region gene product by responder BALB/c cells that could account for functional deletion of the BALB/c-specific GLT helper T cell subset.

On the other hand, one *can* explain this observation by a mechanism involving responses against self-specific *CI* molecules in the following manner: As shown schematically in Fig. 3, if a nonresponder individual displays that phenotype because, for whatever reason, exposure to GLT evokes a very strong (and early) anti-*CI* molecule response, this would, in turn, blunt any possible response to GLT from developing [for details, see Katz (8)]. Exposure of an individual of a

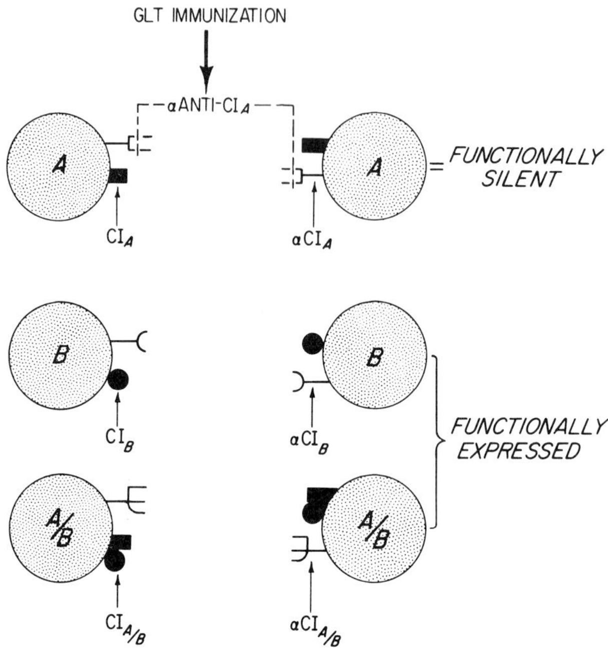

FIGURE 3. Exposure of an ($A \times B$) F_1 hybrid to GLT induces anti-αCI_A responses which render the nonresponder *A* subset functionally silent. Depicted are the 3 minimal subsets of potential self-specific interacting partner cells in heterozygous ($A \times B$) F_1 individuals. Subsets *A* and *B* correspond to the inherited *CI* specificities of the respective parental *A* and *B* donor mice, while subset *A/B* represents a unique F_1-specific subset of interacting cells. The corresponding CI_A, CI_A, and $CI_{A/B}$ target molecules and the corresponding receptors for such molecules (αCI_A, αCI_B, and $\alpha CI_{A/B}$) are depicted. In response to a conventional antigen such as KLH, all 3 subsets of interacting cells would presumably be activated thus explaining the indiscriminate cooperative phenotype of F_1 T cells with partner cells of either parental type or of F_1 type. In contrast, in response to GLT (to which the parent *A* strain is a nonresponder) the model proposes that there develops a rather immediate anti-αCI_A response which renders that particular subset functionally silent; the remaining *B* and *A/B* subsets are functionally expressed hence leading to the phenotype of effective cooperation by GLT-specific F_1 cells for partner cells of parent *B* and ($A \times B$) F_1 type, but no cooperative activity for partner cells of parent *A* type.

responder phenotype to GLT, conversely, would not elicit this type of anti-*CI* molecule response under normal circumstances, and hence the environment of such an individual would be permissive for responses to GLT.

Why, then, does cohabitation of responder cells with nonresponder cells result in nonpermissiveness for the population of responder self-specific cells? This is explained quite simply by the fact that a state of mutual immunological tolerance exists between the cohabitating parental lymphoid cell populations in such chimeras (33). A consequence of such mutual tolerance is the emergence within each parental lymphoid cell population of interacting subsets reciprocally specific (in terms of *CI* molecules expressed and recognized) for the *CI* phenotype of the other parental population (8, 15). Indeed, this point has been experimentally verified (30). It follows from this, therefore, that, for whatever reason GLT evokes a self-specific anti-*CI* response in the nonresponder individual, the state of mutual tolerance in the mixed parental chimeric environment would allow GLT to evoke a comparable response against the *CI* molecules displayed by the corresponding responder-specific subset reactive to GLT that originates from the responder stem cell pool.

The fact that GLT-specific responder helper T cells capable of interacting with B cells of conventional F_1 donor origin were induced in such chimeras implies the existence of (a) an F_1-specific subset of T cells originating from the responder parental lymphoid population and, likewise, (b) a subset of F_1-specific partner B cells (distinct from the subsets corresponding in cooperating specificity for each of the two parental *CI* types) within the conventional CAF_1 partner B-cell population. Moreover, the presence of F_1-specific subsets of T and B cells within the mixed parental chimera explains why such chimeras produced circulating anti-GLT antibodies *in situ* (not shown) despite the absence of detectable GLT-specific helper T cells of BALB/c-specific cooperating potential.[4] The existence of F_1-specific cooperating helper T cells has recently been found in studies performed by Sproviero *et al.* (31) and from our own laboratory (19). The data presented by group IV in Fig. 2 represent, to our knowledge, the first indication of a comparable subset of F_1-specific cooperating B cells.

Recently, Pierce *et al.* (25) reported studies on the helper T-cell repertoires of responder and nonresponder parental and (responder × nonresponder) F_1 mice using the GLΦ (3) system. Using the splenic-fragment culture system, Pierce *et al.* were able to identify three distinct modes of helper T-cell collaborative potential termed, respectively, homologous, isologous, and heterologous [for definitions, see Pierce *et al.* (25)]. They showed that responder mice developed GLΦ-specific T cells capable of interacting homologously with their own syngeneic responder partner B cells as well as isologously (*i.e.*, in a syngeneic fashion) with allogeneic responder B cells in response to DNP-GLΦ. In contrast, nonresponder mice developed GLΦ-specific helper T cells, but only of the type that can interact isologously with partner B cells of the allogeneic responder type; no GLΦ-specific helper T cells displaying homologous interaction capabilities for syngeneic nonresponder partner B cells were observed. Lastly, F_1 mice developed a subset of isologous cooperating cells capable of interacting with partner B cells of the responder parent

[4]*Likewise, the existence of F_1-specific subsets of interacting T and B cells may also explain the observations of Press and McDevitt (26) that mixed (responder + nonresponder) parental → F_1 chimeras display the responder phenotype in response to (T,G)-A-L, although the limitation of the anti-(T,G)-A-L response to antibodies of only responder allotype must reflect an additional mechanism yet to be defined.*

(as well as homologous cooperating cells that could interact with F_1 partner cells), but no subset capable of interacting isologously with partner B cells of nonresponder parent type. Pierce *et al.* concluded that the *Ir* gene mechanism in the GLΦ system involved a functional deletion of a subset of GLΦ-specific helper cells capable of cooperating with partner B cells in a syngeneic fashion. More importantly, as originally shown in our first DNP-GLT experiments (12), their F_1 data demonstrate that the helper T-cell population with potential for collaboration with nonresponder B cells is deleted (functionally) presumably as a result of the presence of the nonresponder MHC gene products in the F_1 environment. We believe that this represents yet another manifestation of responses against self-specific *CI* molecules just as such responses best explain the present data obtained in the *Ir-GLT* system.

An immediate question arises in consideration of these speculations, namely, why must they remain speculations based on indirect evidence? We have no answer for this at present, and it is true that we have had considerable difficulty in obtaining direct experimental evidence proving the existence of such self-specific anti-*CI* molecule responses. Attempts with cell-transfer experiments and searches for circulating molecules (antibodies or otherwise) with the predicted specificities have provided ambiguous results thus far, but are being continued with great vigor. It is noteworthy, in this regard, that Smith and Miller (29) demonstrated quite clearly the presence of a haplotype-specific suppressive mechanism within the chimeric environment of $F_1 \rightarrow$ parent chimeras; however, this suppressive mechanism could only be observed within the chimeric environment and could not be demonstrated by passive transfer of chimeric cells. Preliminary evidence in our own laboratory, again in the *Ir-GLT* system, indicates that the postulated anti-*CI* molecule suppressive mechanism discussed above is acutely radiosensitive, although it recovers in time following exposure to irradiation. Further experiments along such lines should ultimately be successful in clarifying the nature of these phenomena.

ACKNOWLEDGMENTS

The author is grateful to Ms. Rebecca Mead for excellent assistance in the preparation of this manuscript, to Robert F. Bargatze for expert technical assistance in these studies, and to Dr. Paul Maurer, Lee Katz, and Cheryl Bogowitz who collaborated on the original investigations.

REFERENCES

1. Benacerraf, B. and McDevitt, H. O. Histocompatibility-linked immune response genes. *Science 175*, 273 (1972).

2. Billings, P., Burakoff, S. J., Dorf, M. E., and Benacerraf, B. Genetic control of cytolytic T-lymphocyte responses. II. The role of the host genotype in parental → F_1 radiation chimeras in the control of the specificity of cytolytic T-lymphocyte responses to trinitrophenyl modified syngeneic cells. *J. Exp. Med. 148*, 352 (1978).

3. Dorf, M. E. and Benacerraf, B. Complementation of *H-2*-linked *Ir* genes in the mouse. *Proc. Natl. Acad. Sci. U.S.A. 72*, 3671 (1975).

4. Hedrick, S. M. and Watson, J. Genetic control of the immune response to collagen. II. Antibody responses produced in fetal liver restored radiation chimeras and thymus reconstituted F_1 hybrid mice. *J. Exp. Med. 150*, 646 (1979).

5. Kappler, J. W. and Marrack, P. The role of *H-2*-linked genes in helper T-cell function. IV. Importance of T-cell genotype and host environment in *I*-region and *Ir* gene expression. *J. Exp. Med. 148*, 1510 (1978).

6. Katz, D. H. The role of histocompatibility gene complex in lymphocyte differentiation. *Transplant. Proc. 8*, 305 (1976).

7. Katz, D. H. The role of the histocompatibility gene complex in lymphocyte differentiation. *Cold Spring Harbor Symp. Quant. Biol. 41*, 611 (1977).

8. Katz, D. H. Adaptive differentiation of lymphocytes: Theoretical implications for the mechanisms of cell-cell recognition and regulation of immune responses. *Adv. Immunol. 29*, 137 (1980).

9. Katz, D. H. and Benacerraf, B. Genetic control of lymphocyte interactions and differentiation. *In* "The Role of Products of the Histocompatibility Gene Complex in Immune Responses" (D. H. Katz and B. Benacerraf, eds.), p. 355. Academic Press, New York, 1976.

10. Katz, D. H., Hamaoka, T., and Benacerraf, B. Cell interactions between histoincompatible T and B lymphocytes. II. Failure of physiologic cooperative interactions between T and B lymphocytes from allogeneic donor strains in humoral response to hapten-protein conjugates. *J. Exp. Med. 137*, 1405 (1973).

11. Katz, D. H., Hamaoka, T., Dorf, M. E., and Benacerraf, B. Cell interactions between histoincompatible T and B lymphocytes. III. Demonstation that the *H-2* gene complex determines successful physiologic lymphocyte interactions. *Proc. Natl. Acad. Sci. U.S.A. 70*, 2624 (1973).

12. Katz, D. H., Hamoaka, T., Dorf, M. E., Maurer, P. H., and Benacerraf, B. Cell interactions between histoincompatible T and B lymphocytes. IV. Involvement of the immune response (*Ir*) gene in the control of lymphocyte interactions in responses controlled by the gene. *J. Exp. Med. 138*, 734 (1973).

13. Katz, D. H., Graves, M., Dorf, M. E., DiMuzio, H., and Benacerraf, B. Cell interactions between histoincompatible T and B lymphocytes. VII. Cooperative responses between lymphocytes are controlled by genes in the *I*-region of the *H-2* complex. *J. Exp. Med. 141*, 263 (1975).

14. Katz, D. H., Chiorazzi, N., McDonald, J., and Katz, L. R. Cell interactions between histoincompatible T and B lymphocytes. IX. The failure of histoincompatible cells is not due to suppression and cannot be circumvented by carrier-priming T cells with allogeneic macrophages. *J. Immunol.* *117*, 1853 (1976).

15. Katz, D. H., Skidmore, B. J., Katz, L. R., and Bogowitz, C. A. Adaptive differentiation of murine lymphocytes. I. Both T and B lymphocytes differentiating in $F_1 \rightarrow$ parental chimeras manifest preferential cooperative activity for partner lymphocytes derived from the same parental type corresponding to the chimeric host. *J. Exp. Med.* *148*, 727 (1978).

16. Katz, D. H., Katz, L. R., Bogowitz, C. A., and Skidmore, B. J. Adaptive differentiation of murine lymphocytes. II. The thymic microenvironment does not restrict the cooperative partner cell preference of helper T cells differentiating in $F_1 \rightarrow F_1$ thymic chimeras. *J. Exp. Med.* *149*, 1360 (1979).

17. Katz, D. H., Katz, L. R., Bogowitz, C. A., and Maurer, P. H. Adaptive differentiation of murine lymphocytes. IV. (Responder × nonresponder) F_1 T cells can be taught to preferentially help nonresponder, rather than responder, B cells. *J. Exp. Med.* *150*, 20 (1979).

18. Katz, D. H., Katz, L. R., and Bogowitz, C. A. Orchestration of partner cell preferences of cooperating T and B lymphocytes derived from primed conventional F_1 mice. *J. Immunol.* *125*, 1109 (1980).

19. Katz, D. H., Katz, L. R., and Bogowitz, C. A. Cell interaction (CI) molecules on immunocompetent lymphocytes: Development of antiparent CI receptor reactions in F_1 hybrid mice and evidence for a unique F_1 hybrid subset of interacting cells. *J. Exp. Med.* *153*, 407 (1981).

20. Katz, D. H., Katz, L. R., Bogowitz, C. A., and Bargatze, R. F. The major influence on helper T cell cooperative partner cell preferences is exerted by the extrathymic environment. *J. Immunol.* *124*, 1750 (1980).

21. Katz, D. H., Katz, L. R., Bogowitz, C. A., and Maurer, P. H. Plasticity of the immune response phenotype: Evidence that responses against cell interaction molecules may determine the immune response phenotype in a given host environment. *J. Immunol. 127,* 1103 (1981).

22. Kindred, B. and Shreffler, D. C. *H-2* dependence of cooperation between T and B cells *in vitro*. *J. Immunol. 109,* 940 (1972).

23. Longo, D. L. and Schwartz, R. H. Gene complementation. Neither *Ir-GLΦ* gene need be present in the proliferative T cell to generate an immune response to poly($Glu^{55}Lys^{36}$ Phe^{9})n. *J. Exp. Med. 151,* 1452 (1980).

24. Miller, J. F. A. P. Restrictions imposed on T lymphocyte reactivities by the major histocompatibility complex: Implications for T cell repertoire selection. *Immunol. Rev. 42,* 76 (1978).

25. Pierce, S. K., Klinman, N. R., Maurer, P. H., and Merryman, C. F. Role of the major histocompatibility gene products in regulating the antibody response to dinitrophenylated poly(*L*-Glu^{55}, *L*-Ala^{36}, *L*-Phe^{9})n. *J. Exp. Med. 152,* 336 (1980).

26. Press, J. L. and McDevitt, H. O. Allotype-specific analysis of anti-(Tyr, Glu)-Ala-Lys antibodies produced by *Ir-1A* high and low responder chimeric mice. *J. Exp. Med. 146,* 1815 (1977).

27. Rosenthal, A. S. and Shevach, E. M. Function of macrophages in antigen recognition by guinea pig T lymphocytes. I. Requirement for histocompatible macrophages and lymphocytes. *J. Exp. Med. 138,* 1194 (1973).

28. Shevach, E. M. and Rosenthal, A. S. Function of macrophages in antigen recognition by guinea pig T lymphocytes. II. Role of the macrophage in the regulation of genetic control of the immune response. *J. Exp. Med. 138,* 1213 (1973).

29. Smith, F. I. and Miller, J. F. A. P. Suppression of T cells specific for the nonthymic parental *H-2* haplotype in thymus-grafter chimeras. *J. Exp. Med. 151,* 246 (1980).

30. Sprent, J. and von Boehmer, H. T-helper function of parent → F_1 chimeras. Presence of a separate T-cell subgroup able to stimulate allogeneic B cells but not syngeneic B cells. *J. Exp. Med. 149*, 387 (1979).

31. Sproviero, J. F., Imperiale, M. J., and Zauderer, M. Clonal analysis of F_1 hybrid helper T cells restricted to parental or F_1 hybrid major histocompatibility determinants. *J. Exp. Med. 152*, 920 (1980).

32. von Boehmer, H., Haas, W., and Jerne, N. K. Major histocompatibility complex-linked immune-responsiveness is acquired by lymphocytes of low-responder mice differentiating in thymus of high-responder mice. *Proc. Natl. Acad. Sci. U.S.A. 75*, 2439 (1978).

33. von Boehmer, H., Sprent, J., and Nabholz, M. Tolerance to histocompatibility determinants in tetraparental bone marrow chimeras. *J. Exp. Med. 136*, 455 (1975).

Immunopathology: VIIIth International Symposium, 1980

UNIDIRECTIONAL T LYMPHOCYTE INDUCTION OF MONOCYTE PROCOAGULANT MOLECULES[1]

Thomas S. Edgington
Bradford S. Schwartz
Gary A. Levy
Daryl S. Fair

Department of Molecular Immunology,
Research Institute of Scripps Clinic,
La Jolla, California

I. INTRODUCTION[2]

An essential biological requirement for survival is the capacity of the organism to recognize specific stimuli and respond appropriately. Survival of higher organisms requires recognition of infectious agents, neoplastic cells, and trauma as well as organization of an effective host response. Selectional pressures during evolution have led to a wide variety of cellular and molecular mechanisms which provide the diverse

[1]*This is publication number 2404 from the Immunology Departments. This work was supported by NIH research grants CA-28166, HL-16411, and HL-07195. GAL is a fellow of the MRC, Canada.*

[2]*Abbreviations: LPS, bacterial lipopolysaccharide; PCA, procoagulant activity, PBM, peripheral blood mononuclear cells.*

ISBN 0-12-218320-7

functions required to maintain biological fidelity. Indeed, host response mechanisms, exemplified by the antibody response, the generation of cytolytic cells, and the enzymatic sequences of the complement and coagulation systems possess discriminating recognitive molecules, sophisticated regulatory circuits, and selective effectors. Only when the integrity of the host is preserved by both specific recognition of stimuli and effective regulatory networks can host defense mechanisms serve their appropriate biological roles to the benefit of the host. Disease in many circumstances may result from misdirection of these same pathways, thus threatening or violating the very survival of the organism.

A major component of the host defense network is embodied in the cells of the monocyte series. These cells serve as phagocytic effectors and may be induced by lymphocyte products to differentiate to cytolytic cells (28, 30) or by appropriate stimuli to secrete mediators (42-44). Whereas certain responses of monocytes, such as phagocytosis, appear to be direct reactions to stimuli (36), other responses require either the effects of lymphokines (4, 27, 28, 30) or direct cellular collaboration (23, 37). These latter responses, in which the recognitive functions of the T lymphocyte are first invoked and subsequently lead to the production of initiators of the coagulation system, have been only partially characterized (14, 15, 23, 37) and are the subject of this study. The specific response to be addressed involves the synthesis and biological expression of two initiators of the coagulation pathways, one entirely new.

The products of the coagulation network serve as participants in immunologic tissue lesions and may influence cells of the immune system. A participatory role of the monocyte or derivative cells, such as the macrophage, in initiating coagulation is illustrated by the studies of Colvin *et al.* (8).

The induration characteristic of delayed cutaneous hypersensitivity reactions is a direct result of local fibrin deposition. This interpretation has been further substantiated by the lack of induration in the delayed cutaneous hypersensitivity reactions elicited in individuals with hereditary afibrinogenemia (14).

In another example, administration of antimacrophage antisera to rabbits with acute immune complex glomerulonephritis has been shown to prevent the hypercellularity characteristic of this lesion (20). This and the attenuation of glomerular dysfunction by defibrinogenation (21) indicates a direct causal role of not only the monocyte but also the direct participation of fibrin formation in the mediation of immunologically mediated glomerular injury. It has been observed also that attenuation of tumor growth and metastasis follows defibrinogenation of animals (5), suggesting that products of the coagulation system play some role in the host response to tumors. In this regard, Dvorak *et al.* (11) have suggested that fibrin formed at the surface of tumor cells may serve as a physical barrier to effective cellular immune attack. Other evidence for initiation of coagulation pathways during the active phase of some immunologic diseases is supported by the observations in systemic lupus erythematosus of an increase of plasma fibrinopeptide A, which is related to disease activity (10). Furthermore, the high mortality of BxSB mice, a strain of hybrid mice with autoimmune immune complex disease and coronary artery thrombosis, illustrates the association of thrombosis with immune processes (1). Although pathogenetic implications require further analysis, the procoagulant pathways evoked by products of the immune response may serve effector functions as well as modify the responses of the lymphoid system (12, 19).

Among mechanisms that may account for activation of the coagulation pathways in immunologic responses are observations that a number of immunologically interesting stimuli evoke procoagulant activity (PCA) in human peripheral blood mononuclear cells *in vitro*. Stimuli such as bacterial lipopolysaccharide (23, 29, 32), allogeneic cells (35), immune complexes, and aggregated IgG (34, 37) have evoked marked increases in cellular PCA. Based on the effects of anticoagulation on antigen-induced delayed cutaneous hypersensitivity reactions (6, 13) and observations in our laboratory of antigen stimulation, there is evidence to support the contention that PCA is a product of the immune response to antigen.

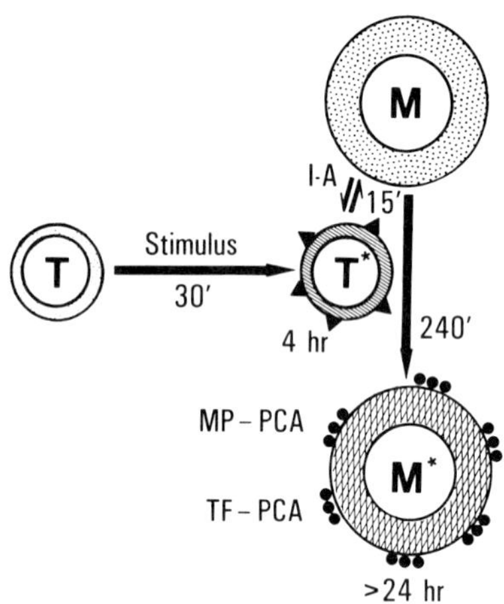

FIGURE 1. Basic scheme for T-cell induction of monocyte procoagulant molecules. T cells (T) are stimulated within 30 min to the "triggered" state (T^*). These cells are stable in this state for 4 hr. Cells induce monocytes or macrophages (M) via an I-A dependent collaboration within 15 min. During the following 4-6 hr, there is full expression of procoagulant activity (PCA). One of two types of PCA are induced, one is tissue factor and the other a novel monocyte prothrombinase. Expression of PCA persists unchanged from 16-72 hr following induction.

The present study addresses the cellular pathways responsible for procoagulant expression of PCA by cells of the monocyte/macrophage series, drawing from selected observations of the responses of murine and human cells elicited by eight stimuli *in vitro* and *in vivo*. We suggest the existence of what appears to be a common unidirectional pathway (Fig. 1) by which (1) T lymphocytes are triggered directly by a variety of stimuli, (b) these triggered T cells rapidly induce monocytes or macrophages, and (c) these cells selectively produce one of two cell membrane-associated procoagulant molecules. This proposed pathway embodies features distinct from lymphokine-mediated pathways, and we believe it may play a role in the pathogenesis of certain immunologic lesions.

II. INDUCTION OF PROCOAGULANT ACTIVITY

Human or murine peripheral blood mononuclear cells (PBM) were used to represent migratory cells that are the source of cellular infiltrates in immunologic tissue lesions. Two selected stimuli are representative: (a) bacterial lipopolysaccharide (LPS) derived from *E. coli* 0111:B4 and (b) soluble immune complexes of human serum albumin and purified specific antibody formed at a 4:1 ratio in antigen excess. In contrast to a number of other immune complex-mediated events, small soluble complexes are more stimulatory than larger complexes (26). LPS was optimally stimulatory to PBM in culture at about 10 ng/ml in the absence of serum or 10 μg/ml in 10% fetal bovine serum. The higher LPS requirement in the presence of serum appears to reflect the binding of LPS by serum high density lipoproteins (41). Soluble immune complexes were used at 70-100 μg/ml, a maximally stimulatory dose. PBM were incubated at 1×10^6 cells/ml for 6-24 hr at 37°C, with or without stimuli as indicated, to examine the cellular requirements, kinetics, and products of this pathway.

When immediately isolated, PBM, as well as splenic lymphoid cells, exhibit little measurable PCA. Viable cells exhibited about 15-20% of the PCA of disrupted cells, indicating that most endogenous PCA is present within the cells with little expressed at the cell surface. After culture for 4-6 hr this increased some; however, addition of appropriate stimuli increased activity markedly. The assay of PCA involved mixing washed viable or disrupted cells at the termination of culture with normal citrated plasma and recalcifying to initiate coagulation. The value of log time required for clot formation was proportional to log PCA based on a rabbit brain thromboplastin standard. In Table I the procoagulant

TABLE I. Induction of Procoagulant Activity in Human and Murine Lymphoid Cells

Cell population*	Stimulus**	Viable cells (mU PCA/10^6)	Disrupted cells (mU PCA/10^6)	Stimulation index***
Human PBM	LPS	562 ± 60	3150 ± 400	17.5
Human PBM	Ag:Ab	905 ± 56	3850 ± 300	22
Murine PBM	LPS	488 ± 44	2417 ± 30	22
Murine PBM	Ag:Ab	684 ± 28	3150 ± 132	15

**Isolated over ficoll-hypaque and cultivated at 1×10^6 cells/ml in the presence of stimulus for 6 hr.*

**E. coli *0111:B4 LPS at 10 μg/ml or Ag:Ab at 70-100 μg/ml.*

****Ratio of 6-hr stimulated total cellular PCA of disrupted cells.*

activity of viable and of disrupted human and murine PBM is given as well as the relative degree of stimulation compared to the basal cell concentration of PCA at zero time. There was a 15- to 22-fold stimulation of cellular PCA. The level of induced PCA was comparable for both species and stimuli. Stimulation was maximal within 6 hr and remained relatively constant for 24 hr.

III. THE PCA POSITIVE CELL

The cellular locus of PCA has been identified first by assay of lymphocytes and of monocytes which had been isolated by adherence. Virtually all PCA induced by either LPS or Ag:Ab complexes was resident in the adherent cell population (Table II). Although consistent with localization to monocytes, the possibility that the PCA positive cell might be a novel cell or represent a minor subpopulation of monocytes was resolved in a second set of experiments using a cytologic assay in which the cells were suspended in plasma agarose (23). The PCA positive cells were identified by the pericellular deposition of fibrin. Whereas unstimulated populations of cells contained few PCA positive cells, most monocytes from stimulated PBM were PCA positive. It was also observed that a few lymphocytes (1-10%) appeared weakly positive. Thus, most monocytes can be induced to produce PCA, and they account for most of the increment in PCA that is induced. It was not possible to assess the quantitative contribution of *individual* monocytes to the PCA, although the possibility that a subset of monocytes might contribute the majority of observed PCA cannot be excluded. Apart from these unresolved aspects, observations were similar with human and murine cells and for a variety of stimuli.

TABLE II. Localization of Procoagulant Activity to Stimulated Human Peripheral Blood Mononuclear Cells

Cell subpopulation	LPS		Ag:Ab	
	$mU/10^6$ cells	Stimulation index*	$mU/10^6$ cells	Stimulation index*
PBM	3,250 ± 250	13	3,600 ± 300	10.3
Monocytes**	27,083 ± 1667	9.3	30,000 ± 1875	9.0
Lymphocytes***	370 ± 42	1.2	410 ± 53	1.1

**Stimulation index is the ratio of stimulated cell PCA at 6 hr to basal cellular PCA at zero time.*

***Monocytes (>98% esterase positive) isolated from stimulated PBM by adherence to plastic.*

****Lymphocytes (<2% esterase positive) isolated from stimulated PBM by nonadherence to plastic.*

IV. CELLULAR COLLABORATION

Attempts at direct stimulation of isolated lymphocytes or monocytes led to no increase of cellular PCA (Table III), even when incubated for 24 hr. When the two cell populations were reconstituted the response of both murine and human cells to stimuli was recapitulated. Induction of PCA was not observed when medium clarified by ultracentrifugation from stimulated lymphocytes was added to monocytes.

The cellular stoichiometry of collaboration was next examined. Isolated lymphocytes were stimulated directly for 6 hr, washed, and added at varying ratios to monocytes at 37°C. Six hours later, the cells were harvested and assayed for total cellular PCA. At 2:1 lymphocytes to monocytes or higher, there there was induction of PCA (Fig. 2). The cell ratios were similar for different stimuli with human and murine cells.

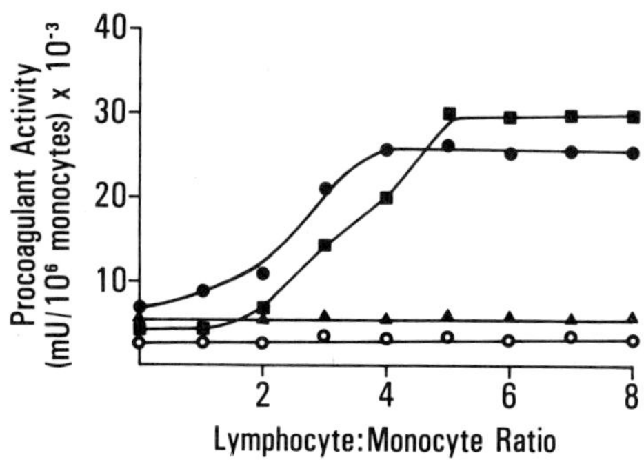

FIGURE 2. Lymphocyte collaboration is required for the generation of monocyte procoagulant activity. Human lymphocytes were first triggered with Ag:Ab (■) or LPS (●), washed, and added in increasing numbers to 1×10^5 monocytes. After 6-hr incubation the monocytes were washed and assayed for PCA. Monocytes alone were stimulated with LPS or Ag:Ab (▲), incubated for 6 hr, washed, and assayed for PCA. Untriggered lymphocytes were added in increasing numbers to 1×10^5 mono- (○) as above and monocyte PCA was assayed.

TABLE III. Direct Stimulation of Isolated Lymphocytes and Monocytes by LPS or Ag:Ab Complexes Does Not Induce Procoagulant Activity

	LPS*		Ag:Ab**	
Cell population	$mU/10^6$ cells	Stimulation index	$mU/10^6$ cells	Stimulation index
PBM	3100 ± 250	6.9	1575 ± 37	4.1
Monocytes***	3750 ± 208	1.4	3550 ± 232	1.0
Lymphocytes****	551 ± 284	1.1	39 ± 1.4	1.1

*6-hr incubation with E. coli *0111:B4 LPS at 10 μg/ml.*

***6-hr incubation with 100 μg Ag:Ab.*

****>98% esterase positive.*

*****<1% esterase positive.*

Collaboration must be mediated by direct contact or by a labile mediator. Addition of clarified medium from lymphocytes 4-6 hr after stimulation, homogenates of stimulated lymphocytes, or lymphocytes flash-fixed 5 min at 0°C with 0.15% glutaraldehyde were without effect. Evidence consistent with a direct contact-mediated collaboration follows from observations that neither cycloheximide nor actinomycin D, at concentrations sufficient to abolish protein and RNA synthesis, respectively, influenced LPS or Ag:Ab triggering of lymphocytes. Similarly, these inhibitors had no effect on the capacity of the triggered lymphocytes to induce PCA when added to monocytes. This effectively argues against newly synthesized lymphokines but does not preclude release of preformed short-lived mediators from the lymphocytes.

V. GENETIC RESTRICTION OF COLLABORATION

Collaborative restriction of the interaction between triggered lymphocytes and monocytes appears to be rigorous. There was no induction of PCA when lymphocytes and monocytes were first triggered by appropriate stimuli and then added to monocytes, when murine lymphocytes and monocytes were of different *H-2* haplotype. This requirement was apparent also when human lymphocytes and monocytes from different individuals were mixed. Using recombinant mice of defined *H-2* haplotype, the genetic requirements for collaboration were defined. Splenic and peripheral blood lymphoid cells from various strains were separated by adherence into lymphocytes and monocytes/macrophages, mixed and stimulated by LPS. Normal PCA responses were observed when both cell classes shared *H-2* of the same haplotype (Table IV). The requirement was contained within *H-2* as indicated by crosses 2 and 5 (Table IV); and the induction of full PCA responses indicated no additional requirement

TABLE IV. Genetic Requirements for Cellular Collaboration in the Induction of Murine Monocyte Procoagulant Activity

Cellular cross	Mouse strains*	Compatibility at *H-2*									PCA induction by LPS
		K	I-A	I-B	I-J	I-E	I-C	S	G	D	
1.	BALB/c	d	d	d	d	d	d	d	d	d	+
	BALB/c	d	d	d	d	d	d	d	d	d	
2.	A	k	k	k	k	k	d	d	d	d	+
	C3H	k	k	k	k	k	k	k	k	k	
3.	A	k	k	k	k	k	d	d	d	d	0
	BALB/c	d	d	d	d	d	d	d	d	d	
4.	A.TL	s	k	k	k	k	k	k	k	d	+
	A	k	k	k	k	k	d	d	d	d	
5.	A.TL	s	k	k	k	k	k	k	k	d	+
	C3H	k	k	k	k	k	k	k	k	k	
6.	A.TL	s	k	k	k	k	k	k	k	d	0
	BALB/c	d	d	d	d	d	d	d	d	d	
7.	A.TL	s	k	k	k	k	k	k	k	d	0
	B10.S(7R)	s	s	s	s	s	s	s	s	d	
8.	B10.A(4R)	k	k	b	b	b	b	b	b	b	+
	C3H	k	k	k	k	k	k	k	k	k	
9.	B10.A(4R)	k	k	b	b	b	b	b	b	b	0
	C57Bl/6	b	b	b	b	b	b	b	b	b	
10.	B10.A(5R)	b	b	b	k	k	d	d	d	d	0
	C3H	k	k	k	k	k	k	k	k	k	
11.	B10.A(5R)	b	b	b	k	k	d	d	d	d	+
	C57Bl/6	b	b	b	b	b	b	b	b	b	

**Spleen lymphocytes from one strain were mixed at 8:1 with adherent macrophages from the other, stimulated with 10 μg LPS per ml in complete medium for 6 hr at 37°C and the PCA of washed and disrupted cells was determined.*

outside the major histocompatibility complex. Limited compatibility at only K and I-A for cross 8 with mixing of [C3H] and [B10.A(4R)] cells was sufficient to generate a full response, although compatibility at K alone as for the cross 7 between [A.TL] and [B10.S(7R)] cells was ineffective. These and the variety of other crosses given in Table IV indicate the requirement for only I-A compatibility.

This restriction is particularly intriguing in light of the Ia positivity of a high proportion of circulating monocytes and the requirement for Ia-positive monocytes/macrophages in the presentation of antigen to T helper cells in the immune response (3). It is not yet known whether the I-A gene product must be expressed by both lymphocyte and monocyte/macrophage.

VI. GENETIC RESTRICTION OF THE RESPONSE

When LPS or Ag:Ab complexes were employed as probes for genetic restrictions of the PCA response in mice, very little difference was seen between mice of different strains, with little variation within a single strain. In contrast, when murine peripheral blood mononuclear cells were exposed *in vitro* to murine hepatitis virus, strain MHV-3, for 4-24 hr there was a strain-dependent difference in the magnitude of the PCA response (Table V). A strain mice were unresponsive to this positive polarity single strand RNA coronavirus; whereas C3H mice responded as they did to LPS. C3H mice develop acute viral hepatitis but hepatic injury progresses to chronic hepatitis, whereas A mice are resistant to injury. When PBM from BALB/c mice were exposed to MHV-3, a response of unparalleled magnitude was observed. This strain is highly susceptible to the virus, infection with 100 pfu consistently resulting in acute fulminant hepatitis with death in 6-7 days.

TABLE V. Murine Hepatitis Virus Induction of PCA

Species	*In vitro* PCA ($mU/10^6$ cells)			*In vivo* PCA ($mU/10^6$ cells)			Histopathology
	Control	LPS*	MHV-3**	Control	LPS***	MHV-3****	
A strain mouse	940	4250	740	220	3900	150	No pathology
C3H strain mouse	810	4100	2,850	180	4250	3,100	Chronic hepatitis
BALB/c strain mouse	780	3850	74,560	250	3700	41,500	Fulminant hepatic necrosis
Human	680	3250	800				

* *PBM assayed for PCA 24 hr after exposure to LPS at 10 μg/ml.*

** *10^6 pfu/ml MHV-3. PBM analyzed 24 hr after exposure to MHV-3* in vitro.

*** *10 μg LPS intraperitoneal. PBM isolated and assayed for PCA 24 hr later.*

**** *10^6 pfu MHV-3 intraperitoneal. PBM isolated 12 hr later and analyzed directly for PCA.*

When these mice were infected *in vivo* and their PBM and spleen cells assayed 0.5 - 24 hr later for PCA, the activation of monocyte PCA *in vivo* preceded the onset of histologically or biochemically documented hepatic injury and was of a magnitude and pattern comparable to that observed *in vitro*. Of interest, is the close parallel observed between the *in vitro* PCA response and the viral disease. This introduces a number of intriguing speculations regarding the potential significance and role of this pathway in the pathogenesis of disease and the role of fibrin deposition in the lesions.

Of particular interest, these observations with MHV-3 suggest a genetic restriction of the PCA response similar to the Ir gene restriction of immune responses (3). Recognition seems species-restricted since human cells do not respond to MHV-3. This is in contrast to what might be expected if triggering resulted from a simple lipid exchange or a nonspecific interaction. Within the murine system the strain specificity is of interest in that A and BALB/c are compatible with *H-2* to the right of I-E yet they differ profoundly in this response. The *H-2* incompatibility between these two strains falls within K through I-E, the Ir gene region. A and C3H strains are *H-2* compatible for K through I-E, yet they also differ in the degree of the PCA response and severity of disease. These observations suggest that more than one genetic locus may influence the response or the genetic restriction may be prescribed by a gene outside *H-2*. Until more detailed mapping is conducted, definitive answers cannot be provided. Available data do however suggest restriction at other than I-A. Although not yet mapped this additional restriction in the PCA response must be considered within the scheme outlined in Fig. 1. Whether these same genes also specify susceptibility of mouse macrophages to MHV (2) is not known.

VII. KINETICS AND METABOLIC REQUIREMENTS

The kinetics of the PCA response by both human and murine cells were comparable, as illustrated in Fig. 3. LPS or Ag:Ab triggered lymphocytes were added in excess to monocytes, and the cells assayed. In about 2 hr PCA increased reaching a maximum within 4-6 hr (Fig. 3A). This amount of PCA was

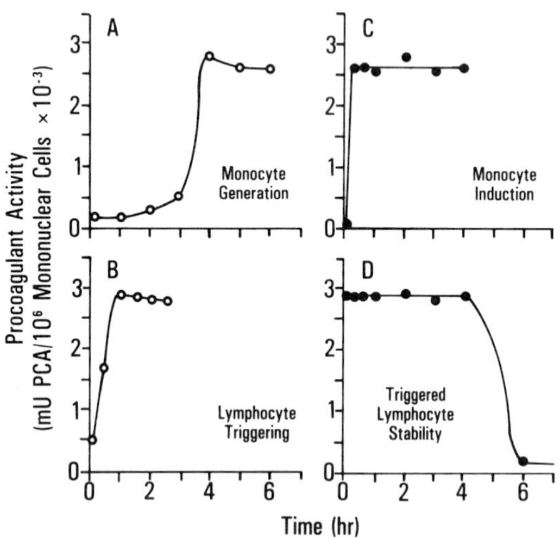

FIGURE 3. Kinetics of lymphocyte instructed monocyte PCA response. (A) Time course for generation of monocyte PCA. 1×10^6 LPS-triggered autologous lymphocytes were added to 1×10^5 human monocytes and PCA was assayed at various time intervals. (B) Time course for LPS triggering of lymphocytes. Lymphocytes (1×10^6 in 1 ml) were incubated with 10 μg LPS for the indicated intervals, washed, and added to 1×10^5 monocyte PCA was then assayed. (C) Temporal requirement for induction of monocytes. LPS-triggered lymphocytes were washed and added to autologous monocytes for intervals of 10 min to 4 hr. They were subsequently removed and the monocytes were incubated for an additional 6 hr and assayed for total PCA. (D) Stability of the triggered state of the lymphocyte. Lymphocytes were triggered for 30 min with LPS, washed, and held in culture for periods of 15 min to 10 hr. They were then assayed for their ability to trigger monocytes. The lymphocytes and monocytes were admixed and 6 hr later the cells were assayed for PCA.

equivalent to greater than 90% PCA-positive monocytes by cytologic assay. Further studies demonstrated that incubation of the monocytes in 10 μg actinomycin D per milliliter or 10 μg cycloheximide per milliliter abolished the increase of PCA, suggesting that the PCA is probably newly synthesized in the monocyte.

When lymphocytes were exposed for variable periods to LPS or Ag:Ab, washed, and added to monocytes for 6 hr partial triggering of lymphocytes occurred in 15 min and was complete within 30 min (Fig. 3B). Adding either LPS or Ag:Ab complexes to the monocytes did not induce the PCA response. The unidirectional aspect of the pathway was repeatedly confirmed for a number of stimuli with human and murine cells by the subsequent addition of untriggered lymphocytes to the stimulated and washed monocytes. In no experiment did this result in triggering of the lymphocytes so as to induce monocyte PCA. Thus, the pathway appeared unidirectional (as illustrated in Fig. 1) and appears to represent a novel cellular sequence different from a proposed lymphokine induction of PCA as described by Edwards and Rickles in a lectin-driven system (15). Presentation of antigen to T lymphocytes by macrophages in the immune response (3) is a well-known pathway that functions in the opposite direction; however, the T lymphocyte once perceiving antigen on the macrophage can induce secondary macrophage responses as well (17).

Two additional kinetic details of the collaborative response are of interest. First, the induction of monocytes by triggered lymphocytes is unusually rapid (Fig. 3C). LPS-triggered lymphocytes were added to adherent monocytes for intervals of 10 min to 4 hr removed, and the monocytes assayed 6 hr later. Within less than 10 min of mixing the monocytes were induced to produce PCA, and induction was complete within 15 min. This also suggests a transient contact-mediated event.

Triggered lymphocytes could be recovered after inducing a first set of monocytes, and these lymphocytes retained full capacity to repeatedly trigger additional aliquots of monocytes, thus the system embodies amplification. Finally, lymphocytes once triggered by stimulus remained triggered for about 4 hr (Fig. 3D), after which they returned to the basal state and subsequently they could be retriggered by the same stimulus.

The metabolic requirements for lymphocyte triggering appear limited. The ability of lymphocytes to become triggered as well as the ability of triggered lymphocytes to induce monocytes was not influenced by inhibitors of protein or RNA synthesis. This suggests that triggering of lymphocytes may involve either a very limited biochemical response or a topographical realignment of lymphocyte surface structures.

VIII. CHARACTERISTICS OF THE LYMPHOCYTE

The collaborating human lymphocyte has been partially characterized. Monocyte-depleted lymphocytes were rosetted with neuraminidase-treated sheep erythrocytes (nE); and the nE^+ (T cells) were separated from nE^- cells (non-T cells) by centrifugation over ficoll-hypaque. Following triggering of these cells with LPS or Ag:Ab only the nE^+ T cells induced isolated monocytes to express PCA (Table VI). These nE^+ cells were separated into T_μ, T_γ, and T_0 by Fc receptors for IgM and and IgG as described by Moretta *et al.* (26). Although not homogeneous, they do represent functionally separated helper cells (T_μ) and suppressor cells (T_γ) for *in vitro* pokeweed mitogen-driven immunoglobulin synthesis. LPS-triggered T_μ cells induced monocyte PCA; however, the resultant concentration of PCA was higher than observed for induction of monocyte PCA by whole LPS-triggered T cells (Table VI). The existence

TABLE VI. Participation of Lymphocyte Classes and Subclasses in the Induction of Monocyte PCA

Lymphocyte class*	Markers	PCA ($mU/10^6$ cells)
T	nE^+	3140
Non-T	nE^-	280
T_γ	nE^+, Fc_γ^+	270
T_μ	nE^+, Fc_μ^+	4170
T_0	nE^+, Fc_μ^-, Fc_γ^-	220

Lymphocytes were triggered with 10 μg/ml LPS for 30 min, washed, and added at a 5.5:1 ratio to autologous monocytes. Six hours later the cells were washed, disrupted, and assayed for PCA.

of suppressor cells was suggested and has since been confirmed. The suppressors are recovered in the T_γ subclass. T cells also serve as inducers for Ag:Ab complex stimulation and viral stimulation; however, it has not yet been determined whether the T subclass functions are comparable.

In the mouse, initial studies of the collaborating lymphocyte have identified it as a θ^+ cell using complement dependent cytolysis with monoclonal anti-θ. Postthymic T cells appear to be required since spleen cells from homozygous BALB/c nude (ν/ν) mice did not respond. These characteristics indicate that a differentiated cell of the T series is required for this pathway and further support the likelihood that direct cell-cell contact mediates collaboration. The C3H/HeJ strain of mice, lacking the gene allele required to respond proliferatively to LPS, respond normally to induction of monocyte PCA (24), indicating independence from this LPS response.

IX. MONOCYTE PROCOAGULANT MOLECULES

Monocyte procoagulant activity was first characterized by dependence on coagulation factors using coagulation factor-deficient plasmas. Both Ag:Ab complex and LPS-stimulated human mononuclear cells expressed full procoagulant activity in Factor VIII or IX deficient plasmas, but were unable to induce coagulation in Factor X, VII, or prothrombin-deficient plasmas (Table VII). The specificity was confirmed by the addition of purified Factor X, VII, or prothrombin, respectively, to deficient plasmas with full reconstitution of the rate of fibrin formation. These data are characteristic of tissue factor induction of blood coagulation, a cell membrane

TABLE VII. Characteristics of PCA Induced in Human and Murine Monocytes by Selected Stimuli

Species PBM	Stimulus	PCA (% of normal plasma) Factor-deficient plasma VIII	IX	VII	X	Prothrombin
Human	LPS*	95	100	7	5	<1
Human	Ag:Ab**	93	100	3	5	<1
Mouse	LPS*	57	55	50	40	<1
Mouse	Ag:Ab**	60	57	55	37	<1
Mouse	MHV***	73	80	98	92	<1

**LPS at 10 μg/ml.*

***Ag:Ab at 4:1 ratio in antigen excess at 100 μg/ml.*

****Murine hepatitis virus, MHV-3 at 10^3 pfu with C3H PBM.*

phospholipo protein that binds and activates Factor VII to VIIa. This is fully consistent with the previous observation of tissue factor induction by LPS in human PBM (33).

The initiation of fibrin formation by stimulated murine monocytes differed (38, 40). Murine monocyte PCA, elicited by LPS or Ag:Ab, induced fibrin formation in all factor-deficient plasmas except for prothrombin deficient plasma (Table VII). Prothrombin-deficient plasmas were able to serve as substrate after reconstitution with purified human prothrombin. Evidence for direct cleavage of prothrombin to a functional thrombin or thrombin-like enzyme was confirmed by use of a simple two protein clotting assay consisting of purified prothrombin and fibrinogen. Murine monocyte suspensions induced a rate of clotting comparable to whole plasma. To confirm the implication that murine monocytes, when induced by LPS or Ag:Ab complex triggered lymphocytes responded by synthesis of a novel prothrombinase, we examined the cleavage of ^{125}I-labeled prothrombin using SDS-PAGE (polyacrylamide gel electrophoresis) analysis. Only after addition of induced murine monocytes was there limited proteolytic cleavage of ^{125}I-labeled prothrombin to yield thrombin-like cleavage products. On the basis of prothrombin cleavage, or by a functional clotting assay, the production of murine monocyte prothrombinase was equivalent to the activity produced by human monocytes, through tissue factor generation.

The inducible monocyte prothrombinase was not consistent with activated plasma Factor X (Xa) based on inhibitor profiles or molecular weight. The enzyme required calcium ions, phospholipid, and was DFP sensitive. It differed from human factor Xa with respect to the higher concentrations of PMSF and lower concentration of DFP required for inhibition. In contrast to plasmin, it was not sensitive to Trasylol. To determine the molecular weight of the murine monocyte

TABLE VIII. Type of Monocyte Procoagulant Activity Induced *in Vitro* and *in Vivo* by Various Agents

Species	Stimulus	Setting	PCA
Mouse	LPS	*In vitro*	Monocyte prothrombinase
Mouse	Ag:Ab	*In vitro*	Monocyte prothrombinase
Mouse	MHV-3*	*In vitro*	Monocyte prothrombinase
Mouse	MHV-3*	*In vivo*	Monocyte prothrombinase
Mouse	MRL/l strain autoimmune disease	*In vivo*	Monocyte prothrombinase
Human	LPS	*In vitro*	Tissue factor
Human	Ag:Ab	*In vitro*	Tissue factor
Human	Viral hepatitis type B	*In vivo*	Monocyte prothrombinase
Human	HB_sAg**	*In vitro*	Monocyte prothrombinase

* *Plaque-purified murine hepatitis virus.*

** *22-nm particles of human hepatitis B virus.*

prothrombinase, membrane-rich fractions of induced murine monocytes were subject to SDS-PAGE. The gel was then sliced and the enzyme eluted and renatured in 1% Triton X-100. The specific activity was recovered from slices at a migration distance equivalent to a molecular weight of approximately 90,000, considerably larger than purified Factor Xa protein (48,000).

More recent studies have indicated that there is a human monocyte counterpart to the murine monocyte prothrombinase. This can be induced by high density and by intermediate density plasma lipoproteins (39), and in this system lymphocyte collaboration is also required (25). Other studies have indicated that certain other stimuli, for example human hepatitis B virus surface antigen (22-nm particles, HBsAg), can induce the monocyte prothrombinase in cells of immune individuals

(Edgington and Levy, unpublished observations). In Table VIII the types of PCA induced by a variety of stimuli are given. The genetically restricted expression of procoagulant molecules in response to murine hepatitis virus (MHV-3) by murine PBM or spenic cells both *in vitro* or *in vivo* is equivalent and results in the production of a monocyte prothrombinase in both circumstances.

X. SUMMARY: CELLULAR PATHWAY OF T-CELL INSTRUCTED GENERATION OF PROCOAGULANT MONOKINES

The elucidation of the PCA pathway has developed from original observations that endotoxin could induce procoagulant activity in blood leukocytes (22, 31). These observations have been extended to include a variety of stimuli, as well as to demonstrate that the pathway appears to have many common features in at least two species. Although not presented here, the same observations pertain to splenic cells (23). This pathway draws upon the role of certain T lymphocytes as recognitive units. These cells are generally perceived as the discriminating recognitive element for the initiation of a variety of humoral and cellular immune responses. In the pathway described here, T cells are demonstrated to have a broader recognitive role. In contrast to the requirement for macrophage presentation of antigen to the lymphocyte in conventional immune responses, the pathway for PCA induction does not include such a role on the part of the macrophage or monocyte. Rather, the lymphocyte functions as the accessory cell and the monocyte/macrophage as the effector cell. A helper T cell recognizes at least two disparate stimuli, LPS and Ag:Ab complexes, and can then induce monocytes or macrophages to produce procoagulant activity. This communication appears to be unidirectional, extremely rapid, and I-A restricted for collaboration, as schematically depicted in Fig. 1. The T cell requires neither protein nor RNA synthesis to accomplish this task.

These studies have led to the characterization of a new pathway of initiation of the coagulation system, separate from both the intrinsic and extrinsic pathways. The monocyte prothrombinase, though induced by different stimuli in mouse as contrasted to human cells, can be produced in either species. The lack of sensitivity to heparin-ATIII introduces new problems in evaluating the use of anticoagulants to dissect the *in vivo* pathophysiology of the PCA pathway. The alternative procoagulant activity results from generation and cell surface expression of tissue factor, the classical initiator of the extrinsic coagulation pathway (Fig. 4).

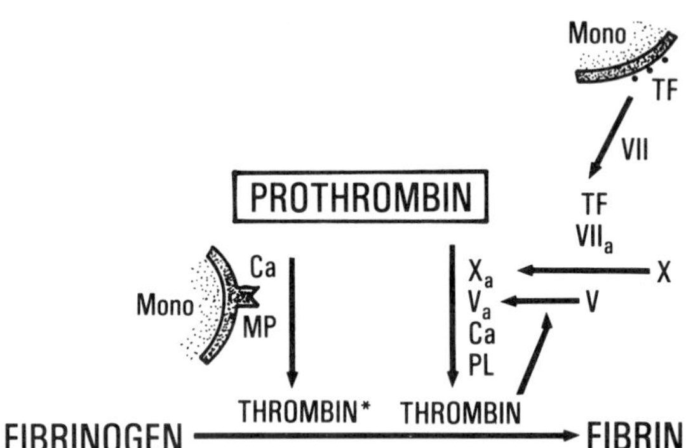

FIGURE 4. Initiation of coagulation by monocytes and macrophages. Monocytes can activate the coagulation system either through the extrinsic pathway of activation with the expression of tissue factor (TF) or by direct cleavage of prothrombin with the monocyte prothrombinase (MP). In both mechanisms functional thrombin is produced which converts fibrinogen to fibrin.

There appears to be not only inducer T cells but also suppressor T cells for this pathway, thus exhibiting classical circuit design. In addition the initial evidence for genetic restrictions in the response to stimuli such as murine hepatitis virus may be similar to the Ir gene restrictions of the immune response. This cellular pathway is distinct from lymphokine activation of monocytes and macrophages with respect both to generation of procoagulant monokines and to other forms of macrophage activation.

XI. PATHOGENETIC SIGNIFICANCE

The pathogenetic implications of the lymphoid PCA response remain to be fully explored. There are a variety of correlations between the features of a number of immunologic tissue lesions and the generation of lymphoid procoagulant activity which could be mediated via either direct cellular collaboration or a proposed lymphokine-mediated pathway (16).

Fibrin is commonly deposited in immunologic tissue lesions. The induration characteristic of the delayed cutaneous hypersensitivity reaction is a result of local deposition of fibrin (7, 8), such that these lesions in afibrinogenemic individuals lack induration (9). Defibrinogenation of experimental animals precludes glomerular injury and proteinuria due to experimental immune complex glomerulonephritis (21). Fibrin deposited at the site of immunologic tissue lesions may have a variety of effects. Not only may it interfere with effective cellular attack of neoplastic cells or infected cells through a "barrier" effect (11); but it may induce platelet activation, microthrombi, vascular injury, and resultant ischemia. The effects of fibrin deposition and subsequent fibrinolysis have only been partially explored, but the latter appears to include suppression of lymphocyte function (12, 19) and local increased vascular permeability (18), both of which are produced by discrete peptides released from fibrin by the fibrinolytic process.

The role of the monocyte and macrophage in basic host defense mechanisms has long been described and appreciated. Due to the functional diversity or potential for diversity, it has been difficult to define narrowly the function of these cells as encountered in various types of tissue lesions. Long suspected, the specifically induced macrophage or monocyte is clearly a source of procoagulant activity, which for the first time is recognized to result from the synthesis of either of two molecules and pathways as outlined schematically in Fig. 4. Other functions that may also be induced in a linked manner remain to be defined. However, increasing knowledge about these cells at the forefront of host defenses and evidence for activation of this pathway *in vivo* during many states of disease promise to clarify the pathogenesis of such diseases.

ACKNOWLEDGMENTS

The authors appreciate the initial discussions of these studies with Dr. Celso Bianco (Department of Pathology, SUNY Downstate, Brooklyn, New York), the dedicated assistance of Patsy Larson and Mary Gortmaker in preparation of the manuscript, the provision of purified bacterial lipopolysaccharides by Dr. David Morrison (Department of Microbiology and Immunology, Emory University, Atlanta, Georgia), and the provision of human Hepatitis B virus particles by Dr. John Gerin (Department of Microbiology and Immunology, Georgetown University, Washington, D.C.).

REFERENCES

1. Accinni, L. and Dixon, F. J. Degenerative vascular disease and myocardial infarction in mice with lupus-like syndrome. *Am. J. Pathol. 96*, 477 (1979).

2. Bang, F. B. and Warwick, A. Mouse macrophages as host cells for the mouse hepatitis virus and the genetic basis of their susceptibility. *Proc. Natl. Acad. Sci. U.S.A. 46*, 1065 (1960).

3. Benacerraf, B. and Germain, R. N. The immune response genes of the major histocompatibility complex. *Immunol. Rev. 38*, 70 (1978).

4. Buchmuller, Y. and Manuel, J. Studies on the mechanisms of macrophage activation. II. Parasite destruction in macrophages activated by supernates from concanavalin A-stimulated lymphocytes. *J. Exp. Med. 150*, 359 (1979).

5. Chmielewska, J., Poggi, A., Janik, P., Latallo, Z. S., and Donati, M. B. Effect of defibrination with batroxobin on growth and metastases of JW sarcoma in mice. *Eur. J. Cancer 16*, 919 (1980).

6. Cohen, S., Benacerraf, B., McCluskey, R. T., and Ovary, Z. Effect of anticoagulants on delayed hypersensitivity reactions. *J. Immunol. 98*, 351 (1967).

7. Colvin, R. B. and Dvorak, H. F. Role of the clotting system in cell mediated hypersensitivity. II. Kinetics of fibrinogen/fibrin accumulation and vascular permeability changes in tuberculin and cutaneous basophil hypersensitivity reactions. *J. Immunol. 14*, 377 (1975).

8. Colvin, R. B., Johnson, R. A., Mihn, M. C., and Dvorak, H. F. Role of the clotting system in cell mediated hypersensitivity. *J. Exp. Med. 138*, 686 (1973).

9. Colvin, R. B., Mossesson, M. W., and Dvorak, H. F. Delayed-type hypersensitivity skin reactions in congenital afibrinogenemia lack fibrin deposition and induration. *J. Clin. Invest. 63*, 1302 (1979).

10. Cronlund, M., Hardin, J., Burton, J., Lee, L., Haber, E., and Block, K. J. Fibrinopeptide A in plasma of normal subjects and patients with disseminated intravascular coagulation and systemic lupus erythematosus. *J. Clin. Invest. 58*, 142 (1976).

11. Dvorak, H. F., Orenstein, N. S., Carvalho, A. C., Churchhill, W. H., Dvorak, A. M., Galli, S. J., Feder, J., Bitzer, A. M., Rypysc, J., and Giovcinco, P. Induction of a fibrin-gel investment: an early event in line 10 hepatocarcinoma growth mediated by tumor-secreted products. *J. Immunol. 122*, 166 (1979).

12. Edgington, T. S., Curtiss, L. K., and Plow, E. F. The immunosuppressive activity of plasmic degradation products of human fibrinogen. *Thromb. Haemostasis 38*, 170 (1977).

13. Edwards, R. L. and Rickles, F. R. Delayed hypersensitivity in man: effects of systemic anticoagulation. *Science 200*, 541 (1978).

14. Edwards, R. L. and Rickles, F. R. On the origin of leukocyte procoagulant activity. *Thromb. Res. 13*, 307 (1978).

15. Edwards, R. L. and Rickles, F. R. The role of human T cells and T cell products for monocyte tissue factor generation. *J. Immunol. 125*, 606 (1980).

16. Edwards, R. L. and Rickles, F. R. The role of monocyte tissue factor in the immune response. *Lymphokine Rep. 1*, 181 (1980).

17. Farr, A. G., Wechter, W. J., Kiely, J.-M., and Unanue, E. R. Induction of cytocidal macrophages following *in vitro* interactions between Listeria-immune T cells and macrophages — role of H-2. *J. Immunol. 122*, 2405 (1979).

18. Gerdin, B. and Saldeen, T. Effect of fibrin degradation products on microvascular permeability. *Thromb. Res. 13*, 995 (1978).

19. Girmann, G., Rees, H., Schwarze, G., and Scheurlen, P. G. Immunosuppression by micromolecular fibrinogen degradation products in cancer. *Nature (London) 59*, 399 (1975).

20. Holdsworth, S. R., Neale, T. J., and Wilson, C. B. Abrogation of macrophage-dependent injury in experimental glomerulonephritis in the rabbit. Use of an antimacrophage serum. *J. Clin. Invest. 68*, 686 (1981).

21. Holdsworth, S. R., Thomson, N. M., Glasgow, E. F., and Atkins, R. C. The effect of defibrination on macrophage participation in rabbit nephrotoxic nephritis: studies using glomerular culture and electron microscopy. *Clin. Exp. Immunol. 37*, 38 (1979).

22. Lerner, R. G., Goldstein, R., and Cummings, G. Stimulation of human leukocyte thromboplastic activity by endotoxin. *Proc. Soc. Exp. Biol. Med. 138*, 145 (1971).

23. Levy, G. A. and Edgington, T. S. Lymphocyte cooperation is required for amplification of macrophage procoagulant activity. *J. Exp. Med. 151*, 232 (1980).

24. Levy, G. A. and Edgington, T. S. Lymphoid procoagulant activity and mitogenesis in the C3H/HeJ mouse: discordant response to LPS (lipopolysaccharide) stimulation. *J. Immunol. 124*, 2665 (1980).

25. Levy, G. A., Schwartz, B. S., Curtiss, L. K., and Edgington, T. S. Plasma lipoprotein induction and suppression of the generation of cellular procoagulant activity *in vitro*. Requirements for cellular collaboration. *J. Clin. Invest. 67*, 1614 (1981).

26. Moretta, L., Webb, S. R., Grossi, G. E., Lydyard, P. M., and Cooper, M. D. Functional analysis of two human T cell subpopulations: help and suppression of B cell responses by T cells bearing receptors for IgM and IgG. *J. Exp. Med. 146*, 184 (1977).

27. Nathan, C. F., Karnovsky, M. L., and David, J. R. Alterations of macrophage functions by mediators from lymphocytes. *J. Exp. Med. 133*, 1356 (1971).

28. Nathan, C. F. and Root, R. K. Hydrogen peroxide release from mouse peritoneal macrophages. Dependence on sequential activation and triggering. *J. Exp. Med. 146*, 1648 (1977).

29. Niemetz, J. and Fani, K. Role of leukocytes in blood coagulation and the generalized Schwartzman reaction. *Nature (London), New Biol. 232*, 247 (1971).

30. Piesseus, W. F., Churchill, W. H., and David, J. R. Macrophages activated *in vitro* with lymphocyte mediators kill neoplastic but not normal cells. *J. Immunol. 114*, 293 (1975).

31. Rapaport, S. I. and Hjort, P. F. The blood clotting properties of rabbit peritoneal leukocytes *in vitro*. *Thromb. Diath. Haemorrh. 17*, 222 (1967).

32. Rickles, F. R., Levin, J., Hardin, J. A., Barr, C. F., and Conrad, M. F., Jr. Tissue factor generation by human mononuclear cells: effects of endotoxin and dissociation of tissue factor generation from mitogenic response. *J. Lab. Clin. Med. 89*, 792 (1977).

33. Rickles, F. R. and Rick, P. D. Structural features of salmonella typhimurium lipopolysaccharide required for activation of tissue factor in human mononuclear cells. *J. Clin. Invest. 59*, 1188 (1977).

34. Rothberger, H., Zimmerman, T. S., Spiegelberg, H. L., and Vaughan, J. H. Leukocyte procoagulant activity. Enhancement of production *in vitro* by IgG and antigen-antibody complexes. *J. Clin. Invest. 59*, 549 (1977).

35. Rothberger, H., Zimmerman, T. S., and Vaughan, J. H. Increased production and expression of tissue thromboplastin-like procoagulant activity *in vitro* by allogeneically stimulated human leukocytes. *J. Clin. Invest. 62*, 649 (1978).

36. Schnyder, J. and Baggiolini, M. Role of phagocytosis in the activation of macrophages. *J. Exp. Med. 148*, 1449 (1978).

37. Schwartz, B. S. and Edgington, T. S. Lymphocyte collaboration is required for induction of murine monocyte procoagulant activity by immune complexes. *J. Immunol. 127*, 438 (1981).

38. Schwartz, B. S., Levy, G. A., Fair, D. S., Curtiss, L. K., and Edgington, T. S. A novel prothrombin activator is expressed by human circulating monocytes exposed to certain plasma lipoproteins. *Circulation 62*, 279 (1980).

39. Schwartz, B. S., Levy, G. A., Fair, D. S., Curtiss, L. K., and Edgington, T. S. Plasma lipoprotein induction and suppression of the generation of cellular procoagulant activity *in vitro*. I. Two procoagulant activities are produced by peripheral blood mononuclear cells. *J. Clin. Invest. 67*, 1650 (1981).

40. Schwartz, B. S., Levy, G. A., Fair, D. S., and Edgington, T. S. Murine monocytes produce a novel prothrombin activator in response to Ag:Ab or LPS stimulated lymphocytes. *Fed. Proc. 40*, 1055 (1981).

41. Ulevitch, R. J., Johnston, A. R., and Weinstein, D. B. New function for high density lipoproteins. Their participation in intravascular reactions of bacterial lipopolysaccharides. *J. Clin. Invest. 64*, 1516 (1979).

42. Unkeless, J. C., Gordon, S., and Reich, E. Secretion of plasminogen activator by stimulated macrophages. *J. Exp. Med. 139*, 834 (1974).

43. Werb, Z. and Gordon, S. Elastase secretion by stimulated macrophages. Characterization and regulation. *J. Exp. Med. 142*, 361 (1975).

44. Werb, Z. and Gordon, S. Secretion of a specific collagenase by stimulated macrophages. *J. Exp. Med. 142*, 346 (1975).

Immunopathology: VIIIth International Symposium, 1980

REGULATION OF CONTACT SENSITIVITY AND TOLERANCE

Henry N. Claman
Stephen D. Miller
John W. Moorhead

Departments of Medicine,
Microbiology, and Immunology,
University of Colorado School of Medicine,
Denver, Colorado

It is now quite clear that immunologic responses are highly regulated. The type, magnitude, and duration of any response represents the net balance of a number of variables. These variables include type and dose of antigen, route of presentation, genetic makeup of the responder, etc. It seems likely that complete understanding of the immunological system will show that it is indeed a network of interacting forces as postulated by Jerne (13). Mechanisms of control can be seen in a variety of systems, and we have chosen to study contact sensitivity.

I. THE CONTROL OF CONTACT SENSITIVITY

Contact sensitivity is an example of delayed hypersensitivity (DH) mediated primarily by T cells T_{DH}. [Although antibody to the contactant may be produced in some situations,

ISBN 0-12-218320-7

this is a modifying factor and not the primary pathophysiologic process (4).] We have found it convenient to distinguish two arms of this response: the afferent and the efferent limbs. The afferent limb includes the events following epicutaneous sensitization with antigen and involves the proliferation and maturation of the T cells responsible for delayed hypersensitivity T_{DH}. The efferent limb is activated when sensitized cells or animals are reexposed to specific antigens. The T_{DH} produce and release lymphokines which, in turn, attract and activate nonspecific cells such as macrophages and other lymphocytes. The entire collection of cells that accumulate over a 24-48 hr period makes up the inflammatory reaction characteristic of delayed hypersensitivity. A number of investigations in experimental contact sensitivity in animals has shown that this process of contact sensitization is highly regulated. The regulation can be seen when one explores a number of variables such as (a) antigen presentation, (b) antigen dose, (c) genetic restrictions, and (d) duration of the sensitized state.

A. Antigen Presentation in Contact Sensitivity

An effective contact sensitizer is one able to couple covalently to self components. Much of the experimental work has used chemically reactive haptens such as dinitrofluorobenzene (DNFB). Thus, the "real" antigen is actually contactant-coupled-to-self formed *in vivo*. It is likely that the complete antigen in the skin is formed by the conjugation of contactant to Langerhans cells in the epidermis (4). This antigen-cell complex is then recognized by the appropriate clone of T_{DH} lymphocytes. This supposition is based on the following findings: (a) T cells recognize antigens best when they are presented on a membrane containing Ia molecules of the major histocompatibility complex (MHC), and Langerhans cells have such molecules; (b) DNFB applied to skin sites that are relatively deficient in Langerhans cells does not sensitize well [and in fact can induce tolerance (43)]. The sensitization phase is complete when T_{DH} cells recognize the antigenic complex, multiply, and recirculate throughout the body.

In contrast to contactants presented on the skin, the same molecules given intravenously or intraperitoneally, tip the balance toward unresponsiveness, at least in part via the production of suppressor cells (see Section II). Thus, the *manner* of presentation is crucial for determining the extent of sensitization and the degree of tolerance.

B. *Antigen Dose in Contact Sensitivity*

Contact sensitization with DNFB is, like all immunologic phenomena, dose related. As one increases the antigen dose, the degree of sensitization increases to an optimal point. Beyond this point, *supra*optimal doses of DNFB actually induce lesser amounts of sensitivity. In fact, animals painted with supraoptimal DNFB show some hyporesponsiveness or tolerance. This phenomenon is mediated by an excess of suppressor cells which are activated by supraoptimal doses of antigen (perhaps escaping "processing" by Langerhans cells)(34). This kind of regulation thus provides a limit to the degree of clonal expansion of delayed hypersensitivity T cells that might otherwise be excessive when driven by larger and larger doses of antigen. It is not clear why the net response actually goes down instead of leveling off.

C. *Genetic Restrictions*

Immunologic reactions are genetically controlled, and T-cell responses involve recognition of antigen and of portions of the MHC (7). This is true of contact reactions as well, although the precise locus of the control mechanisms has not been entirely clarified (4) and is beyond the scope of this chapter.

D. *Duration of Contact Sensitivity Is Controlled by Antiidiotypic Antibody*

The duration of the sensitized state also turns out to be a highly regulated phenomenon. Whereas contact sensitivity to DNCB in guinea pigs lasts for months, mice sensitized with epicutaneous DNFB lose sensitivity with time. After an optimal state of sensitization 5-6 days after DNFB painting, sensitivity wanes; mice challenged at 9-15 days after sensitization show little evidence of DNFB sensitivity. Zembala *et al.* (45) showed that B lymphocytes at this later time were able to suppress recipient mice. Studies in our laboratory followed this up. We showed that sensitized mice had in their serum (during the waning of sensitization) a factor that was suppressive to DNFB sensitization. We called this "suppressive immune serum" (SIS). SIS was (a) antigen-specific, (b) immunoglobulin, (c) not anti-DNP, and (d) not DNP (36). It was, however, able to combine with mouse anti-DNP (but not rabbit anti-DNP), and could block the passive transfer of contact sensitivity by cells from DNFB immune donors. By all these criteria, SIS appeared to be an antibody directed to receptors on T cells responsible for the passive transfer of DNFB contact sensitivity. It would thus qualify as an antiidiotypic antibody as its target is presumably the receptor for DNP-self on T cells. This interpretation is confirmed by the fact that SIS appears to be similar or identical to an antibody raised by immunizing mice with lymph node cells taken 4 days after sensitization with DNFB. Such cells are enriched for T cells mediating contact sensitivity to DNFB, and the antiserum they provoke (after absorption) can be considered to be an "anti-T_{DH}" serum (J. W. Moorhead, unpublished observations).

The significance of this finding lies in its accord with the Jerne network hypothesis. It can be summarized by saying that during the course of normal contact immunization with DNFB, the magnitude and duration of the apparent sensitized state is limited and down-regulated by the induction of an antibody against the idiotype recognizing DNP-self. Presumably, the expanded clone of specific T_{DH} perturbs the network by triggering cells making antiidiotypic antibodies (SIS), and these substances exert a negative regulatory effect.

II. THE REGULATION OF CONTACT SENSITIVITY BY SUPPRESSOR CELLS

Early experiments by Sulzberger, Chase, and deWeck showed that tolerance to contact sensitivity could be induced by prior injection of cogeners of the sensitizing compund (4). The mechanisms for this tolerance were not understood. In the early 1970s, Gershon and Kondo showed that suppressor cells, particularly suppressor T cells (Ts) were important in the induction and maintenance of immunologic tolerance (10). Contact sensitivity systems have proved to be a fruitful model for elucidating the manner in which various suppressive circuits operate. This section will briefly describe the role of Ts in tolerance to and regulation of the DNFB contact sensitivity response.

A. *Suppressor T Cells Induced by DNBS*

Hapten-specific tolerance to DNFB contact sensitivity is easily induced by the iv injection of water-soluble $DNBSO_3$ (29). The unresponsiveness develops gradually over a period of 7 days and is mediated in part by an antigen-specific Ts. The non-MHC restricted Ts are demonstable in both lymph node and spleen, but not in the thymus of injected mice. The Ts are Ia^- and the precursors are not sensitive to adult thymectomy, indicating that they are in the long-lived population of T cells. Ts induced by DNBS inhibit the afferent limb of sensitivity (23) as they specifically depress cell proliferation in draining lymph nodes of recipient mice following sensitization, and they are suppressive only if transferred to recipients directly before or shortly after the latter are sensitized. The suppressive activity of these Ts is inhibited by pretreatment with rabbit or mouse anti-DNP serum (27). This finding was originally interpreted to mean that the Ts had accessible DNP on their cell membranes, but more recent experiments (J. W. Moorhead, unpublished) have indicated that a subset of the anti-DNP antibodies is reacting with an anti-idiotype receptor on the DNBS-induced Ts.

B. *Suppressor T-Cell Networks Induced by DNP-Modified Syngeneic Spleen Cells*

Following the initial observation of Battisto and Bloom (1), we found that the iv injection of minute amounts of DNFB coupled to syngeneic spleen cells (DNP-SC) leads to profound and efficient unresponsiveness to DNFB contact sensitivity (17). Since then, this method has been demonstrated in other contact sensitivity systems (12) and in delayed hypersensitivity to complex protein antigens (22, 32). The tolerance induced by DNP-SC appears to be mediated by two pathways:

clone inhibition and activity of Ts (19). Tolerance develops within 1 day of injection and lasts 6-8 weeks, but Ts are only demonstrable from 4-21 days after tolerization. The Ts appear as two distinct waves of suppression. The first suppressor (Ts-1) is found in the spleen and lymph nodes of tolerant donors from 3 to 9 days post tolerization. The precursors of Ts-1 are sensitive to 100-200 mg/kg of cyclophosphamide (19) and short-term adult thymectomy and arise primarily from the spleen (37). These cells bear the classic suppressor phenotype in that they are $Lyt\text{-}2^+$ and $I\text{-}J^+$.

The target of Ts-1 has been shown to be the efferent (elicitation) phase of the contact sensitivity response (21), and may well involve hapten-MHC components passively bound to T_{DH} (see Section III,B). Ts-1 can suppress previously sensitized recipients if transferred one day prior to ear challenge. Furthermore, cotransfer of Ts-1 and DNFB-immune T_{DH} to normal recipients blocks the passive transfer of contact sensitivity. This efferent suppression of syngeneic DH by Ts-1 requires a third cell which we have termed Ts-auxiliary (Ts-aux). Ts-aux is present in lymph node populations from DNFB-sensitized mice and is sensitive to cyclophosphamide (T_{DH} is not). Ts-aux is also sensitive to short-term adult thymectomy and bears I-J determinants (35). Ts-1 and Ts-aux interact via allotype-linked interactions to suppress the effector function of T_{DH}. This network is shown in Fig. 1. Thus, T-T interactions, perhaps idiotype/antiidiotype in nature, are required for the expression of the suppressive activity of Ts-1 and appear to be similar to both the feedback suppression system of Eardley *et al.* (8) and the carrier-specific suppressor system of Tada and Okumura (38).

The use of DNP-SC provided an excellent model to ask whether MHC restrictions were involved in Ts induction or expression. We had observed that only those DNP congeners

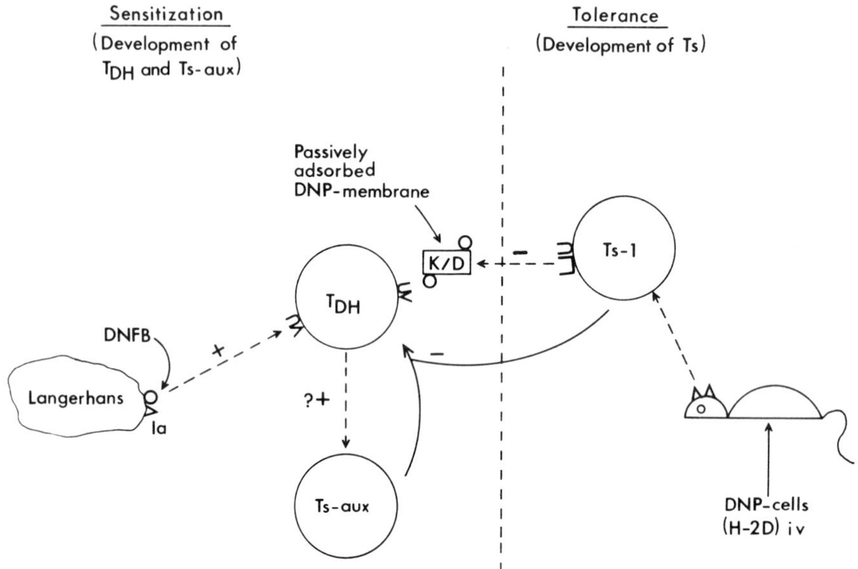

FIGURE 1. A schematic representation of sensitization to to DNFB and down-regulation (tolerance) by efferent-acting Ts-1 induced in another animal (other regulatory cells are omitted). DNFB is painted on the skin and couples to Ia-positive Langerhans cells. This complex expands the clone of T_{DH} which bear receptors for DNP and for Ia. These T_{DH} also carry passively adsorbed membrane (from macrophages?) carrying DNP and K/D. Painting with DNFB also induces a Ts-auxiliary cell (Ts-aux) which may be stimulated by T_{DH}. In tolerance (on the right), iv injection of DNP-cells bearing H-2D induce efferent-acting Ts-1. These cells, when mixed with T_{DH} (*and* in the presence of Ts-aux) inhibit T_{DH}.

that covalently couple to self proteins were able to induce tolerance and Ts in the DNFB contact sensitivity system (3, 4). Compounds such as monovalent DNP-lysine and DNP-γ2a and DNP-D-G,L, which are potent DNP-specific B-cell tolerogens (11, 15), were found neither to stimulate Ts directly nor to block their subsequent stimulation by DNP-SC, indicating that Ts are induced by DNP coupled to self membranes (18). Studies with congenic resistant mice showed that DNP-MHC determinants, specifically DNP-H-2D, were in fact essential for the induction of Ts-1 (20). In contrast to the requirement for H-2D region compatibility for Ts-1 induction, these Ts were found to be non-MHC restricted in their expression. Blocking experiments using DNP-SC lysates showed that the wave of MHC-nonrestricted Ts consisted of a polyclonal wave of suppressor activity composed of distinct MHC-restricted Ts. That is, some of the clones were specific for DNP-syngeneic determinants and other clones recognized DNP-allogeneic determinants (16). Recent experiments have shown that if the spleen cells are modified with limiting concentrations of DNFB, the Ts-1 induced appear to be MHC restricted to H-2K and/or H-2D region determinants (S. D. Miller, unpublished). We have invoked a two-receptor model of Ts activation to explain these observations (5). Thus, Ts-1 appears to recognize DNP-modified MHC determinants and inhibits efferent sensitivity.

About 14 days after tolerization with syngeneic DNP-SC, Ts are still demonstrable in the spleen, but can no longer be detected in the lymph nodes. In contrast to the first wave of suppression, we have recently shown that this second-order Ts (Ts-2) appears to inhibit the afferent (induction) phase of sensitivity. Thus, Ts-2 inhibits normal post-DNFB sensitization cell proliferation in the draining lymph nodes of recipient mice, but has no effect on passive transfer of sensitization upon cotransfer with DNFB-immune T_{DH} cells. Also, in contrast to Ts-1, Ts-2 is MHC restricted in the expression of its suppressive properties. We feel that Ts-2 is antiidiotypic in nature since (a) it can be inhibited by treatment with anti-DNP serum, but not with DNP-SC lysates and (b) Ts-2 appears to neutralize the efferent suppressive properties of Ts-1 when both Ts are transferred to normal recipients together with DNFB-immune T_{DH} cells (S. D. Miller and H. N. Claman, unpublished). Thus, the injection of DNP-modified syngeneic cells appears to lead to the induction of a complex Ts network. A similar situation has been recently demonstrated in DH to azobenzenearsonate (33), where the injection of an idiotype-positive suppressor factor with antigen-binding properties into normal mice leads to the induction of an antiidiotypic second-order Ts.

III. SUPPRESSOR FACTORS IN CONTACT SENSITIVITY

In addition to Ts, contact sensitivity reactions are also regulated by suppressor factors (6, 24, 26, 44, 45). In this section, we will describe some of the properties and characteristics of a "soluble suppressor factor" (SSF) which regulates the effector limb of contact sensitivty to DNFB. For a detailed discussion of suppressor factors that regulate humoral immunity and other types of cell-mediated responses, the reader is referred to recent comprehensive review articles (9, 38).

A. *Induction, Characteristics, Specificity, and Mode of Action of Soluble Suppressor Factor*

1. Induction. T cells that produce SSF are induced by the iv injection of the reactive hapten DNBS (750 mg/kg). Triggering of SSF production, however, requires additional cell stimulation, which is achieved by epicutaneous application of DNFB 5 days after tolerization by the DNBS (24). This secondary stimulation is obligatory for SSF production and is hapten specific (24). Sixteen to twenty-four hours after painting the tolerant mice with DNFB, lymph node cells are placed in culture for 48 hr, during which time the factor is released into the culture medium. The nature of the secondary triggering stimulus *in vivo* is unknown. However, recent *in vitro* studies indicate that factor-production is stimulated by the specific interaction of the DNBS-primed T cells with DNP in association with H-2K and/or H-2D gene products (J. W. Moorhead, unpublished observations).

2. *Characteristics*. This suppressor factor has been partially characterized by column and affinity chromatography. Based on the elution profile of activity from Sephadex G-100 columns, the factor appears to have a molecular weight of between 35,000 and 60,000. It is not known whether it exists as a single molecule or has subunit structure. Affinity chromatography studies have shown that the factor does not bear antigenic determinants of immunoglobulin heavy or light chains nor does it have the hapten DNP associated with it (25). Rather, the factor expresses determinants encoded by genes in the MHC (25) which appear to map to the I-E/C subregion. Thus, this factor belongs to a family of suppressor molecules that have also been shown to carry determinants endoded by I region genes (14, 28, 30, 40-42).

3. *Specificity*. Suppression by SSF is hapten specific, i.e., it suppresses contact sensitivity to DNFB but not to TNCB (24). In addition, the factor is adsorbed by, and can be recovered from, affinity columns conjugated with DNP proteins (24). Other columns conjugated with TNP proteins do not adsorb the factor. These findings suggest that the specificity of suppression by SSF is based, at least in part, on its ability to discriminate between DNP and TNP. This would indicate that recognition of hapten is an essential step in factor-mediated suppression.

4. *Mode of Action*. Regulation of contact sensitivity by SSF is limited to suppressing effector functions of DNFB-immune T cells. In other words, the factor suppresses the ability of immune T cells to transfer contact sensitivity

in vivo (24) or to produce MIF *in vitro* (J. W. Moorhead, unpublished observations). SSF appears to have no effect on the induction of immune T cells and thus far, repeated injection of SSF into normal mice has not induced Ts. This latter finding is in contrast to the studies of Greene, *et al.* (12) which showed that injection of TNCB suppressor factor-induced specific Ts which regulated effector functions of TNCB-immune T cells.

B. Genetic Restrictions for SSF-Mediated Suppression

In addition to having hapten specificity, suppression by SSF is also genetically restricted by genes that map in the MHC. However, unlike other factors that carry I region determinants and require I region identity with their target cells (9, 38, 39), suppression by SSF requires identity at the H-2K and/or H-2D region between the factor-producing strain and the donor of immune cells (25). It follows then that gene products of these loci serve as target or interacting molecules for the suppressor factor. We established this point by adsorbing suppressor supernatants with a variety of normal or immune LN cell populations. These studies clearly showed that the target or acceptor molecules for SSF are expressed only on DNFB-immune T cells (26). Furthermore, in order for the T cells to adsorb the factor, they must share with the factor-producing strain either the H-2K or H-2D region of the MHC (26).

The essential role of these histocompatibility determinants was further shown by antiserum blocking studies. Immune T cells treated with antibodies specific for H-2K or H-2D determinants no longer adsorb the factor (26). Treating the cells with antibodies directed against Ia antigens has no effect. However, further studies showed that histocompatibility antigens alone were not the target molecules for SSF. Treating immune T cells with affinity-purified anti-DNP antibodies also blocks adsorption of the factor (26). Thus, the target molecules on DNFB-immune T cells for SSF are histocompatibility antigens associated with the hapten DNP. However, it does not appear that this target complex, i.e., DNP-H-2K or H-2D, is formed by the covalent binding of DNFB with the histocompatibility antigens expressed by the T cells. Rather, the complex appears to be passively adsorbed to the T_{DH} cells since short-term incubation of the immune T cells *in vitro* in serum-free medium renders them insensitive to SSF-mediated suppression and incapable of adsorbing the suppressor factor. We believe that during this *in vitro* incubation, the complex is shed from the surface of the T_{DH} cells. The source of the DNP-H-2 complex is not known although it most likely comes from membrane material shed by antigen-presenting cells (macrophages?). Although speculative at this time, it is possible that the DNP-H-2K/H-2D complex recognized by SSF represents the same or similar determinants which are recognized by cytotoxic T cells induced *in vitro* to hapten-modified autologous lymphocytes (2, 31). The meaning of this similarity with respect to the mechanism of suppression by SSF remains to be determined, but the experiments so far allow a tentative model, as shown in Fig. 2.

At the present time, exactly how the factor interacts with the DNP-H-2K/H-2D complex is not known. The ability of either anti-H-2 or anti-DNP antibodies alone to block adsorption suggests that the factor must bind or recognize both moieties simultaneously. We do not know, however, whether the factor is monovalent and recognizes a neoantigen produced by the association of DNP and H-2, i.e., altered self, or whether it is bi- or multivalent and recognizes the two as independent

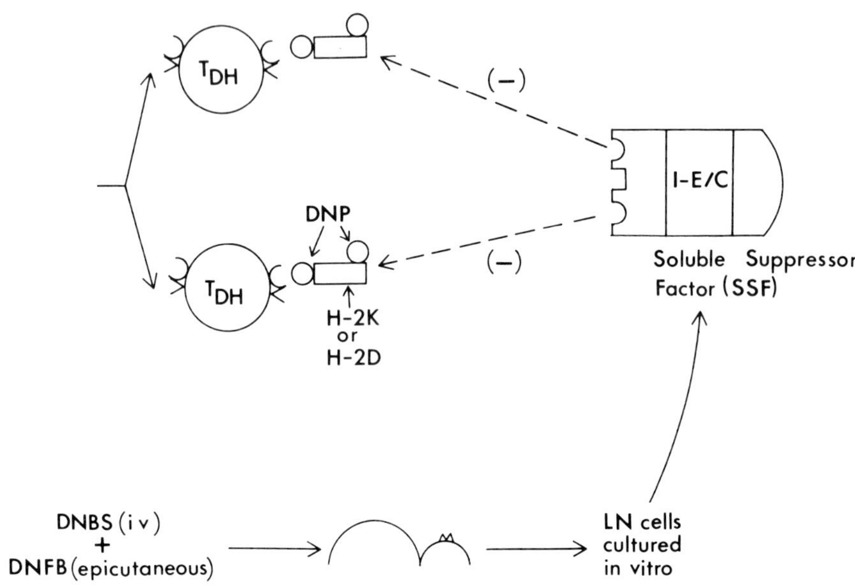

FIGURE 2. The action of soluble suppressor factor (SSF) raised by a combination of DNBS iv and DNFB epicutaneously. This factor has affinity for the passively adsorbed DNP-K/D on T_{DH}, and also bears I-E/C determinants. It down-regulates the T_{DH}.

structures. It seems unlikely that the factor is directed against a neoantigen since it is adsorbed by DNP affinity columns where such a determinant would not be present. Rather, we believe the factor is at least bivalent, expressing one receptor site specific for DNP and one site specific for self H-2K or H-2D determinants. Confirmation of this model must await biochemical analysis of the factor.

IV. SUMMARY

The work outlined above shows that contact sensitivity reactions are controllable at virtually every stage. The sensitization process is regulated by antiidiotypic antibody. Tolerance to contact sensitivity can be deliberately induced prior to sensitization by "free" hapten or hapten coupled to cells. This tolerance is effected by a variety of mechanisms including suppressor cells, suppressor factors, and probably some other nonsuppressive mechanisms. It seems reasonable that such mechanisms operate in all instances of T-cell responses.

REFERENCES

1. Battisto, J. R. and Bloom, B. R. Dual immunological unresponsiveness induced by cell membrane coupled hapten or antigen. *Nature (London) 212*, 156 (1966).

2. Burakoff, S. J., Germain, R. D., Dorf, M. E., and Benacerraf, B. Inhibition of cell-mediated cytolysis of TNP-derivitized target cells by alloantisera directed to products of the K and D loci of the H-2 complex. *Proc. Natl. Acad. Sci. U.S.A. 73*, 625 (1976).

3. Claman, H. N. Tolerance and contact sensitivity to DNFB in mice. V. Induction of tolerance with DNP compounds and with free and membrane-associated DNFB. *J. Immunol. 116*, 704 (1976).

4. Claman, H. N., Miller, S. D., Conlon, P. J., and Moorhead, J. W. Control of experimental contact sensitivity. *Adv. Immunol. 30*, 121 (1980).

5. Claman, H. N., Miller, S. C., and Sy, M. A. Suppressor cells in tolerance to contact sensitivity active against hapten-syngeneic and hapten-allogeneic determinants. *J. Exp. Med. 146*, 19 (1977).

6. Claman, H. N., Miller, S. D., Sy, M. S., and Moorhead, J. W. Suppressive mechanisms involving sensitization and tolerance in contact allergy. *Immunol. Rev. 50*, 105 (1980).

7. Doherty, P. C., Gotze, D., Trinchieri, G., and Zinkernagel, R. M. Models for recognition of virally modified cells by immune thymus-derived lymphocytes. *Immunogenetics 3*, 517 (1976).

8. Eardley, D. D., Shen, F. W., Cantor, H., and Gershon, R. K. Genetic control of immunoregulatory circuits: genes linked to the Ig locus govern communication between regulatory T-cell sets. *J. Exp. Med. 150*, 44 (1979).

9. Germain, R. N. and Benacerraf, B. Helper and suppressor T cell factors. *Springer Semin. Immunopathol. 3*, 93 (1980).

10. Gershon, R. K. and Kondo, K. Infectious immunological tolerance. *Immunology 21*, 903 (1971).

11. Golan, D. T. and Borel, Y. Nonantigenicity and immunologic tolerance: the role of the carrier in the induction of tolerance to the hapten. *J. Exp. Med. 134*, 1046 (1971).

12. Greene, M. I., Pierres, A., Dorf, M. E., and Benacerraf, B. The I-J subregion codes for determinants on suppressor factor(s) which limit the contact sensitivity to picrylchloride. *J. Exp. Med. 146*, 293 (1977).

13. Jerne, N. K. Toward a network theory of the immune system. *Ann. Immunol. (Paris) 125*, 373 (1974).

14. Kapp, J. A., Pierce, C. W., DeLaCroix, F., and Benacerraf, B. Immunosuppressive factor(s) extracted from lymphoid cells of nonresponder mice primed with L. glutamic acid-L-alanine-L-tyrosine (GAT). I. Activity and antigenic specificity. *J. Immunol. 116*, 305 (1976).

15. Katz, D. H., Davie, J. M., Paul, W. E., and Benacerraf, B. Carrier function in anti-hapten antibody responses. IV. Experimental conditions for the induction of hapten-specific tolerance or for the stimulation of anti-hapten anamnestic responses by "nonimmunogenic" hapten-polypeptide conjugates. *J. Exp. Med. 134*, 201 (1971).

16. Miller, S. D. Suppressor T cell mechanisms in contact sensitivity. III. Apparent non-major histocompatibility complex restriction is a result of multiple sets of MHC-specific suppressor T cells induced by syngeneic 2,4-dinitrophenyl-modified lymphoid cells. *J. Exp. Med. 150*, 676 (1979).

17. Miller, S. D. and Claman, H. N. The induction of hapten-specific T cell tolerance using hapten-modified lymphoid cells. I. Characteristics of tolerance induction. *J. Immunol. 117*, 1519 (1976).

18. Miller, S. D., Conlon, P. J., Sy, M. S., Moorhead, J. W., Colon, S., Grey, H. M., and Claman, H. N. Nature of hapten-modified determinants involved in induction of T cell tolerance and suppressor T cells to DNFB contact sensitivity. *J. Immunol. 124*, 1187 (1980).

19. Miller, S. D., Sy, M. S., and Claman, H. N. The induction of hapten-specific T cell tolerance using hapten-modified lymphoid cells. II. Relative roles of suppressor T cells and clone inhibition in the tolerant state. *Eur. J. Immunol. 7*, 165 (1977).

20. Miller, S. D., Sy, M. S., and Claman, H. N. Genetic restrictions for the induction of suppressor T cells by hapten-modeified lymphoid cells in tolerance to DNFB contact sensitivity: role of the H-2D region of the major histocompatibility complex. *J. Exp. Med. 147*, 788 (1978).

21. Miller, S. D., Sy, M. S., and Claman, H. N. Suppressor T cell mechanisms in contact sensitivity. I. Efferent blockade by syninduced suppressor T cells. *J. Immunol. 121*, 265 (1978).

22. Miller, S. D., Wetzig, R. P., and Claman, H. N. The induction of cell-mediated immunity and tolerance with protein antigens coupled to syngeneic lymphoid cells. *J. Exp. Med. 149*, 758 (1979).

23. Moorhead, J. W. Tolerance and contact sensitivity to DNFB in mice. VI. Inhibition of afferent sensitivity by suppressor T cells in adoptive tolerance. *J. Immunol. 117*, 802 (1976).

24. Moorhead, J. W. Soluble factors in tolerance and contact sensitivity to DNFB in mice. I. Suppression of contact sensitivity by soluble suppressor factor released *in vitro* by lymph node cells containing specific suppressor cells. *J. Immunol. 119*, 315 (1977).

25. Moorhead, J. W. Soluble factors in tolerance and contact sensitivity to DNFB in mice. II. Genetic requirements for suppression of contact sensitivity by soluble suppressor factor. *J. Immunol. 119*, 1773 (1977).

26. Moorhead, J. W. Soluble factors in tolerance and contact sensitivity to DNFB in mice. III. Histocompatibility antigens associated with the hapten DNP serve as target molecules on DNFB-immune T cells for soluble suppressor factor. *J. Exp. Med. 150*, 1432 (1979).

27. Moorhead, J. W. and Scott, D. W. Tolerance and contact sensitivity to DNFB in mice. VII. Functional demonstration of cell-associated tolerogen in lymph node cell populations containing specific suppressor cells. *Cell. Immunol. 28*, 443 (1977).

28. Perry, L., Benacerraf, B., and Greene, M. I. Regulation of the immune response to tumor antigens. IV. Tumor antigen-specific suppressor factor(s) bear I-J determinants and induce suppressor T cells *in vivo*. *J. Immunol. 121*, 2144 (1978).

29. Phanuphak, P., Moorhead, J. W., and Claman, H. N. Tolerance and contact sensitivity to DNFB in mice. III. Transfer of tolerance with "suppressor T cells." *J. Immunol. 113*, 1230 (1974).

30. Rich, S. S., David, C. S., and Rich, R. R. Regulatory mechanisms in cell-mediated immune responses. VII. Presence of I-C subregion determinants on mixed lymphocyte reaction suppressor factor. *J. Exp. Med. 149*, 114 (1979).

31. Schmitt-Verhulst, A. M., Sachs, D. H., and Shearer, G. M. Cell-mediated lympholysis of TNP-mediated autologous lymphocytes: confirmation of the genetic control of response to TNP-modified H-2 antigens by the use of anti-H-2 and anti-Ia antibodies. *J. Exp. Med. 143*, 211 (1976).

32. Sherr, D. H., Cheung, N. K. V., Heghinian, K., Benacerraf, B., and Dorf, M. E. Immune suppression *in vivo* with anti-modified syngeneic cells. II. T cell-mediated nonresponsiveness to fowl gamma globulin. *J. Immunol. 122*, 1899 (1979).

33. Sy, M. S., Dietz, M. H., Germain, R. N., Benacerraf, B., and Greene, M. I. Antigen and receptor driven regulatory mechanisms. IV. Idiotype-bearing I-J^+ suppressor T cell factors induce second-order suppressor T cells which express antiidiotypic receptors. *J. Exp. Med. 151*, 1183 (1980).

34. Sy, M. S., Miller, S. D., and Claman, H. N. Immune suppression with supraoptimal doses of antigen in contact sensitivity to DNFB. *J. Immunol. 119*, 240 (1977).

35. Sy, M. S., Miller, S. D., Moorhead, J. W., and Claman, H. N. Active suppression of 1-fluoro-2,4-dinitrobenzene-immune T cells: requirement of an auxiliary T cell induced by antigen. *J Exp. Med. 149*, 1197 (1979).

36. Sy, M. S., Moorhead, J. W., and Claman, H. N. Possible role of anti-receptor antibodies in regulation of contact sensitivity to DNFB in mice. *J. Immunol. 123*, 2593 (1979).

37. Sy, M. S., Miller, S. D., Kowach, H. B., and Claman, H. N. A splenic requirement for the generation of suppressor cells. *J. Immunol. 119*, 2095 (1977).

38. Tada, T. and Okumura, K. The role of antigen-specific T cell factors in the immune response. *Adv. Immunol. 28*, 1 (1979).

39. Tada, T., Taniguchi, M., and David, C. S. Properties of the antigen-specific suppressive T cell factor in the regulation of antibody responses in the mouse. IV. Special subregion assignment of the gene(s) that codes for the suppressive T cell factor in the H-2 histocompatibility complex. *J. Exp. Med. 144*, 713 (1976).

40. Tada, T., Taniguchi, M., and David, C. S. Suppressive and enhancing T-cell factors as I-region gene products: properties and the subregion assignment. *Cold Spring Harbor Symp. Quanit. Biol. 41*, 119-127 (1977).

41. Taniguchi, M. and Miller, J. F. A. P. Specific suppression of the immune response by a factor obtained from spleen cells of mice tolerant to human γ-globulin. *J. Immunol. 120*, 21 (1978).

42. Theze, J., Waltenbaugh, C., Germain, R. N., and Benacerraf, B. Immunosuppressive factor(s) specific for L-glutamic acid-L-tyrosine. IV. *In vitro* activity and immunochemical properties. *Eur. J. Immunol. 7*, 705 (1977).

43. Toews, G. B., Bergstresser, P. R., and Streilein, J. W. Epidermal Langerhans cell density determines whether contact hypersensitivity or unresponsiveness follows skin painting with DNFB. *J. Immunol. 124*, 445 (1980).

44. Zembala, M. and Asherson, G. L. T cell suppression of contact sensitivity in the mouse. II. The role of soluble suppressor factor and its interaction with macrophages. *Eur. J. Immunol. 4*, 799 (1974).

45. Zembala, M., Asherson, G. L., Noworolski, J., and Mayhew, B. Contact sensitivity to picryl chloride: the occurrence of B suppressor cells in the lymph node and spleen of immunized mice. *Cell. Immunol. 25*, 266 (1976).

Immunopathology: VIIIth International Symposium, 1980

CELL-CELL INTERACTIONS IN THE EXPRESSION OF HISTAMINE-INDUCED SUPPRESSOR CELL ACTIVITY

Dennis J. Beer
Charles A. Dinarello
Lanny J. Rosenwasser
Ross E. Rocklin

The Divisions of Allergy and Immunology
and Experimental Medicine,
Department of Medicine,
Tufts-New England Medical Center Hospital,
Boston, Massachusetts

The role of cells that regulate immune responses has recently been the focus of many studies both in animal models and in man. For example, an abnormal number or state of activation of suppressor T cells has been demonstrated in some patients with agammaglobulinemia (7, 33) or with isolated immunoglobulin deficiency (34), as well as in animal models of agammaglobulinemia (4). Non-T cell suppressors have also been detected in the polyclonal immunodeficiency associated with multiple myeloma (6), the anergy associated with Hodgkin's disease (32), and widespread granulomatous infections (10). Suppressor cells have also been implicated in the immunological enhancement of tumor growth (12). At the other end of the spectrum in immunological response, loss of suppressor cell

ISBN 0-12-218320-7

activity has been implicated in the pathogenesis of autoimmune disorders studied in animal models and in autoimmune disease of man (2, 13).

These regulatory or suppressor cells have a number of surface membrane structures by which they can be identified. In the mouse, T-cell populations may be distinguished by virtue of their Ly phenotype (8). Antisera to the Ly-2,3$^+$ phenotype eliminates specific and nonspecific T-cell suppressor activity (8, 17). Human suppressor cells may also be identified by the presence of receptors for the Fc portion of IgG or receptors for vasoactive amines such as histamine on their membranes (18, 22, 28).

The histamine receptor-bearing T lymphocyte has been of particular interest to this laboratory. Experiments in a number of species have suggested that vasoactive amines may play an important role in regulating immune responses both *in vivo* and *in vitro* (5, 27, 37). Histamine is of particular interest because of its inhibitory effects *in vivo* on the expression of delayed cutaneous hypersensitivity and *in vitro* on T cell-mediated cytotoxicity, lymphocyte proliferation, and lymphokine production (3, 16, 19, 20, 26, 36). An analysis of the mechanism of suppression by histamine *in vitro* revealed that the amine did not affect macrophage responses to migration inhibitory factor (MIF) or antigen presentation to lymphocytes (22). Instead, it was found that lymphocytes chromatographed on histamine-affinity columns produced MIF and proliferated normally on challenge with antigen or mitogen, even in the presence of histamine. The latter observation suggested the possibility that the histamine-responsive cells exerted a regulatory influence on T-cell effector responses. This subsequently led to the finding that lymphocytes stimulated by histamine elaborate a soluble factor, termed histamine-induced suppressor factor or HSF, with immunosuppressive properties (21). The cells that produce HSF have been partially characterized. Human blood T- and B-cell populations, separated by affinity chromatography with rabbit antihuman $F(ab')_2$, were examined for their ability to make HSF. Highly purified populations of T cells, but not B cells, produced HSF in response to varying concentrations of histamine (24). When human mononuclear cells were chromatographed over columns containing conjugates of insolublized histamine, the nonretained cells did not produce significant amounts of HSF. In addition, it was shown that cells synthesizing HSF predominantly express histamine-type 2 receptors because 4-methylhistamine (H_2 agonist), but not 2-methylhistamine (H_1 agonist), was capable of inducing HSF production. Furthermore, cimetidine (H_2 antagonist), but not chlorpheniramine (H_1 antagonist), could abrogate the histamine-induced generation of HSF. Studies employing rosette formation with IgG (T_γ) or IgM (T_μ)-coated ox red cells revealed that cells with histamine receptors compromise approximately 50% of the T_γ subpopulation, but are not found in the T_μ subpopulation (24).

Sufficient information has now been accumulated to postulate a model for the regulatory role of histamine in cellular immune reactions (23). Histamine might serve as a negative-feedback regulator of lymphocyte function, as depicted in Fig. 1. Release of histamine from tissue mast cells or basophils may result from an IgE-mediated mechanism or through the action of a recently described lymphokine, histamine-releasing factor (31). Once released, histamine presumably activates the suppressor limb of the immune reaction and dampens the response by decreasing production or release of MIF, lymphocyte blast transformation, and possibly other lymphocyte functions. The possible simultaneous release of diverse lymphokines such as MIF, which enhance cellular immune reactions,

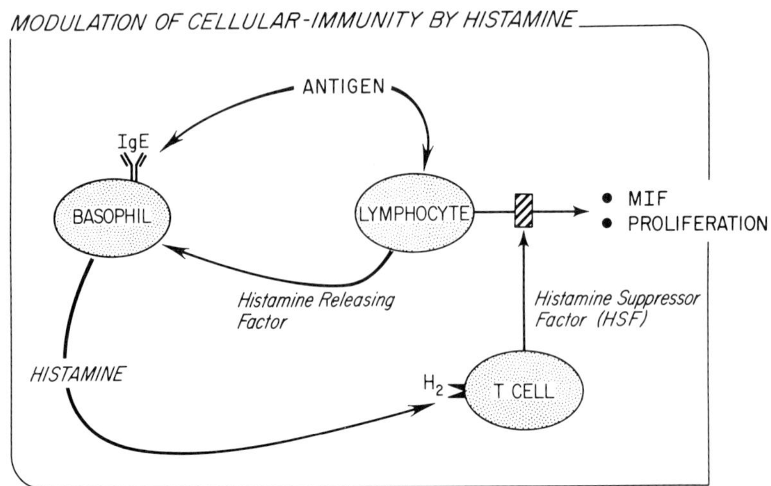

FIGURE 1. A proposed model to explain the regulatory role of histamine as part of a negative feedback mechanism on cellular immune phenomenon. See text for explanation.

and histamine-releasing factor, which via subsequent histamine release and consequent generation of HSF serves to dampen these responses, would make the balance of local environmental considerations an important factor in determining the extent or character of an immune reaction resulting in any given situation.

Employing an *in vitro* co-culture technique, we have investigated certain basic biological aspects of the histamine-induced suppressor cell system. The generation of suppressor cells using histamine and their assay is similar to that described for concanavalin A (Con A) (29). Human blood mononuclear cells were isolated from healthy volunteers by means of density centrifugation in a ficoll-Hypaque gradient. The cells were cultured at a concentration of 6×10^5 ml in medium Tc-199 (containing 15% AB serum and antibiotics) in the absence or presence of histamine (10^{-5} *M* to 10^{-3} *M*) for 24 hr at 37°C in a 5% CO_2-95% humidified atmosphere. Indicator cells from the same subject were cultured separately in the absence of any stimulant in culture medium. Following incubation, the control or histamine-activated suppressor cells were mitomycin treated (50 μg/ml) for 1 hr at 37°C, washed three times with TC-199 and mixed with autologous indicator cells at a 1:2 ratio. The cell mixture was then stimulated by 10 μg/ml of Con A and placed in microtiter plates (2×10^5 cells/well) for three days. Eighteen hours prior to terminating the cultures, 1 μCi/well of [^{3}H]thymidine was added. Incorporation of [^{3}H]thymidine into cellular DNA was determined by harvesting the cultures in a MASH II harvester and the radioactivity recorded by liquid scintillation counting. The degree of suppression of [^{3}H]thymidine incorporation was determined by the following formula:

$$\%\ \text{suppression} = 1 - \frac{\text{C.P.M. in presence of histamine}}{\text{C.P.M. in absence of histamine}} \times 100$$

The mean C.P.M. was determined from quadruplicate wells, with the variability of any one quadruplicate being less than 10%. An example of the suppressor cell activity obtained using mononuclear cells from healthy volunteers is summarized in Fig. 2. Blood mononuclear cells from three subjects when precultured with histamine (10^{-5} to 10^{-3} *M*) and subsequently combined with autologous indicator cells inhibited the proliferative response to Con A in a dose-dependent fashion.

Several investigators have demonstrated in murine systems that adherent accessory cells are required for the *in vitro* activation of splenic T cells by Con A (1, 11). Using 3-g nylon wool columns to deplete human peripheral blood mononuclear cells (PBMC) of adherent cells (predominantly macrophages and B cells), we have recently demonstrated that the remaining nonadherent T-cell enriched (NWNA-T) population was not triggered by histamine to express its regulatory function. Esterase staining of the NWNA-T population showed fewer than 1% esterase-positive cells. The data from three experiments

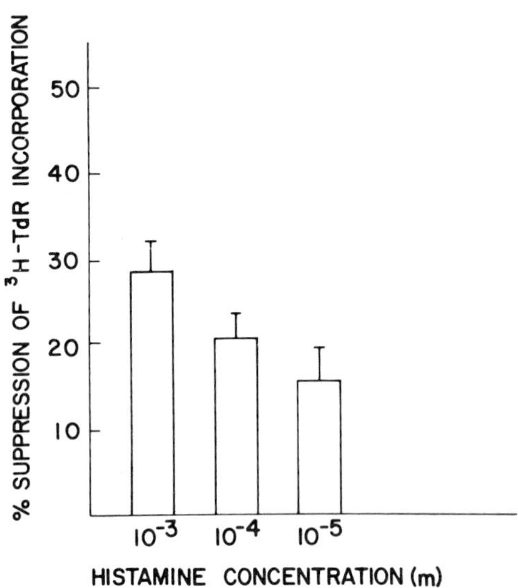

FIGURE 2. Histamine-induced suppression of the proliferative response using a co-culture technique. Mononuclear cells from three individuals were cultured for 18 hr with 10^{-5} to 10^{-3} *M* histamine and then co-cultured with autologous indicator cells that were then stimulated to concanavalin A. The data are expressed as percent suppression of tritiated thymidine incorporation ±SEM. Histamine caused a dose-dependent suppression of proliferation.

are summarized in Table I. Suppression of [^{3}H]thymidine uptake at each of two concentrations of histamine (10^{-3} *M* and 10^{-4} *M*) is expressed as the mean % ±SEM. Addition of 10% autologous glass adherent cells or 20% sheep red blood cell (E) rosette-negative autologous cells was sufficient to restore histamine-induced suppressor activity to the NWNA-T cell population. Autologous E rosette-positive cells were unable to restore histamine-induced suppressor activity to the NWNA-T population.

Having established that adherent cells (macrophages/monocytes) subserve an accessory function in the activation of histamine-induced suppressor cells, we investigated the role of soluble products derived from monocytes in replacing the

TABLE I. Requirement for Monocytes in the Activation of Histamine-Induced Suppressor T Cells*

Cell population	% Suppression of [^{3}H]thymidine incorporation	
	10^{-3} *M* histamine	10^{-4} *M* histamine
Peripheral blood mononuclear cells (PBMC)	26 ± 3	21 ± 2
Nylon wool nonadherent T-cell enriched (NWNA-T)	5 ± 1	0 ± 4
NWNA-T + 20% E rosette negative cells	31 ± 4	20 ± 1
NWNA-T + 10% monocytes	25 ± 3	20 ± 1

*****Suppression of tritiated thymidine incorporation at each of two concentrations of histamine is expressed as the mean percent ±SEM for three separate experiments. Peripheral blood mononuclear cells depleted of nylon-wool adherent cells were unable to express suppressor activity when stimulated with histamine. Reconstitution of this T-cell-enriched population with autologous monocytes either in the form of E rosette-negative cells or glass adherent cells restored histamine-induced suppressor activity to the NWNA-T cell population.*

adherent cell requirement for the generation of histamine-induced T-suppressor cells. As shown in Table II, crude monocyte supernatants generated from human allogeneic monocytes that have phagocytized heat-killed *Staphylococcus albus* were capable of reconstituting the histamine-stimulated suppressor activity of NWNA-T cells.

Prior investigations have demonstrated that purified human leukocytic pyrogen (LP) partially replaced the macrophage requirement for murine thymus (T) lymphocyte recognition of specific antigens (25) and that LP and leukocyte-activating factor (LAF, Interleukin-I) are the same molecule (9, 25). We therefore attempted to identify the biochemical and functional

TABLE II. Ability of Monocyte Factors to Replace the Adherent Cell Requirement for the Generation of Histamine-Induced Suppressor T-Cells*

Cell population	% Suppression of [^{3}H]thymidine incorporation	
	10^{-3} *M* histamine	10^{-4} *M* histamine
Peripheral blood mononuclear cells (PBMC)	26 ± 3	21 ± 2
Nylon wool nonadherent T-cell enriched (NWNA-T)	5 ± 1	0 ± 4
NWNA-T + crude monocyte supernatant	26 ± 4	19 ± 1
NWNA-T + 40,000 MW fraction	28 ± 4	22 ± 3
NWNA-T + 15,000 MW fraction	31 ± 4	30 ± 3

Suppression of tritiated thymidine incorporation at each of two concentrations of histamine is expressed as the mean percent ±SEM for three separate experiments. Crude monocyte supernatant was capable of reconstituting the histamine-stimulated suppressor activity of NWNA-T cells. The activity was confined to 40,000- and 15,000-daltons moieties within the crude supernatant.

properties of that moiety in crude monocyte supernatant capable of reconstituting histamine-inducible suppressor activity of NWNA-T cells.

Crude monocyte-derived supernatants were fractionated on Sephadex G-50 gels. Two peaks of pyrogenic activity were identified with apparent molecular weights of approximately 40,000 and 15,000 (9). These peak fractions were capable of reconstituting NWNA-T histamine-activated suppressor activity (see Table II). Neither the crude monocyte supernatant nor the 40,000 and 15,000 molecular weight species were themselves able to activate suppressor cells nonspecifically. Since the active fractions had an apparent MW similar to that of LP, the 15,000-dalton fraction was applied to a rabbit antihuman LP Sepharose-4B immunoabsorbant. The nonretained material was unable to reconstitute NWNA-T histamine-activated suppressor cell activity. Reconstitutive activity was recovered from the immunoabsorbant column following elution with citric acid. In addition to reconstituting histamine-induced suppressor activity to human NWNA-T cells, these fractions were capable of producing fever in female white rabbits and were able to enhance the proliferative response of murine thymic cells (T) to PHA (data not shown). The latter assay system is used to measure LAF activity.

Since monocytes have been shown to act as regulatory cells, capable of inhibiting lymphocyte proliferation by a mechanism that may involve prostaglandin synthesis (15), it was of particular interest to determine whether histamine-induced suppressor activity was sensitive to the effects of indomethacin (a prostaglandin synthetase inhibitor). The use of the co-culture technique permitted us to divide the histamine-induced suppressor cell system into a generation phase and an effector phase. When indomethacin was added to the generation phase of the suppressor cell assay at a concentration of 1 μg/ml, there was no enhancement or decrement in the generation of histamine-induced suppressor cells (Table III). However, when indomethacin (1 μg/ml) was added at the time of the co-culture of histamine-triggered suppressor cells and autologous indicator cells, there was a significant abrogation of suppressor cell activity. In other words, the inhibitory action of histamine-induced suppressor cells could be partially blocked by adding a prostaglandin synthetase inhibitor to the mitogen-stimulated cultures.

TABLE III. Effect of Indomethacin on Histamine-Induced Suppressor T-Cell activity*

Cell population	% Suppression of [^{3}H]thymidine incorporation	
	10^{-3} *M* histamine	10^{-4} *M* histamine
Peripheral blood mononuclear cells (PBMC)	26 ± 3	21 ± 2
PBMC and indomethacin added to generation phase	29 ± 4	17 ± 4
PBMC and indomethacin added to effector phase	10 ± 5	6 ± 2

**Suppression of tritiated thymidine incorporation at each of two concentrations of histamine is expressed as the mean percent ±SEM for three separate experiments. Indomethacin at a concentration of 1 μg/ml had no effect on histamine-induced suppression when added during the generation phase of a co-culture experiment. When indomethacin (1 μg/ml) was added during the effector phase of the co-culture there was significant abrogation of suppressor cell activity.*

The above data partially characterize the cell-cell interactions involved in histamine-generated suppressor activity. Afferent and efferent limbs of suppressor activity involve many steps linked by T cell-monocyte cooperation. The monocyte is required as an accessory cell for the triggering of T cells by histamine, and as an effector cell to mediate suppression. The generation phase of histamine-induced suppressor T lymphocytes requires the presence of monocytes or a monokine derived from mononuclear phagocytes. This monokine has physicochemical, biological, and antigenic properties similar to leukocytic pyrogen. The soluble factor derived from monocytes that subserves the accessory adherent cell function in the generation of HSF-secreting T lymphocytes can be labeled "semi-purified" LP. We are in the process of producing highly purified LP by a sequence of immunoabsorption followed by citric acid elution and sequential gel filtration on Sephadex G-50, Sephadex G-15, and finally ion exchange over DEAE (9). The moiety thus isolated, which then produces fever in rabbits and demonstrates LAF activity in the mitogen-stimulated murine thymocyte assay, will be tested for its ability to reconstitute the NWNA-T cell response to histamine. We suggest that HSF may stimulate mononuclear phagocytic cells to secrete inhibitory protaglandins which diminish lymphocyte proliferation.

Reduction in immune reativity *in vitro* can result from exposure to a large number of biological agents. In addition to histamine, prostaglandins of the E series (PGE), Con A, hydrocortisone, isoproterenol, and interferon can all suppress a wide variety of immunologic reactions (5, 14, 15, 35). The existence of many immunosuppressive substances raises the question of their mechanisms of action and whether or not there may be a common denominator responsible for their suppressive effects. In this regard, Staszak and Goodwin (30) have recently shown a link between the synthesis of prostaglandin and the ability of histamine to inhibit the *in vitro* lymphocyte proliferative response to mitogen. Their evidence for this is as follows: First, inhibition of mitogenesis by PGE_2 was significantly correlated with inhibition by histamine. If histamine and PGE_2 show a common inhibitory pathway, then inhibition by any single agent should correlate with inhibition by the other. Second, indomethacin partially blocked inhibition by histamine. Inhibition by histamine was also blocked by RO 20-5720, whose only known action is reversible inhibition of prostaglandin synthetase. Lastly, histamine lost its ability to inhibit PHA-stimulated [^{3}H]thymidine incorporation in peripheral blood mononuclear cells after removal of nylon-wool adherent cells. The latter effect could be explained either by the requirement of monocytes for suppressor cell activation and/or production of PGE by monocytes during the effector stage of suppression.

Our recent studies are in basic agreement with the findings of Staszak and Goodwin. The co-culture technique that we employed permits an expansion of their findings. The generation phase of histamine-induced suppressor cells was not affected by the addition of indomethacin. Rather, the effector phase of histamine-induced suppression was abrogated. This loss of histamine-induced suppression at the effector phase by indomethacin suggests that the T-cell-induced suppressive mediator HSF (25,000-40,000 daltons) stimulates another cell, probably a monocyte to synthesize prostaglandins. The latter may directly inhibit T-cell proliferation or lymphokine production.

The observation that histamine is unable to inhibit mitogen-induced proliferation of mononuclear cells after removal of nylon-wool adherent cells can best be explained by understanding Fig. 3. We depict a model of the cell-cell interactions required for the expression of histamine-induced suppression. Histamine, in the presence of monocytes or their secretory product (lymphocyte activating factor = leukocytic pyrogen = Interleukin-I), stimulates a subpopulation of T lymphocytes to secrete histamine-suppressor factor. This lymphokine in turn stimulates mononuclear phagocytes to synthesize inhibitory prostaglandins which suppress a given immune response. The secretion and activity of LP is unaffected by a prostaglandin synthetase inhibitor, whereas the secretion of inhibitory prostaglandins promoted by HSF is inhibitable by such a compound. Of course, HSF could work by other means and its activity not necessarily be limited to the one pathway shown.

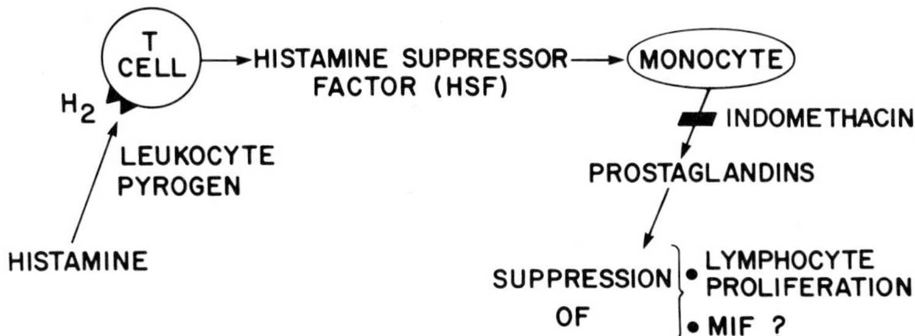

FIGURE 3. A proposed model of the cell-cell interactions required for the expression of histamine-induced suppression. See text for discussion.

In summary, we have shown that certain cell-cell interactions are involved in the activation and expression of histamine-induced suppression of T-cell proliferation. The generation of histamine-triggered suppressor T lymphocytes requires the presence of a secretory product from monocytes which biochemically appears to resemble leukocytic pyrogen. The effector phase of histamine-induced suppression requires monocytes capable of synthesizing inhibitory prostaglandins.

REFERENCES

1. Ahmann, G. B., Sachs, D. H., and Hodes, R. J. Requirement for an Ia-bearing accessory cell in Con A-induced T cell proliferation. *J. Immunol. 121*, 1981 (1978).

2. Allison, A. C., Denman, A. M., and Barnes, R. D. Cooperating and controlling functions of thymus-derived lymphocytes in relation to autoimmunity. *Lancet ii*, 135 (1971).

3. Ballet, J. J. and Merler, E. The separation and reactivity *in vitro* of a subpopulation of human lymphocytes which bind histamine. Correlation of histamine reactivity with cellular maturation. *Cell. Immunol 24*, 250 (1976).

4. Blaese, R. M., Weiden, P. L., Koski, I., and Dooley, N. Infectious agammaglobulinemia: Transmission of immunodeficiency with grafts of agammaglobulinemia cells. *J. Exp. Med. 140*, 1097 (1974).

5. Bourne, H. R., Lichtenstein, L. M., Melmon, K. L., Henney, C. S., Weinstein, Y., and Shearer, G. M. Modulation of inflammation and immunity by cyclic AMP. *Science 184*, 19 (1974).

6. Broder, S., Humphrey, R., Durm, M., Blackman, M., Meade, B., Goldman, C., Strober, W., and Waldmann, T. Impaired synthesis of polyclonal (non paraprotein) immunoglobulins by circulating lymphocytes from patients with multiple myeloma: Role of suppressor cells. *N. Engl. J. Med. 293*, 887 (1975).

7. Broom, B. C., DeLaConcha, E. G., Webster, A. D. B., Janossy, G. J., and Asherson, G. L. Intracellular immunoglobulin production *in vitro* by lymphocytes from patients with hypogammaglobulinemia and their effect on normal lymphocytes. *Clin. Exp. Immunol. 23*, 73 (1976).

8. Cantor, H., Shen, F. W., and Boyse, E. A. Separation of helper T cells from suppressor T cells expressing different Ly components. II. Activation by antigen: After immunization antigen-specific suppressor and helper activities are mediated by distinct T-cell subclasses. *J. Exp. Med. 143*, 1391 (1976).

9. Dinarello, C. A. and Rosenwasser, L. J. Lymphocyte activating properties of human leukocytic pyrogen. *In* "Advances in Immuno-Pharmacology" (J. W. Hadden, L. Chedid, T. Mullen, and F. Spreasico, eds.), 419-425, Pergamos, Oxford, 1981.

10. Ellner, J. J. Suppressor adherent cells in human tuberculosis. *J. Immunol. 121*, 2573 (1978).

11. Frelinger, J. A. Ia-bearing cells promote the concon-navalin A mitogenic response of Ia-negative T cells. *Eur. J. Immunol. 7*, 447 (1977).

12. Fujimoto, J., Greene, M. I., and Sehan, A. H. Regulation of the immune response to tumor antigens. I. Immunosuppressor cells in tumor-bearing hosts. *J. Immunol. 116*, 791 (1976).

13. Gerber, H. L., Hardin, J. A., Chused, T. M., and Steinberg, A. D. Loss with age in NZB/W mice of thymic suppressor cells in the graft-vs-host reaction. *J. Immunol.* *113*, 1618 (1974).

14. Goodwin, J. S., Messner, R. P., and Williams, R. C., Jr. Inhibitions of T-cell mitogenesis: Effect of mitogen dose. *Cell. Immunol.* *45*, 303 (1979).

15. Goodwin, J. A. and Webb, D. R. Regulation of the immune response by prostaglandins. *Clin. Immunol. Immunopathol.* *15*, 106 (1980).

16. Henney, C. S., Bourne, H. R., and Lichtenstein, L. M. The role of cyclic 3′, 5′ adenosine monophosphate in the specific cytolytic activity of lymphocytes. *J. Immunol.* *108*, 1526 (1972).

17. Jandinski, J., Cantor, H., Tadakuma, T., Peavy, D. L., and Pierce, C. W. Separation of helper T cells from suppressor T cells expressing Ly components. I. Polyclonal activation: Suppressor and helper activities are inherent properties of distinct T-cell subclasses. *J. Exp. Med.* *143*, 1382 (1976).

18. Moretta, L., Webb, S. E., Grassi, C. E., Lydyard, P. M., and Cooper, M. D. Functional analysis of two human T-cell subpopulations: Help and suppression of B-cell responses by T-cells bearing receptors for IgM or IgG. *J. Exp. Med.* *146*, 184 (1977).

19. Plaut, M., Lichtenstein, L. M., Gillespie, E., and Henney, C. S. Studies on the mechanism of lymphocyte-mediated cytolysis. IV. Specificity of the histamine receptor on effector T cells. *J. Immunol.* *111*, 389 (1973).

20. Rocklin, R. E. Modulation of cellular-immune responses *in vivo* and *in vitro* by histamine receptor-bearing lymphocytes. *J. Clin. Invest.* *57*, 1051 (1976).

21. Rocklin, R. E. Histamine-induced suppressor factor (HSF): Effect on migration inhibitory factor (MIF) production and proliferation. *J. Immunol.* *118*, 1734 (1977).

22. Rocklin, R. E., Greineder, D., Littman, B. H., and Melmon, K. L. Modulation of cellular immune function *in vitro* by histamine receptor-bearing lymphocytes: Mechanism of action. *Cell. Immunol.* *37*, 162 (1978).

23. Rocklin, R. E., Greineder, D. K., and Melmon, K. L. Histamine-induced suppressor factor (HSF): Further studies on the nature of the stimulus and the cell which produces it. *Cell. Immunol. 44*, (1978).

24. Rocklin, R. E., Breard, J., Gupta, S., Good, R. A., and Melmon, K. L. Characterization of the human blood lymphocytes that produce a histamine-induced suppressor factor (HSF). *Cell. Immunol. 51*, 226 (1980).

25. Rosenwasser, L. J., Dinarello, C. A., and Rosenthal, A. S. Adherent cell function in murine T lymphocyte antigen recognition. IV. Enhancement of murine T cell antigen recognition by human endogenous pyrogen. *J. Exp. Med. 150*, 709 (1979).

26. Schecter, B., Segal, S., and Feldman, M. Generation of suppressor lymphocytes during sensitization in culture against a syngeneic tumor: Affinity chromatography on insolubilized histamine. *J. Immunol. 120*, 1268 (1978).

27. Schwartz, A., Askenase, P. W., and Gershon, R. K. The effect of locally injected vasoactive amines on the elicitation of delayed-type hypersensitivity. *J. Immunol. 118*, 159 (1977).

28. Shearer, G. M., Melmon, K. L., Weinstein, Y., and Sela, M. Regulation of antibody response by cells expressing histamine receptors. *J. Exp. Med. 136*, 1302 (1972).

29. Shou, L., Schwartz, S. A., and Good, R. A. Suppressor cell activity after conconavalin A treatment of lymphocytes from normal donors. *J. Exp. Med. 143*, 1100 (1976).

30. Staszak, C. and Goodwin, J. S. Is prostaglandin a mediator for the inhibitory action of histamine, hydrocortisone and isoproterenol? *Cell. Immunol. 54*, 351 (1980).

31. Thueson, D. O., Speck, L. S., Left-Brown, M. A., and Grout, J. A. Histamine releasing activity (HRA): I. Production by mitogen-or antigen-stimulated human mononuclear cells. *J. Immunol. 123*, 626 (1979).

32. Twomey, J. J., Laughter, A. H., Farrow, S., and Douglas, C. C. Hodgkin's disease: An immunodepleting and immunosuppressive disorder. *J. Clin. Invest. 56*, 467 (1975).

33. Waldmann, T. A., Durm, M., Broder, S., Blackman, M., Blaese, R. M., and Strober, W. Role of suppressor T cells in pathogenesis of common variable hypogammaglobulinemia. *Lancet ii*, 609 (1974).

34. Waldmann, T. A., Broder, S., Krakauer, R., Durm, M., Meade, B., and Goldman, C. Defects in IgA secretion and in IgA specific suppressor cells in patients with isolated IgA deficiency. *Clin. Res. 24*, 483A (1976).

35. Wallen, W. C., Dean, J. H., Gauntt, C., and Lucas, D. O. Suppression of lymphocyte stimulation in mouse spleen cells by interferon preparations. *In* "Effects of Interferon on Cells, Viruses and the Immune System" (A. Geraldes, ed.), 355-365, Academic Press, New York, 1975.

36. Wang, S. R. and Zweiman, B. Histamine suppression of human lymphocyte responses to mitogens. *Cell. Immunol. 36*, 28 (1978).

37. Weinstein, Y. and Melmon, K. L. Control of immune responses by cyclic AMP and lymphocytes that adhere to histamine columns. *Immunol. Commun. 5*, 401 (1976).

Immunopathology: VIIIth International Symposium, 1980

IMMUNOGLOBULIN SUBCLASSES AND B-CELL SUBPOPULATIONS[1]

John H. Slack[2]
John P. McKearn[2]
Jeff W. Paslay[2]
Moon Nahm[3]
Andrzej Stanisz
Joseph M. Davie

Department of Microbiology and Immunology,
Washington University School of Medicine,
St. Louis, Missouri

I. INTRODUCTION

Most immunologists believe that T cells differentiate in the thymus along separate pathways leading to distinctly different and noninterchangeable subpopulations. In a teleological sense, this is simplest because it limits the options of an individual cell; a T cell can be a suppressor or a helper, but not both. Therefore, antigen functions to activate a T

[1] *Supported by U.S.P.H.S. Grants AI-11635, AI-05599, and AI-15353.*
[2] *Supported by Training Grant CA-09118.*
[3] *Supported by Training Grant GM-07157.*

ISBN 0-12-218320-7

cell to perform the one task that it was precommitted to perform. On the other hand, current thinking about B lymphocytes demands a great deal of plasticity from a single clone of cells. Not only must a single B-cell clone have the ability to produce any of 8-10 different antibody classes or subclasses, it must do so in response to different kinds of signals, recognizing the characteristics of the antigen and influences by such accessory cells as T cells and macrophages.

It is clear now that heterogeneity exists among B-lymphocyte populations. The B-cell populations stimulated by thymus-independent (TI) and thymus-dependent (TD) antigens differ morphologically (9), have variations in cell surface immunoglobulin receptors (19), have distinct differentiation antigens (1, 11), and in some cases can be distinguished by limiting dilution analysis (12, 18). Although their relationships are not proven, these B-cell populations have been thought to appear sequentially as a single B-cell lineage.

The ability of different antigenic forms to trigger distinct B-cell populations has been attributed by Cambier *et al.* (5) to a quality common to an antigen group, such as a mitogenicity of the TI antigens, or through a T-cell mechanism common to TD antigens, both properties of antigens independent of antigenic determinants. For a group of antigens to trigger different B-cell populations through antigenic determinants alone would require a nonrandom distribution of variable region receptors among B-cell subpopulations.

This issue is of major importance to an observation recently made by us (16). We found that a number of carbohydrate antigens, including dextran, the phosphocholine (PC)-containing C polysaccharide of pneumococcus (PC-vaccine) and group A streptococcal vaccine (GA-vaccine) stimulate IgG antibody responses dominated by the mouse IgG3 subclass. This observation was particularily intriguing because IgG3 makes up only a minor portion of normal serum IgG. As we will show, we believe that this association is the result of the fact that these antigens preferentially stimulate a subpopulation of B cells that may be restricted to production of certain immunoglobulin subclasses.

II. THE SUBCLASS-SPECIFIC NATURE OF THE CBA/N IMMUNODEFICIENCY

Normally, B-cell populations predominantly express surface IgM soon after birth and change to IgD predominance in adult animals (20). Furthermore, the IgD-predominant cells express distinctive differentiation antigens not found on B cells from neonatal animals (1, 11). The B cells produced by the CBA/N strain of mice continue to express features characteristic of the earliest appearing B cells, suggesting an arrest or delay in maturation. The responsiveness of mice possessing this defect has distinguished two groups of TI antigens; the deficiency permits CBA/N mice to respond to TI-1 antigens but not to TI-2 antigens (13, 15). TI-1 antigens are molecules that are mitogenic for B cells, whereas TI-2 antigens include dextran, PC-vaccine, and GA-vaccine, the antigens that stimulate IgG responses restricted to IgG3.

This observation suggested the possibility that the CBA/N deficiency may involve a B-cell population responsible for IgG3 expression. Indeed, this possibility was confirmed in recent experiments (17). The relative proportions of each serum isotype and of spleen cells secreting each isotype in defective mice compared to nondefective mice are shown in Fig. 1. Mice bearing the CBA/N defect differ little from normal mice except with respect to the ability to produce IgM and IgG3. Furthermore, the IgM and IgG3 deficiency is not

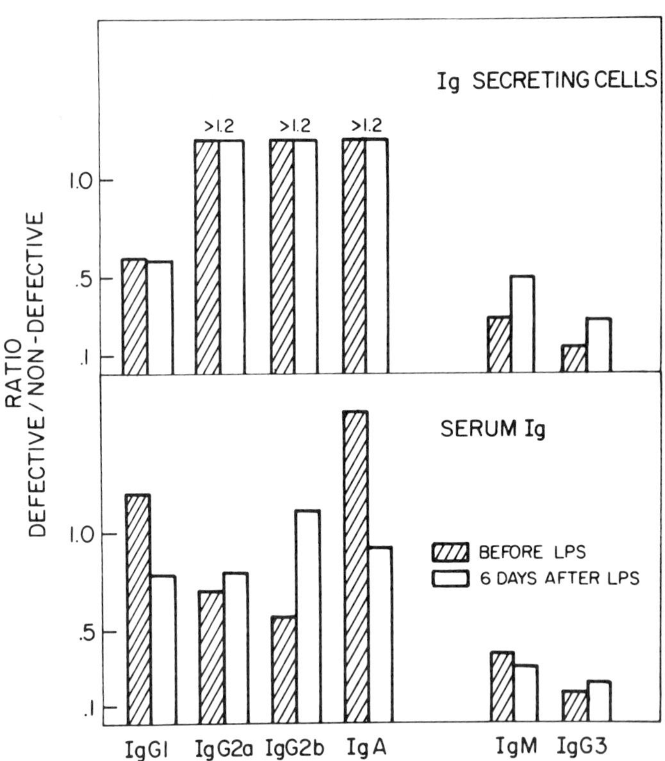

FIGURE 1. Relative levels [defective (CBA/N × DBA/2) F_1 males compared to nondefective (DBA/2 × CBA/N) F_1 male mice] of immunoglobulin-secreting spleen cells (upper panel) and of serum isotypes (lower panel) before (▨) and 6 days after (□) LPS stimulation. Spleen cells secreting antibody of a particular isotype were detected by a reverse plaque assay using protein A-coated SRBC and subclass-specific facilitating antisera. Specificities of the facilitating antisera used in the reverse-plaque assay and in an antigen-specific plaquing system (Fig. 2) were determined with panels of cell lines secreting monoclonal antibody of each major mouse Ig subclass. Immunoglobulin serum levels were determined by an isotype-specific RIA. [Adapted from Perlmutter *et al.* (17).]

corrected by stimulation with the B-cell mitogen, lipopolysaccharide (LPS). Clearly the deficiency is IgG subclass associated, involving a B-cell population that has most of the IgG3 precursor lymphocytes as well as a related IgM precursor population. Whether the defect of CBA/N is a selective deficiency in cells committed to production of IgM and IgG3 or is a result of a more central deficiency is not resolved. What is clear is that B lymphocytes generating all IgG subclasses with the exception of IgG3 develop normally.

III. DIFFERENT ANTIGEN CATEGORIES (TI-1, TI-2, AND TD) STIMULATE DIFFERENT IgG SUBCLASS RESPONSES

If the inability of CBA/N to respond to TI-2 antigens reflects the dominance by the IgG3 portion of the response, the ability to respond to the TI-1 and TD antigens may indicate that these antigens generate responses involving IgG subclasses other than IgG3. The IgG plaque-forming cell responses to TI-1, TI-2, and TD antigens were thus determined in the normal BALB/c mouse (21) (Fig. 2). All the major antigen groups generate IgG as well as IgM antigen-specific plaques. Furthermore, each antigen group generates a distinctive response pattern of IgG isotypes. The TI-1 antigens elicit responses with two major IgG components, IgG3 and IgG2, in similar amounts. The TI-2 responses show almost a complete domination by IgG3 with little IgG2. TD antigens, on the other other hand, stimulate a major IgG1 response with small amounts of IgG3 and IgG2.

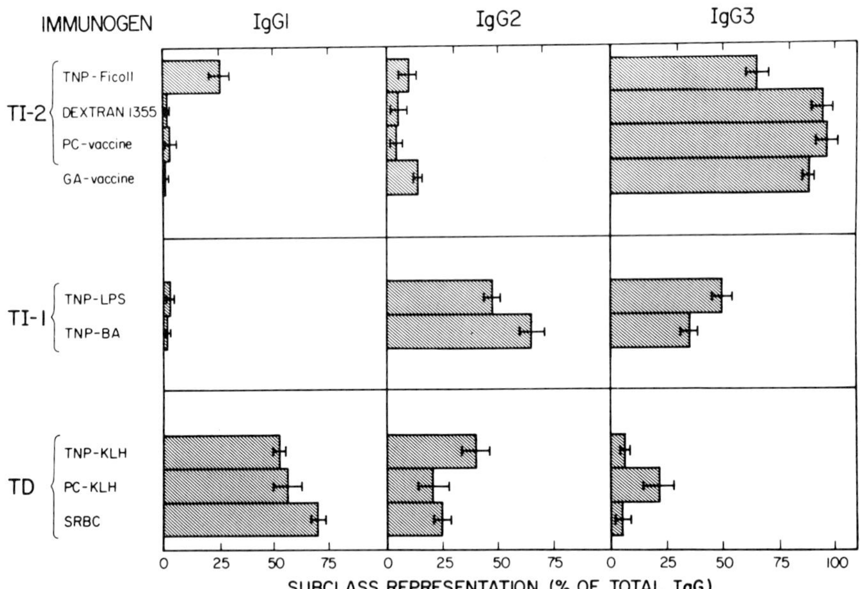

FIGURE 2. Antibody isotype distribution to TI-1, TI-2, and TD immunogens. Animals in groups of five were given a single injection of TNP-LPS, TNP-Ficoll, α-(1 → 3)-dextran (all 100 μg IP), TNP-BA and PC-vaccine (10^9 and 10^8 organisms IP, respectively), two injections of TNP-KLH and PC-KLH (100 μg in CFA followed in one month by 100 μg in IFA) and with multiple injections of GA-vaccine and SRBC; then plaqued 5-7 days after the last administration of antigen. Shown here are the geometric means and standard errors of the antigen-specific PFC facilitated with anti-γ1, -γ2 (2a + 2b), and -γ3 antisera normalized to the total indirect PFC response. To measure only the indirect plaques IgM (direct) plaques were suppressed with an anti-M104E (IgM) antiserum (21).

IV. ABSENCE OF IgG3 ANTIGEN SPECIFIC RESPONSES IN THE CBA/N MOUSE STRAIN

Although it is clear that TI-1, TI-2, and TD antigens stimulate different patterns of response, all antigen groups stimulate IgG3. Since the immunodeficiency of the CBA/N strain of mice is reflected chiefly in the ability to express IgG3, it was of particular interest to examine the subclass distribution of the antibodies made by CBA/N mice to TI-1 and TD antigens as a further test of the association of the deficiency with IgG3 production. Shown in Table I are the responses to TI-1, TI-2, and TD antigens by (CBA/N × BALB/c) F_1 male mice, which express the defect, compared to those of (BALB/c × CBA/N) F_1, nondefective males. The results clearly show that the defective animals have selective deficiencies in IgG3 antibody responses to all classes of antigens. Thus, IgG3 responses to TI-1, TI-2, and TD antigens are reduced 80-90% in defective animals, whereas IgG1 and IgG2 components are essentially normal.

V. MITOGENS STIMULATE DIFFERENT PATTERNS OF IgG RESPONSES

The association of a particular B-cell subpopulation with responses to certain antigens and with responses involving a rare IgG subclass suggests specialization of B cells with regard to isotype production. Since the known B-cell subpopulations have several surface antigen differences (1, 11), it was possible that B-cell subpopulations might differ in their expression of mitogen receptors (8) and in their ability to be stimulated by mitogens (10). We therefore examined the IgG isotypes produced in response to several B-cell mitogens (12a) (Fig. 3). It is clear that the responses to the three

TABLE I. The IgG PFC Response to TI-1, TI-2, and TD Antigens in Normal (BALB/c × CBA/N) F_1 Males and (CBA/N × BALB/c) F_1 Males Expressing an X-Linked Immunodeficiency

Immunogen (type)*	Isotype				Defective** (CBA/N × BALB/c) F_1 (PFC/$10^{6\Delta}$)	Nondefective (BALB/c × CBA/N) F_1 (PFC/$10^{6\Delta}$)	Ratio defective/nondefective	p value
	IgG3	IgG2	IgG1	IgM				
TNP-LPS (TI-1)	+				7(1.4)	230(1.2)	0.03	<0.001
		+			80(1.2)	116(2.1)	0.70	N.S.
				+	220(1.1)	330(1.0)	0.67	N.S.
TNP-BA (TI-1)	+				3(1.5)	34(1.4)	0.09	<0.001
		+			40(1.2)	38(1.3)	1.0	N.S.
				+	80(1.3)	78(1.3)	1.0	N.S.
TNP-Ficoll (TI-2)	+				2(2.1)	23(1.3)	0.09	<0.001
				+	2(1.1)	250(1.2)	0.01	<0.001
TNP-BSA (TD)	+				21(2.0)	105(1.7)	0.18	<0.005
		+			109(1.6)	198(1.4)	0.55	N.S.
			+		173(1.2)	253(1.1)	0.68	N.S.
				+	23(2.0)	212(1.1)	0.11	<0.001

**Antigens were administered as described in Fig. 2. Seven days later IgM, IgG1, IgG2, and IgG3 anti-TNP PFC were measured in the spleen.*

***The values shown are geometric means obtained from five individual mice and their standard error factors.*

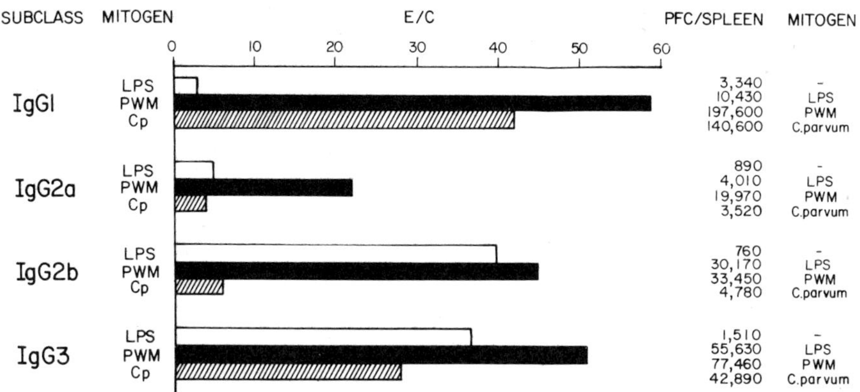

FIGURE 3. Stimulation of IgG isotypes by B-cell mitogens. CBA/J mice in groups of 10-17 received optimal doses of LPS, PWM, or *C. parvum* administered ip. Seven days later, the IgG isotype responses were measured in the spleen.

mitogens studied were different. LPS stimulates chiefly IgG2b and IgG3, PWM stimulates all IgG subclasses, and *C. parvum* elicits IgG1 and IgG3 responses. Other investigators have found unequal isotype responses by different types of mitogenic molecules. Lipoprotein (3) and AVIS, a mitogen from actinomyces (6), stimulate responses identical to that of LPS. Furthermore, activated T cells augment immunoglobulin production only of the IgG1 and IgG2 isotypes (3).

VI. DISCUSSION

It is well established that there are at least two forms of immunocompetent B cells: (a) a B cell that lacks Lyb3,5,7, which appears early after birth, responds to TI-1 and TD antigens, and is expressed in CBA/N mice and (b) a B cell that possesses Lyb3,5,7, which matures later in ontogeny, responds to TI-2 antigens and is absent or defective in CBA/N mice (Table II). Our studies raise the possibility that these populations may also be restricted in the subclasses of

TABLE II. Characteristics of Known B-Cell Subpopulations

Characteristics	B cell type		References
	B_{μ}	B_{δ}	
Ontogeny	Early	Late	(14)
Lyb3,5,7	-	+	(1, 11)
Antigens that stimulate	TI-1, TD	TI-2	(15)
CBA/N	Present	Absent	(1, 11)
Surface Ig	IgM predominant	IgD predominant	(19)

immunoglobulins they produce. It appears that most, if not all, IgG3 is derived from the second type of B cell. It is not possible to say whether other isotypes are restricted to one of the B-cell types at this point. However, it should be possible to answer this once methods are available for readily

TABLE III. IgG Subclass Responses to Different Stimuli

Stimulant	IgG subclass stimulated			References
	IgG1	IgG2	IgG3	
TD antigens	++	++	±	(21)
T cells	++	++	±	(3)
TI-1 antigens	--	++	++	(21)
LPS	--	++	++	(12a)
AVIS	--	++	++	(6)
LP	--	++	++	(3)
TI-2 antigens	--	--	++	(21)
PWM	++	++	++	(12a)
C. parvum	++	±	++	(12a)

separating B-cell subpopulations. However, by summarizing the available data concerning IgG antibody responses, it is possible to discern recurring patterns (Table III). TD antigens and activated T cells both induce IgGl and IgG2 responses. LPS, AVIS, LP, and hapten conjugates of LPS and *B. pertussis* stimulate IgG2 and IgG3. Nonmitogenic polysaccharides stimulate only IgG3. Other mitogens give different patterns.

It is possible to imagine several B-cell subpopulations, each restricted in its capacity to secrete immunoglobulins emerging either from single or multiple lineages (Fig. 4). Mitogens and antigens could be selective in their stimulation of the subpopulations by means of nonrandom distribution of mitogen receptors and/or particular activation requirements of each subpopulation. For example, it seems clear that only antigens or mitogens that also activate T cells are capable of stimulating IgGl antibody production. However, attempts to

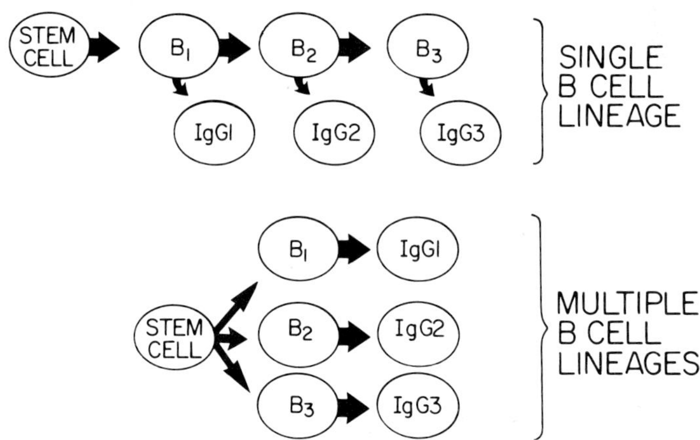

FIGURE 4. A diagram showing two B-cell differentiation schemes. A single lineage model with all the IgG subclasses generated sequentially within a single B-cell population. A multiple-lineage model on the other hand, with populations of B cells that at some time point during differentiation have become developmentally distinct and now give rise to the different IgG subclasses.

alter the isotype of responses to certain antigenic determinants have shown that the quality of the antigen signal is not the only important issue. Thus, coupling streptococcal group A carbohydrate to protein did not change the isotype from IgG3 to IgG1, the response remained as IgG3 (16). This raises the interesting possibility that the B-lymphocyte subpopulations do not represent different stages of maturation of a single lineage of B-lymphocyte development, as shown in the upper portion of Fig. 4, but might represent distinct B-cell lineages. Furthermore, multiple B-cell lineages could be specialized not only to the production of certain C_H regions, but also could be restricted to the expression of certain V_H regions. This could explain why the CBA/N mouse does not produce significant amounts of T15 idiotype when stimulated with PC-KLH, even though substantial amounts of IgG1 anti-PC antibody are produced (Nahm *et al.*, unpublished observations). The association of particular isotypes with specific antigenic determinants is shown clearly in the rat when PC-KLH and PC-vaccine stimulate IgG2c (the rat analog of IgG3) whereas DNP-KLH and ABA-KLH stimulate almost no IgG2, but rather elicit IgG2a responses (7).

Additional evidence in support of precommitted B-cell lineages is provided by recent studies by Burrows and coworkers, who have shown that an Abelson virus-transformed cell line that normally produced IgM can be induced to secrete IgG2b, but not other isotypes (4).

These results are difficult to explain by more conventional models in which a single B-cell clone is capable of producing all isotypes associated with any V_H region. Clearly, much more work will be needed to decide between current models of B-cell differentiation. However, the possible existence of additional, distinctive differentiation antigens on B-cell subsets should allow more definitive studies to be performed.

VII. CONCLUSIONS

1. Different classes of antigens or mitogens stimulate distinct patterns of IgG isotype responses.

2. The ability of antigens to stimulate distinct IgG subclasses seems independent of T-cell influences, route of immunization, adjuvants, or form of the immunogen. As an example, TI-2 antigens include both thymus-independent and thymus-dependent polysaccharide antigens that can be administered as soluble molecules, bacterial vaccines, or coupled to proteins. The names applied to the sets of antigens, TD, TI-1, and TI-2, are not accurate, therefore.

3. Different classes of antigens may stimulate distinct subsets of B cells; in turn, B-cell subsets may be restricted to the production of only certain immunoglobulin classes or subclasses.

REFERENCES

1. Ahmed, A., Scher, I., Sharrow, S. O., Smith, A. H., Paul, W. E., Sachs, D. H., and Sell, K. W. B-lymphocyte heterogeneity. Development and characterization of an alloantiserum which distinguishes B-lymphocyte differentiation alloantigens. *J. Exp. Med. 145*, 101 (1977).

2. Amsbaugh, D. F., Hansen, C. T., Prescott, B., Stashak, P. W., Barthold, D. R., and Baker, P. J. Genetic control of the antibody response to Type III pneumococcal polysaccharide in mice. I. Evidence that an X-linked gene plays a decisive role in determining responsiveness. *J. Exp. Med. 136*, 931 (1972).

3. Augustin, A. A. and Coutinho, A. Specific T helper cells that activate B cells polyclonally. *In vitro* enrichment and cooperative function. *J. Exp. Med. 151*, 587 (1980).

4. Burrows, P. D., Beck, G. B., and Wabl, M. R. Expression of μ and γ immunoglobulin heavy chains in different cells of a cloned mouse lymphoid line. *Proc. Natl. Acad. Sci. U.S.A. 78*, 564 (1981).

5. Cambier, J. C., Vitetta, E. S., Uhr, J. W., and Kettman, J. R. B cell tolerance. II. Trinitrophenyl human gamma globulin-induced tolerance in adult and neonatal murine B cells responsive to thymus dependent and independent forms of the same hapten. *J. Exp. Med. 145*, 778 (1977).

6. Clagett, J., Engel, D., and Chi, E. *In vitro* expression of immunoglobulin M and G subclasses by murine B lymphocytes in response to a polyclonal activator from actinomyces. *Infect. Immun. 29*, 234 (1980).

7. Der-Balian, G. P., Slack, J., Clevinger, B. L., Bazin, H., and Davie, J. M. Subclass restriction of murine antibodies. III. Antigens that stimulate IgG3 in mice stimulate IgG2c in rats. *J. Exp. Med. 152*, 209 (1980).

8. Forni, L. and Coutinho, A. An antiserum which recognizes lipopolysaccharide-reactive B cells in the mouse. *Eur. J. Immunol. 8*, 56 (1978).

9. Gorczynski, R. M. and Feldmann, M. B cell heterogeneity-difference in the size of B lymphocytes responding to T dependent and T independent antigens. *Cell. Immunol. 18*, 88 (1975).

10. Gronowicz, E. and Coutinho, A. Heterogeneity of B cells: direct evidence of selective triggering of distinct subpopulations by polyclonal activators. *Scand. J. Immunol. 5*, 55 (1976).

11. Huber, B., Gershon, R. K., and Cantor, H. Identification of a B-cell surface structure involved in antigen-dependent triggering. Absence of this structure on B-cells from CBA/N mutant mice. *J. Exp. Med. 145*, 10 (1977).

12. Lewis, G. K. and Goodman, J. W. Carrier-directed anti-hapten responses by B-cell subsets. *J. Exp. Med. 146*, 1 (1977).

12a. McKearn, J. P., Paslay, J. W., and Davie, J. M. Subclass restriction of murine antibodies. IV. Preferential stimulation of different IgG antibody subclasses by polyclonal B-cell activators. Submitted.

13. Mond, J. J., Scher, I., Mosier, D. E., Blaese, M., and Paul, W. E. T-independent responses in B cell-defective CBA/N mice to *Brucella abortus* and to trinitrophenyl (TNP) conjugates of *Brucella abortus*. *Eur. J. Immunol. 8*, 459 (1978).

14. Mosier, D. E., Mond, J. J., and Goldings, E. A. The ontogeny of thymic independent antibody responses *in vitro* in normal mice and mice with an X-linked B cell defect. *J. Immunol. 119*, 1874 (1977).

15. Mosier, D. E., Scher, I., and Paul, W. E. *In vitro* responses of CBA/N mice: spleen cells of mice with an X-linked defect that precludes immune responses to several thymus-independent antigens can respond to TNP-lipopolysaccharide. *J. Immunol. 117*, 1363 (1976).

16. Perlmutter, R. M., Hansburg, D., Briles, D. E., Nicolotti, R. A., and Davie, J. M. Subclass restriction of murine anti-carbohydrate antibodies. *J. Immunol. 121*, 566 (1978).

17. Perlmutter, R. M., Nahm, M., Stein, K. E., Slack, J., Zitron, I., Paul, W. E., and Davie, J. M. Immunoglobulin subclass-specific immunodeficiency in mice with an X-linked B-lymphocyte defect. *J. Exp. Med. 149*, 993 (1979).

18. Quintans, J. and Cosenza, H. Antibody response to phosphorylcholine *in vitro*. II. Analysis of T-dependent and T-independent responses. *Eur. J. Immunol. 6*, 399 (1976).

19. Scher, I., Sharrow, S. O., and Paul, W. E. X-linked B-lymphocyte defect in CBA/N mice. III. Abnormal development of B-lymphocyte populations defined by their density of surface immunoglobulin. *J. Exp. Med. 144*, 507 (1976).

20. Scher, I., Sharrow, S. O., Wistar, R., Jr., Asofsky, R., and Paul, W. E. B-lymphocyte heterogeneity: Ontogenetic development and organ distribution of B-lymphocyte populations defined by their density of surface immunoglobulin. *J. Exp. Med. 144*, 494 (1976).

21. Slack, J., Der-Balian, G. P., Nahm, M., and Davie, J. M. Subclass restriction of murine antibodies. II. The IgG plaque-forming cell response to thymus-independent type 1 and type 2 antigens in normal mice and mice expressing an X-linked immunodeficiency. *J. Exp. Med. 151*, 853 (1980).

Immunopathology: VIIIth International Symposium, 1980

ISOTYPE-SPECIFIC REGULATION OF THE IgE RESPONSE BY IgE-BINDING FACTORS[1]

Kimishige Ishizaka
Masaki Suemura
Junji Yodoi
Mitsuomi Hirashima

Department of Medicine and Microbiology,
The Johns Hopkins University School of Medicine
at the Good Samaritan Hospital,
Baltimore, Maryland

I. INTRODUCTION

It is well established that the IgE antibody response is highly dependent on T cells. Differentiation of precursor B cells to IgE-forming cells requires antigen-specific helper T cells, and this process is regulated by antigen-specific suppressor T cells. However, the IgE antibody response does not parallel the IgG response to the same antigen. Many investigators have shown that the IgE antibody response is highly dependent on the nature and dose of immunogen as well as on the

[1]*This work was carried out supported by U.S.P.H.S. grants AI-11202 and AI-14784. This paper is publication No. 412 from the O'Neill Laboratories at the Good Samaritan Hospital.*

ISBN 0-12-218320-7

adjuvant employed [reviewed in Ishizaka (6)]. It became clear also that low dose X-irradiation or cyclophosphamide treatment before immunization enhanced the IgE response without affecting the IgG response. Such dissociation between the IgE antibody response and IgG antibody response under various experimental conditions suggested the possibility that IgE antibody response is controlled by isotype-specific regulatory mechanisms in addition to antigen-specific regulation. Indeed, Watanabe *et al.* (16), as well as Chiorazzi *et al.* (2), provided evidence that enhancement of IgE response by X-irradiation is due to depletion of nonspecific T cells that selectively regulate the IgE response. Subsequently, Katz and associates have shown that a population of such suppressor cells expands after treatment of mice with complete Freund's adjuvant (CFA) (15). They also demonstrated that the serum of CFA-treated mice contained a soluble factor that selectively suppressed the IgE response. The same investigators later demonstrated another soluble factor with opposite (enhancing) biological activity in the serum of CFA-treated mice (8).

Another example of isotype-specific regulation of the IgE response is the nematode infection. It is known that infection of antigen-primed rats with *Nippostrongylus brasiliensis* (Nb) enhances the IgE antibody formation to the priming antigen without affecting the IgG response (1, 10). Jarrett and Ferguson (7) have shown that T cells are essential for the IgE-specific potentiation. These findings strongly suggest that a certain population of T cells selectively regulates the IgE response. However, we had no idea how these T cells or T cell factors recognize precursors of IgE-forming cells. In the past several years, we have studied the mechanisms for isotype-specific regulation of the IgE response in the rat. Our results showed that a subset of activated T cells form soluble factors having affinity for IgE, and that these factors selectively regulate the IgE response. One of the IgE-binding factors selectively enhances the IgE response and another IgE-binding factor selectively suppresses the response. In this chapter, I would like to summarize experimental conditions for the formation of IgE-potentiating factor and IgE-suppressive factor, respectively, and then discuss the possible relationship between the two factors.

II. FORMATION OF IgE-POTENTIATING FACTOR AND IgE-SUPPRESSIVE FACTOR

In order to elucidate the mechanisms for selective enhancement of IgE-response, we took *Nippostrongylus* infection as an experimental model and studied the effect of T cells from Nb-infected rats on the *in vitro* IgE response of DNP-OA primed cells to homologous antigen. Thus, mesenteric lymph node (MLN) cells of DNP-OA primed rats were mixed with T cells from either Nb-infected rats or normal rats, and the mixtures were cultured with DNP-OA for 5 days for IgE- and IgG-forming cell responses. As shown in Fig. 1, T cells from Nb-infected animals selectively enhanced the IgE-forming cell response of DNP-OA primed cells to homologous antigen, whereas T cells from normal animals failed to do so (12). The results indicated that the ratio of IgE to IgG response is determined not only by antigen-specific cell populations but also by bystander T cells. We wondered if T cells from Nb-infected rats may release a soluble factor that can selectively potentiate the IgE response. Indeed, a culture supernatant of MLN cells from Nb-infected rats selectively enhanced the IgE response of DNP-OA primed cells to homologous antigen without affecting the magnitude of the IgG_2 response. However, the same supernatant did not affect either IgE or IgG responses of the same cells to DNP-heterologous carrier, indicating that the

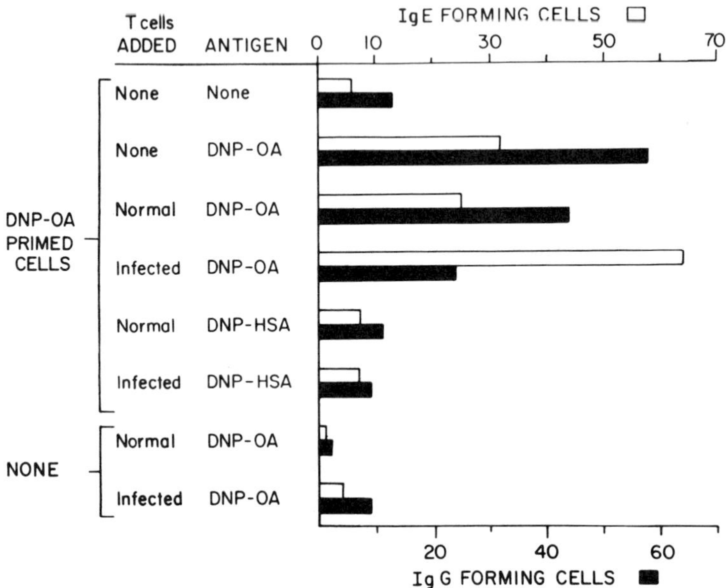

FIGURE 1. Effect of by-stander T cells from Nb-infected rats on the Ig-forming cell response of DNP-OA primed cells. 10^5 DNP-OA primed cells were mixed with an equal number of T cells from either normal or Nb-infected rat, and the cells were cultured with either DNP-OA or DNP-HSA. The figure shows the number of IgE- and IgG_2-forming cells per 10^6 cells seeded.

effective substance is not a T-cell replacing factor. Gel filtration of the culture supernatant indicated that the molecular weight of the IgE-potentiating factor is between 10,000 and 20,000 daltons, significantly smaller than the molecular weight of T-cell replacing factor (12).

Further studies on the IgE-potentiating factor have shown that the factor can be absorbed by B cells but not by T cells. More importantly, the factor has affinity for IgE (13). Thus, it appears that the factor will bind to IgE-bearing B cells through surface IgE and enhance the differentiation of these cells to IgE-forming cells. Since the factor does not have affinity for the other B cells, the effect of this factor is selective for IgE isotype. Because of the affinity for IgE, the IgE-potentiating factor could be absorbed by IgE-Sepharose and was recovered from the beads by elution at acid pH. The purified IgE-binding factor actually enhanced the IgE response. The factor can be detected *in vitro* as well, by inhibition of $Fc_{\varepsilon}R(+)$ cells with IgE-coated ox erythrocytes.

We wondered why T cells from Nb-infected animals release IgE binding factor. Fortunately, separate experiments in our laboratory on Fc_{ε} receptor-bearing lymphocytes revealed the source of IgE-potentiating factor. In normal MLN cells, the proportion of $Fc_{\varepsilon}R(+)$ cells was 2 to 4%. Two weeks after Nb-infection, however, the proportion of $Fc_{\varepsilon}R(+)$ cells increased to 20% or higher. Most of the $Fc_{\varepsilon}R(+)$ cells belong to B cells, but a portion of T cells from the infected animals bore $Fc_{\varepsilon}R$ (17). As the IgE-potentiating factor has affinity for IgE, we anticipated that the factor may be related to $Fc_{\varepsilon}R$. Indeed, the source of IgE-potentiating factor was removed by depletion of $Fc_{\varepsilon}R(+)$ cells in MLN cells (13). Furthermore, evidence was obtained that the factor was derived from cell surface components of $Fc_{\varepsilon}R(+)$ T cells in MLN of Nb-infected rats (20).

Subsequent experiments revealed the presence of IgE-binding factors with an opposite biological function. In the course of experiments on the $Fc_{\varepsilon}R(+)$ lymphocytes, we realized that the proportion of $Fc_{\varepsilon}R(+)$ cells in lymphoid tissues is regulated by the concentration of IgE in the environment (18). In the mesenteric lymph node cells obtained 8 days after Nb-infection, the proportion of $Fc_{\varepsilon}R(+)$ cells was 2 to 3%. If one incubated these lymphocytes with 1 to 10 μg/ml of rat IgE, however, the proportion of $Fc_{\varepsilon}R(+)$ cells increased to 10 to 16% within 16 to 24 hr of culturing. After the culture, the receptors were expressed on both B and T cells. Furthermore, supernatants obtained from the culture contained an IgE-binding factor (19). We wondered whether the factor might have the ability to potentiate the IgE response, but the results of the

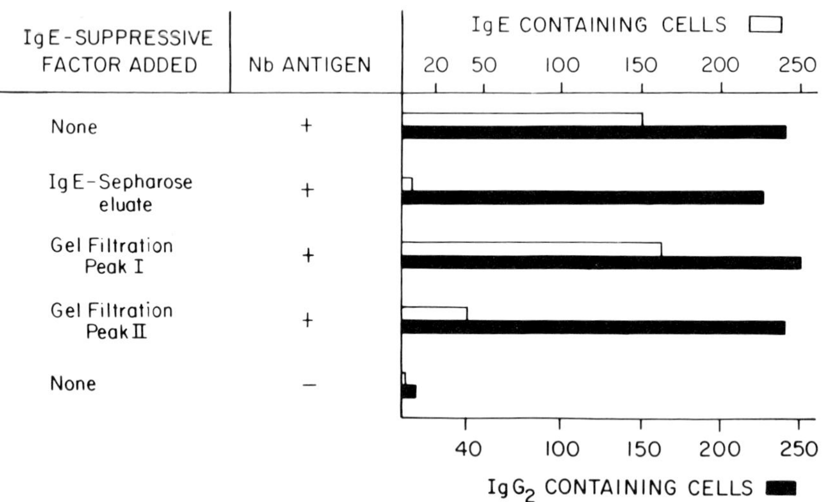

FIGURE 2. The suppressive effect of IgE-binding factors on the IgE response to Nb antigen. MLN cells from Nb-infected rats were obtained 4 weeks after infection, and the cells were cultured with Nb antigen in the presence of IgE-binding factor, which was obtained by culture of MLN cells from the day 8 Nb-infected rats with IgE. Purified IgE-binding factor (i.e., eluate from IgE Sepharose) selectively suppressed IgE response. IgE-binding factors were fractionated on a Sephadex G75 column. The factor was detected in two peaks which corresponded to 25,000 - 45,000 and 10,000 - 20,000 daltons, respectively. Suppressive activity was associated with IgE-binding factors in peak II.

experiments showed that this IgE-binding factor selectively suppressed, rather than enhanced, the IgE response (3).

In the experiment shown in Fig. 2, IgE-binding factors obtained from MLN cells of infected rats on day 8 were purified and added to MLN cells of Nb-infected rats. Incubation of the cells with Nb antigen induced both IgE and IgG responses; however, addition of purified IgE-binding factor to this system selectively suppressed the IgE response. Gel filtration of the IgE-binding factors revealed two different molecules with affinity for IgE. One component has a molecular weight

TABLE I. Comparisons of IgE-Potentiating Factor and IgE Suppressive Factor

	IgE-potentiating factor	IgE-suppressive factor
Origin	$Fc_{\varepsilon}R(+)$ T	T cells
Affinity for IgE	+	+
Molecular weight	10,000 ~ 20,000	10,000 ~ 20,000
Affinity for lentil lectin	+	-
Source	Nb-infected (14 day)	Nb-infected (8 day) + IgE
	B. pertussis	Complete Freund's adjuvant

between 25,000 and 45,000 and the other factor had a molecular weight between 10,000 and 20,000. The ability to suppress the IgE response was associated with the smaller molecules.

The properties of IgE-potentiating factor and IgE-suppressive factor are summarized in Table I. The two factors are comparable with respect to affinity for IgE and molecular weight. The main difference between the two factors is in the carbohydrate moiety. The potentiating factor is bound to lentil lectin Sepharose and was eluted with α-methyl-D-mannoside. In contrast, suppressive factor did not bind to lentil lectin Sepharose or Con A Sepharose.

In the experiments discussed so far, both IgE-binding factors were obtained from lymphocytes of Nb-infected rats. However, more recent experiments showed that the formation of the factors is not confined to the parasite infection. It was found that mesenteric lymph node cells from rats treated with CFA formed IgE-binding factors even when the cells were cultured in the absence of IgE; furthermore, the serum of CFA-treated animals contained IgE-binding factors. The majority of the IgE binding factors in the culture supernatants and serum was identical to IgE-suppressive factor obtained from Nb-infected rats (4). It was also found that an injection of *B. pertussis* vaccine into rats induced the formation of IgE-potentiating factor. Serum of *B. pertussis* vaccine-treated rats contained the potentiating factor and their circulating lymphocytes in peripheral blood released IgE-potentiating factor *in vitro*. We do not yet know how CFA and pertussis vaccine treatment induces the formation of either IgE-suppressive factor or IgE-potentiating factor. It is well known that pertussis vaccine is one of the best adjuvants for the IgE response (9), whereas pretreatment of rodents with CFA suppresses the IgE response (15). The formation of IgE-binding factors with opposite biological function in rats treated with the two different adjuvants strongly suggests that IgE-binding factors are involved in the regulation of IgE responses *in vivo*.

III. RELATIONSHIP BETWEEN IgE-POTENTIATING FACTOR AND IgE-SUPPRESSIVE FACTOR

The fundamental questions to be asked involve the relationship between the IgE-potentiating factor and IgE-suppressive factor, and whether the two factors are derived from distinct subsets of T cells. As both factors were formed by mesenteric lymph node cells of Nb-infected rats, we wondered if activated T cells may respond to IgE for the formation of the factors. In the next experiment, therefore, normal MLN cells were cultured with 1 μg/ml or 10 μg/ml of Con A for 2 to 3 days, and Con A-activated cells were cultured with IgE (Fig. 3). In both cultures, the proportion of $Fc_{\varepsilon}R(+)$ cells increased, and the activated cells released IgE-binding factors into culture medium. However, the nature of IgE-binding factors were different depending on the concentration of Con A

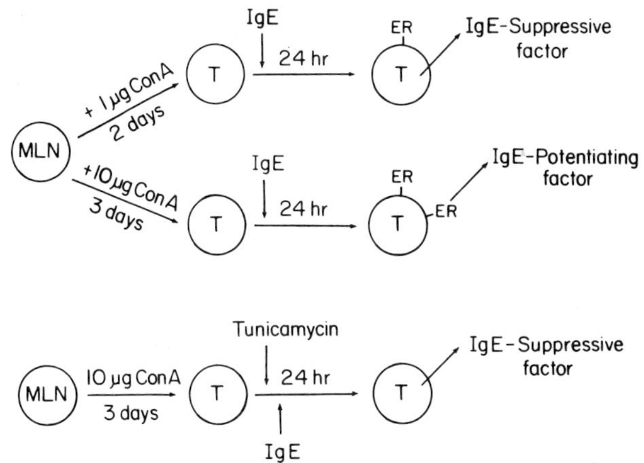

FIGURE 3. Formation of IgE-binding factors by Con A-activated cells. Mesenteric lymph node cells were cultured with either 1 μg/ml Con A or 10 μg/ml Con A, and Con A-activated cells were cultured with IgE for 24 hr. 1-μg/ml Con A-activated cells formed IgE-suppressive factor, whereas 10-μg/ml Con A-activated cells formed IgE-potentiating factor. If 10-μg/ml Con A-activated cells were incubated with IgE in the presence of 1 μg/ml tunicamycin, IgE-binding factors formed by the cells suppressed the IgE response.

for preculture. The majority of IgE-binding factors formed by 1-μg Con A-activated cells did not have affinity for lentil lectin, and this factor selectively suppressed the IgE response. In contrast, essentially all IgE-binding factors formed by 10-μg Con A-activated cells had affinity for lentil lectin Sepharose, and this factor potentiated the IgE response. These data suggested to us the possibility that the nature of IgE-binding factors is decided in the process of biosynthesis. Since IgE-potentiating factor has affinity for lentil lectin, whereas IgE-suppressive factor does not, we wondered if glycosylation of the protein was essential for the formation of IgE-potentiating factors.

In order to test this possibility, 10-μg Con A-activated cells were incubated with IgE in the presence of tunicamycin which inhibits protein glycosylation (14). In the presence of

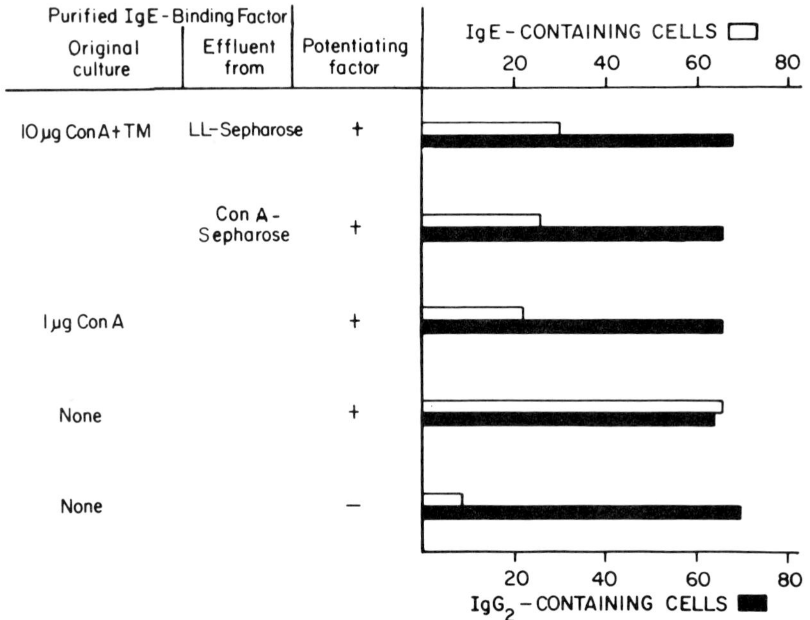

FIGURE 4. The suppressive effect of IgE-binding factors obtained from 10-μg/ml Con A-activated cells in the presence of tunicamycin. 10-μg/ml Con A-activated cells were cultured with IgE in the presence of 1 μg/ml tunicamycin. Purified IgE-binding factors in CF were passed through lentil lectin Sepharose followed by Con A-Sepharose, and the effluent fractions were assessed for their ability to suppress IgE-potentiating factor-enhanced IgE response. Purified IgE-binding factor from 1-μg/ml Con A-activated cells was employed as controls. Preparations of IgE-binding factors were diluted so that the three preparations were comparable with respect to their ability to inhibit rosette formation of $Fc_{\varepsilon}R(+)$ cells with IgE-coated ox erythrocytes.

tunicamycin, $Fc_{\varepsilon}R(+)$ cells were not induced by IgE. This antibiotic did not affect the amount of IgE-binding factors formed, but changed the nature of IgE-binding factors formed by the same cells. The majority of IgE-binding factors formed in the presence of tunicamycin did not have affinity for lentil lectin or Con A, and this factor failed to enhance the IgE response. We wondered if this factor had the ability to suppress the IgE response. Thus, purified IgE-binding factor from tunicamycin-containing culture was absorbed with Con A-Sepharose to remove possible contamination of IgE-potentiating factor, and the fraction was added to DNP-OA primed cells together with IgE-potentiating factor. As shown in Fig. 4, IgE-binding factors formed by tunicamycin-containing culture suppressed the potentiating factor-enhanced IgE response. The suppressive activity of that factor was almost comparable to that of the IgE-suppressive factor formed by 1-μg Con A-activated cells. We do not know whether the IgE-binding factor formed in the presence of tunicamycin is identical to the IgE-suppressive factor. However, the results suggest the possibility that the same cells have the capacity to form either IgE-potentiating factor or IgE-suppressive factor, and that biologic activity of the IgE-binding factors may be decided in the process of glycosylation.

More recent experiments provided evidence that cells forming IgE-potentiating factor may be switched to form suppressive factor by pretreatment with glucocorticoid. The experiments were based on previous findings by Spiegelberg, who showed that the proportion of $Fc_{\varepsilon}R$(+) cells in circulating lymphocytes was extremely low in steroid-treated atopic patients (11). We anticipated that glucocorticoid might prevent the expression of $Fc_{\varepsilon}R$ on the cell surface of B and T cells and might affect the nature of IgE-binding factors formed by T cells. Thus, we prepared 10-μg Con A-activated cells and added 5 μ*M* dexamethasone 12 hr before the termination of Con A culture. Cells were washed and then incubated with IgE. As described, 10-μg Con A-activated cells expressed $Fc_{\varepsilon}R$ and formed IgE-potentiating factor upon incubation with IgE. If the same cells were pretreated with dexamethasone, however,

$Fc_{\varepsilon}R$ expression on the cells was prevented, and IgE-binding factors formed by the cells suppressed, rather than enhanced, the IgE response.

Since dexamethasone might have a similar effect on the expression of $Fc_{\varepsilon}R$ *in vivo*, we injected 0.2 mg dexamethasone into Nb-infected rats 2 weeks after the infection. Two days after the injection, the proportion of $Fc_{\varepsilon}R(+)$ cells in the

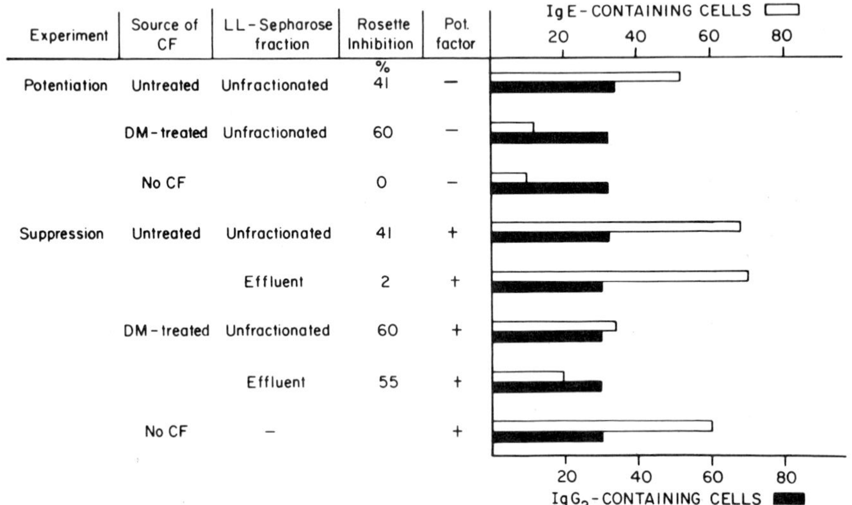

FIGURE 5. Biological activity of IgE-binding factors formed by MLN cells of Nb-infected rats treated with dexamethasone (DM). Nb-infected rats received 0.2 mg dexamethasone at the day 14 of infection. MLN cells of DM-treated and untreated (Nb-infected) rats were incubated for 24 hr to obtain culture filtrates. IgE-binding factors in the culture filtrates were purified by using IgE-Sepharose and assessed the ability to potentiate the IgE response of DNP-OA primed cells (top 3 rows). The IgE-binding factors from DM-treated rats failed to enhance the IgE response. The IgE-binding factors from both untreated and DM-treated rats were absorbed with lentil lectin Sepharose. The majority of the factor from untreated rats was absorbed, while the majority of the factor from DM-treated rats was not bound to lectin (effluent has a high rosette inhibiting activity). IgE-binding factors from DM-treated rats as well as their effluent fraction suppressed IgE response (bottom 5 rows).

mesenteric lymph node cells diminished to 10 to 12%, as compared with 21 to 23% in control animals. Mesenteric lymph node cells from both treated and untreated animals were cultured for 24 hr and culture filtrates fractionated on a lentil lectin Sepharose. As expected, essentially all IgE-binding factor from untreated rats bound to lentil lectin Sepharose and was recovered by elution with α-methyl-D-mannoside. In contrast, the majority of IgE-binding factors formed by the lymphocytes of desamethasone-treated animals failed to bind to lentil lectin. Dexamethasone treatment of Nb-infected rats affected biologic function of IgE-binding factors formed by their lymphocytes. As shown in Fig. 5, IgE-binding factors formed by MLN cells of dexamethasone-treated animals failed to potentiate the IgE response. In fact, the majority of IgE-binding factors, which failed to bind to lentil lectin Sepharose, suppressed the potentiating factor-enhanced IgE response. The same fraction of the culture filtrate of the lymphocytes from untreated animals contained no IgE-binding factor and failed to suppress the IgE response. These results suggested that dexamethasone treatment of Nb-infected animals inhibited glycosylation of IgE-binding factor in their lymphocytes and thereby shifted the formation of IgE-potentiating factor to IgE-suppressive factor. We do not know how dexamethasone affects the glycosylation of such factors. However, our recent experiments suggest that synthesis of phospholipase A_2 inhibitor by dexamethasone (5) is involved in the inhibition of glycosylation.

IV. SUMMARY

Activated rat T lymphocytes form soluble factors having affinity for IgE and selectively regulating the IgE response. Formation of IgE-potentiating factor on the lymphocytes was observed following *Nippostrongylus* infection of rats or treatment with Bordetella pertussis vaccine, which enhanced the IgE synthesis. In contrast, treatment of rats with complete Freund's adjuvant induced the formation of IgE-suppressive factor. Both IgE-binding factors were comparable with respect to their affinity for IgE and molecular weight. The major difference between the two factors was that IgE-potentiating factor had affinity for lentil lectin, whereas IgE-suppressive factor did not. Evidence was obtained that the carbohydrate moiety of IgE-potentiating factors is essential to their biologic activity.

The IgE-binding factors were obtained by exposure of Con A-activated lymphocytes with homologous IgE. Under the experimental conditions employed, the majority of IgE-binding factors formed by 1-μg Con A-activated cells was IgE-suppressive factor, whereas the factors formed by 10-μg Con A-activated cells was IgE-potentiating factor. However, the nature of IgE-binding factors formed by the latter cells changed by preventing protein glycosylation. Tunicamycin prevented the expression of $Fc_{\varepsilon}R$ on the cell surface but did not prevent the formation of IgE-binding factors. However, the IgE-binding factors formed in the presence of tunicamycin suppressed, rather than enhanced, the IgE response. Similar effects on the nature of IgE-binding factors were obtained by pretreatment of lymphocytes with dexamethasone prior to incubation with IgE. Indeed, dexamethasone injected into *Nippostrongylus*-infected rats switched their lymphocytes to form IgE-suppressive factor rather than IgE-potentiating factor. These findings suggest that the same cells have capacities to form both IgE-potentiating factor and IgE-suppressive factor, and that the biological activity of the IgE-binding factors is decided in the process of glycosylation.

REFERENCES

1. Bloch, K., Ohman, J. L., Jr., Waltin, J., and Cyan, R. W. Potentiated reagin response: initiation with minute dose of antigen and alum followed by infection with *Nippostrongylus brasiliensis*. *J. Immunol. 110*, 197 (1973).

2. Chiorazzi, N., Fox, D. A., and Katz, D. H. Hapten specific IgE antibody responses in mice. VI. Selective enhancement of IgE antibody production by low doses of X-irradiation and by cyclophosphamide. *J. Immunol. 117*, 1629 (1976).

3. Hirashima, M., Yodoi, J., and Ishizaka, K. Regulatory role of IgE-binding factors from rat T lymphocytes. III. IgE-specific suppressive factor with IgE-binding activity. *J. Immunol. 125*, 1442 (1980).

4. Hirashima, M., Yodoi, J., and Ishizaka, K. Regulatory role of IgE-binding factors from rat T lymphocytes. IV. Formation of IgE-binding factors in rats treated with complete Freund's adjuvant. *J. Immunol. 125*, 2154 (1980).

5. Hirata, F., Schiffmann, E., Venkatasubramanian, K., Salmon, D., and Axelrod, J. A phospholipase A_2 inhibitory protein in rabbit neutrophils induced by glucocorticoid. *Proc. Natl. Acad. Sci. U.S.A. 77*, 2533 (1980).

6. Ishizaka, K. Cellular events in the IgE antibody response. *Adv. Immunol. 23*, 1 (1976).

7. Jarrett, E. E. E. and Ferguson, A. Effect of T cell depletion on the potentiated reagin response. *Nature (London) 250*, 420 (1974).

8. Katz, D. H., Bargatze, R. F., Bogowitz, C. A., and Katz, L. R. Regulation of IgE antibody production by serum molecules. IV. Complete Freund's adjuvant induces both enhancing and suppressive activities detectable in the serum of low and high responder mice. *J. Immunol. 122*, 2184 (1979).

9. Mota, I. The mechanism of anaphylaxis. I. Production and biological properties of mast cell sensitizing antibody. *Immunology 7*, 681 (1964).

10. Orr, T. S. C., Riley, P. A., and Doe, J. E. Potentiated reagin response to egg albumin in *Nippostrongylus brasiliensis* infected rats. III. Further studies on the time course of the reagin response. *Immunology 20*, 185 (1971).

11. Spiegelberg, H. L., O'Conor, R. D., Simon, R. A., and Mathison, D. A. Lymphocytes with immunoglobulin E. Fc receptors in patients with atopic disorders. *J. Clin. Invest. 64*, 714 (1979).

12. Suemura, M. and Ishizaka, K. Potentiation of IgE response *in vitro* by T cells from rats infected with *Nippostrongylus brasiliensis*. *J. Immunol. 123*, 918 (1979).

13. Suemura, M., Yodoi, J., Hirashima, M., and Ishizaka, K. Regulatory role of IgE-binding factors from rat T lymphocytes. I. Mechanisms of enhancement of IgE response by IgE-potentiating factor. *J. Immunol. 125*, 148 (1980).

14. Takatsuki, A., Arima, K., and Tamura, G. Inhibition of biosynthesis of polyisoprenol sugars in chick embryo microsomes by tunicamycin. *Agric. Biol. Chem. 39*, 2089 (1975).

15. Tung, A. S., Chiorazzi, N., and Katz, D. H. Regulation of IgE antibody production by serum molecules. I. Serum from complete Freund's adjuvant-immune donors suppresses irradiation-enhanced IgE production in low response strain. *J. Immunol. 120*, 2050 (1978).

16. Watanabe, N., Kojima, S., and Ovary, Z. Suppression of IgE antibody production in SJL mice. I. Nonspecific suppressor T cells. *J. Exp. Med. 143*, 833 (1976).

17. Yodoi, J. and Ishizaka, K. Lymphocytes bearing Fc receptors for IgE. I. Presence of human and rat T lymphocytes with Fc_{ε} receptors. *J. Immunol. 122*, 2577 (1978).

18. Yodoi, J., Ishizaka, T., and Ishizaka, K. Lymphocytes bearing Fc receptors for IgE. II. Induction of Fc_{ε} receptor bearing rat lymphocytes by IgE. *J. Immunol. 123*, 455 (1979).

19. Yodoi, J. and Ishizaka, K. Lymphocytes bearing Fc receptors for IgE. IV. Formation of IgE-binding factor by rat T lymphocytes. *J. Immunol. 124*, 1322 (1980).

20. Yodoi, J. , Hirashima, M., and Ishizaka, K. Regulatory role of IgE-binding factors from rat T lymphocytes. II. Glycoprotein nature and source of IgE-potentiating factor. *J. Immunol. 125*, 1436 (1980).

DISCUSSION

DR. H. ISLIKER: Can you change biologic activities of IgE-potentiating factors by removing or splitting carbohydrate?

ANSWER: The IgE-potentiating factors were inactivated by treatment with neuraminidase-coupled Sepharose. The enzyme-treated factors maintained IgE-binding activities but no enhancing activity on the IgE response. It is not established whether the factors can suppress the IgE response.

DR. H. SPIEGELBERG: Can you get IgE-binding factors from human lymphocytes by incubation with human IgE?

ANSWER: Human lymphocytes did not form a detectable amount of IgE-binding factors upon incubation with IgE. However, activated lymphocytes obtained by either antigenic stimulation or by mixed lymphocyte cultures formed IgE-binding factors upon exposure to IgE. We do not know either the physico-chemical properties or biologic activities of human IgE-binding factors.

DR. C. G. COCHRANE: Prevention of an increase in $Fc_{\varepsilon}R(+)$ cells by tunicamycin does not necessarily mean that carbohydrate is essential for the expression of $Fc_{\varepsilon}R$. It is quite possible that unglycosylated $Fc_{\varepsilon}R$ may be expressed on the cell surface but may be degraded or released easily.

ANSWER: I completely agree with your opinion. Since unglycosylated IgE-binding factors were released from the cells, failure of detecting $Fc_{\varepsilon}R$ on these cells may simply mean that receptors may not stay long enough to be detected.

A question was asked whether corticosteroid actually suppresses the IgE antibody response. Dr. K. Ishizaka answered that he does not have any data on *in vivo* experiments. Dr. Roy Patterson commented that a rapid decrease in serum IgE level was observed when patients with aspergylus infection were treated with steroid.

Dr. J. Uhr asked whether the IgE-binding factors are multivalent. Dr. Ishizaka answered that he does not know the valency of the factors, but imagines that they are not multivalent since the molecular weight of the factors is only between 10,000 to 20,000.

Immunopathology: VIIIth International Symposium, 1980

GENETICS OF THE IMMUNE RESPONSE TO THE α-1,6 EPITOPE OF DEXTRAN[1]

Carmen Fernandez
Göran Möller

Department of Immunobiology,
Karolinska Institute, Wallenberglaboratory,
Stockholm, Sweden

I. INTRODUCTION

Dextran B 512 is a thymus-independent antigen that gives rise to a very restricted and homogeneous immune response with regard to antibody affinity (5, 21). Immunogenicity is dependent upon molecular weight and only dextran preparations with a molecular weight of about 70,000 or more are immunogenic (6, 15, 17), the strongest responses being obtained with native dextran (MW 10^7). Dextran is also a potent polyclonal B cell activator for induction of antibody synthesis; and, as expected, only preparations with a molecular weight above 70,000 function as polyclonal activators (2). The capacity to produce antibodies against the α-1,6 epitope of dextran

[1]*This work was supported by grants from the Swedish Cancer Society and the Swedish Medical Research Council.*

ISBN 0-12-218320-7

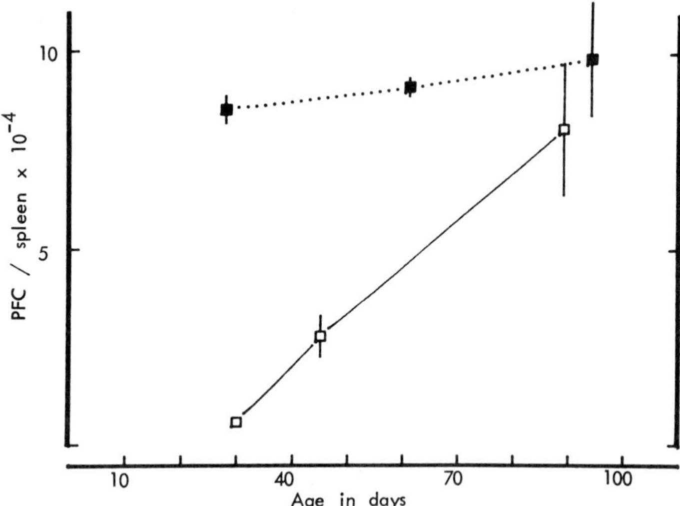

FIGURE 1. The immune response to the α-1,6 epitope of dextran (Dx) (□) or to the hapten FITC (■) in C57BL mice of different ages. The mice were immunized iv with body weight-adjusted doses of native dextran (corresponding to 10 μg/20 g) or FITC-dextran (100 μg/20 g). Five (with dextran) or four (with FITC-dextran) days later the immune response was determined against SRBC coated with 40 μg/10 ml of stearoyl dextran or with 0.5 mg/ml of FITC.

matures late (Fig. 1) and full responsiveness is reached at the age of 3 months (9). The late maturation was not caused by the inability of dextran to function as a polyclonal B cell activator in young mice, but by the failure to express antibodies to dextran, as shown by the inability of LPS to induce the synthesis of antidextran antibodies, whereas antibodies of all other specificities studied were induced by LPS.

II. NONRESPONDER STRAINS

Several mouse strains were found to be high responders to dextran, in particular CBA and C57BL (Table I). Other strains failed to respond or were low responders [e.g., A, A.CA, DBA, and CBA/N (4, 7)]. Since CBA/N mice are immunodeficient with

TABLE I. IgM Responses to the α-1,6 Epitope of Dextran in Different Strains

Strain	H-2 genotype	Igh-C genotype	PFC/spleen
CBA	k	j	33,373
C57BL/10	b	b	51,440
C57BL/6	b	b	29,520
B10.A(4R)	h4	b	33,440
B10.D2	d	b	42,103
B10.A(5R)	i5	b	54,420
B10.S	s	b	30,600
B10.T(6R)	2	b	31,200
A	a	e	2,455
A.CA	f	e	3,930
A.TH	t2	e	4,988
A.TL	tl	e	1,167
A.BY	b	e	1,588
BALB/c	d	a	1,142
C57L	b	a	2,517
DBA	d	c	1,160
AKR	k	d	2,320
A × CBA	a/k	e/j	18,620
A × C57BL	a/b	e/j	23,000
A.CA × CBA	f/k	e/j	19,360
BAB.14	d	b	23,442
CB.20	d	b	74,131
C57BL(lgh-1^{a})	b	a	1,079
CBA (lgh-1^{b})	k	b	35,547
CBA/N	k	j	5

regard to a number of thymus-independent antigens, the mechanism of unresponsiveness was studied separately.

Dextran was found to be a potent polyclonal B cell activator in both A and CBA mice, indicating that the lack of the activating receptor cannot be the mechanism of unresponsiveness in strain A mice. When the hapten FITC was coupled to dextran and the conjugate used to immunize A and CBA mice, equally strong anti-FITC responses were found in both strains (Fig. 2). Thus, dextran can function as an efficient carrier for an antihapten response also in dextran nonresponder strains. However, polyclonally activating concentrations of LPS failed to induce the synthesis of antibodies against the α-1,6 epitope, although antibodies against other antigens were induced, indicating that A mice do not possess or express antibodies against the α-1,6 epitope of dextran (7).

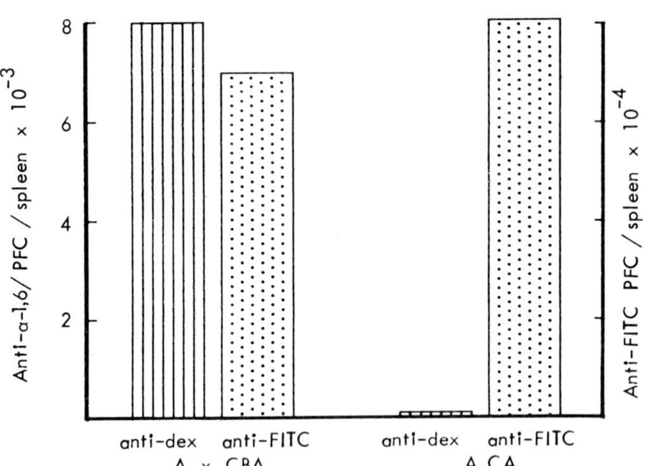

FIGURE 2. Immune response against α-1,6 and FITC in A × CBA F_1 and A.CA mice after immunization iv with 100 μg/mouse of native or FITC-Dx B512. The response was determined at day 5 by using the Jerne plaque assay as modified for the detection of PFC against α-1,6. For detection of anti-α-1,6 PFC, SRBC were conjugated with 40 μg of stearoyl Dx in 10 ml of a 5% suspension of SRBC. Anti-FITC PFC were detected with SRBC conjugated with a solution of 5 mg/ml of FITC.

III. THE ANTI-α-1,6 RESPONSE IS LINKED TO THE Igh-C LOCUS

The ability of about 20 inbred mouse strains to give an IgM response to dextran was tested (4, 7, 13). All strains carrying the $Igh\text{-}1^b$ or the $Igh\text{-}1^j$ allotypes were found to give a significant antidextran response irrespective of their *H-2* genotype (Table I). In contrast, all strains, including recombinant inbred strains, possessing $Igh\text{-}1^c$, $Igh\text{-}1^d$, or $Igh\text{-}1^e$ allotypes were low responders.

In F_1 hybrids between high- and low-responder strains, an IgM plaque-forming cell (PFC) response was always obtained, but the number of plaques was approximately half that found in the high-responder parental strain used in the cross (13).

IV. BACKCROSS SEGREGATION

F_1 mice derived from CBA high-responder and A low-responder mice were backcrossed to the low-responder A strain, and at the age of 3 months 28 of the offspring were immunized with dextran and the IgM PFC response determined. At the same time, serum was collected from individual mice and analyzed for Igh-C locus-determined allotypes.

It was found that responsiveness to the α-1,6 epitope of dextran segregated with the allotype of the high-responder CBA strain (7). Thus, responsiveness to dextran is most likely determined by a variable gene(s) in the heavy-chain locus. This is in agreement with the finding that F_1 hybrids between high- and low-responder strains were always responders, but that the number of PFC obtained was approximately half that obtained with the high-responder parental strain, suggesting allelic exclusion of a gene in the heavy-chain locus.

V. THE CBA/N STRAIN

CBA/N mice are known to be unable to respond to certain thymus-independent antigens, such as ficoll and PVP, but can mount a weak response to other TI antigens, such as LPS (18, 19). CBA/N mice were found to be totally nonresponsive to dextran. Genetically, it is to be expected that CBA/N mice should carry the V gene coding for antibodies against dextran, since the defect in this strain has been mapped to the × chromosome, whereas the dextran gene is localized in the heavy-chain locus. It was actually found that female (CBA/N × DBA) F_1 hybrids expressed the CBA idiotype (see later) on their antidextran antibodies. When CBA/N mice were immunized with FITC-dextran they also failed to respond to the FITC epitope, but they gave a small but definite response to FITC when it was conjugated to horse red cells (7). Thus, dextran failed to function as carrier for an antihapten responses in CBA/N mice, suggesting that the B cells of this strain either lack the activating receptor for dextran or that a subpopulation of B cells capable of responding to dextran has been deleted. It was directly demonstrated that dextran in high (polyclonally activating) concentrations failed to activate B cells from CBA/N mice, whereas LPS induced polyclonal antibody synthesis, although to a smaller degree than in normal CBA mice.

Thus, two different genetic mechanisms can lead to the inability of a mouse strain to produce antibodies against dextran. Several strains lack the Igh-V gene coding for antibodies against dextran and therefore fail to produce antibodies against the α-1,6 epitope, whereas they can respond to haptens coupled to dextran, indicating that their B cells possess the activating receptor for dextran. CBA/N mice that should possess the Igh-V gene fail to respond, because they lack the cells (or the receptors) responding to the activating properties of dextran, and consequently they are also unable to respond to haptens coupled to dextran.

VI. C57BL BUT NOT CBA MICE MAKE AN IgG RESPONSE TO DEXTRAN

Both CBA and C57BL mice possess one (or several linked) Igh-V genes coding for antidextran antibodies, and both give a strong IgM response to the α-1,6 epitope. However, only C57BL gave an IgG PFC response (10) (Fig. 3). Furthermore, nude mice on C57BL background and thymectomized, lethally irradiated and bone marrow repopulated C57BL mice, gave an IgG response to dextran indicating that the IgG response was thymus-independent, as has been found before with two other thymus-independent antigens (1, 20).

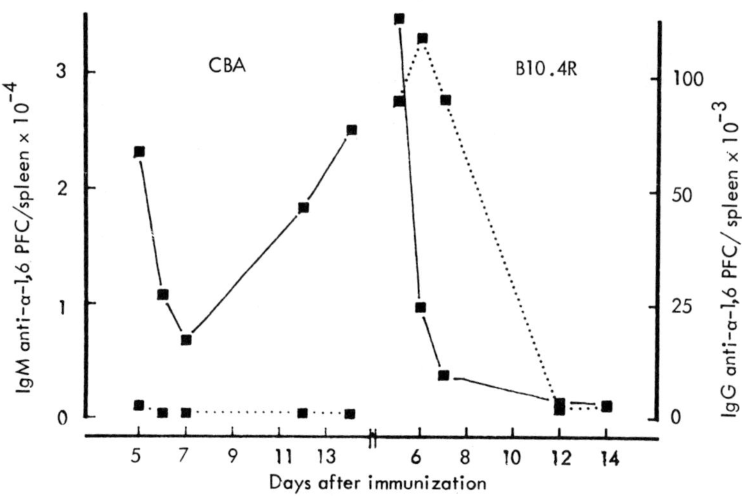

FIGURE 3. Kinetics of the IgM (■———) and IgG (■------) response against the α-1,6 epitope of native dextran B512 in CBA and B10.A(4R) mice. The IgG response represents the total number of plaque-forming cells (PFC) after addition of developing serum. The developing serum caused a 50-95% suppression of the number of IgM PFC.

In the case of immune responses to thymus-dependent antigens under IR gene control it has been found that IgG responses can be obtained by coupling the antigen to an immunogenic carrier. Therefore, we studied whether T-cell dependent forms of dextran could induce an IgG response in CBA mice. Low molecular weight dextran was conjugated to the plant protein edestin and the conjugate shown to have a thymus-dependent antidextran response in CBA mice (16). However, edestin-dextran also failed to induce IgG antibodies to dextran in CBA mice, although it induced IgG antidextran antibodies in C57BL mice.

When FITC-dextran was used to immunize CBA and C57BL mice, both strains gave an IgG response to the FITC epitope. Therefore, the inability of CBA mice to produce IgG antibodies to the α-1,6 epitope appears to be determinant specific, since they fail to produce IgG only against the α-1,6 determinant. It should be pointed out that suppressor T cells or other suppressor cells have not been observed in the immune response to dextran or after tolerance induction (3, 14). Even so, direct experiments were carried out to study whether some suppressor influences could be present in CBA mice preventing an IgG response. In these experiments CBA spleen cells were transferred into irradiated C57BL mice and *vice versa*. CBA cells consistently failed to produce IgG antibodies in C57BL, whereas cells from C57BL mice gave an IgG response in irradiated CBA mice.

Although the mechanism of the inability of CBA mice to give an anti-α-1,6 IgG response is unknown, it seems possible that the translocation of V, D, and J segments to the constant segments in the chromosome and governing heavy-chain synthesis does not occur at random. There are other examples in the dextran system suggesting a regulated V, D, J, and C gene translocation. Thus, the very late ontogenic maturation of the dextran response compared to responses determined by other

Igh-V genes may be explained by regulation of V to C region translocations, although other regulating mechanisms cannot be excluded.

VII. AUTOANTIIDIOTYPIC ANTIBODIES IN THE DEXTRAN RESPONSE

After a primary response to dextran in CBA mice, there is a second spontaneous peak of IgM antidextran antibodies. In the second peak the plaques are smaller and less clear than in the first peak. In C57BL mice there is only one peak of plaque-forming cells and subsequently no plaque-forming cells can be detected. Attempts were made to induce a secondary

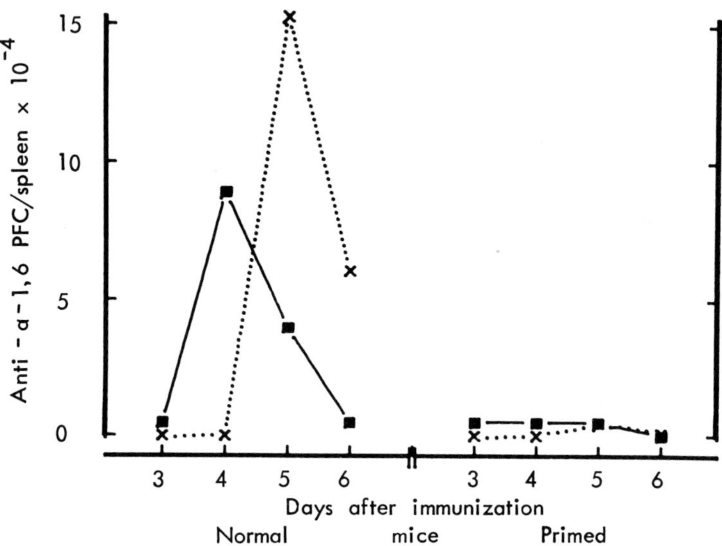

FIGURE 4. Primary and secondary IgM and IgG responses to the α-1,6 epitope of dextran in C57BL mice. Six days after the primary immunization with dextran and horse erythrocytes, the mice and previously untreated controls were given 10 units of dextranase and at day 14 they were immunized with the same antigen mixture. The primary immune responses in previously untreated mice are shown to the left and the secondary response to the right. IgM plaque-forming cells (PFC) are indicated with solid and IgG PFC with dotted lines.

response to dextran in CBA and C57BL mice (Fig. 4). However, a very marked depression in the response as compared to a primary antidextran response was found with regard to both IgM and IgG antibodies (12). It is possible to remove dextran from the Ig receptors *in vivo* by the injection of dextranase (8). When immunized mice were given dextranase followed some days later by an immunogenic dose of dextran there was still no response.

The strong suppression that was induced after a primary response to dextran was specific for the α-1,6 epitope. However, dextran-responsive B cells could be demonstrated in the suppressed mice by transferring them into lethally irradiated untreated syngeneic mice. Nude mice were not suppressed after a primary immunization with dextran, and suppression could be

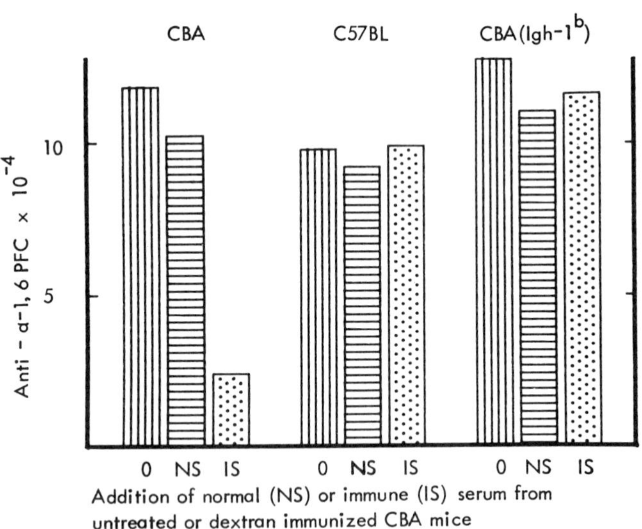

FIGURE 5. Autoantiidiotypic antiserum form CBA mice only suppresses antidextran plaque-forming cells from CBA mice, but not from C57BL or CBA(Igh-1^b) mice. The mice were bled; the antiserum was absorbed 12 days after immunization with dextran, absorbed with dextran, and added to the agar in the plaque assay at a final dilution of 1/1000. Normal CBA serum was used as a control.

passively transferred with serum from primed mice to previously untreated mice. Serum from immunized animals also transferred suppression to untreated mice when the serum was absorbed with dextran, excluding antibody feedback suppression as the responsible mechanism. Finally, it was shown that dextran-absorbed serum from immunized mice suppressed the development of antidextran plaque-forming cells *in vitro* (Fig. 5) and that the suppressive principle was an immunoglobulin of 7S type (11). Thus, during the immune response to dextran both CBA and C57BL mice spontaneously develop autoantiidiotypic antibodies that prevent a subsequent response.

Suppression of the dextran response after priming persists for a very long time and is caused by autoantiidiotypic antibodies. The synthesis of these autoantiidiotypic antibodies is T-cell dependent, since nude mice do not produce them and since nude mice also give a second response after priming.

VIII. THE AUTOANTIIDIOTYPIC ANTIBODIES ARE STRAIN SPECIFIC

Serum-containing autoantiidiotypic antibodies from CBA mice suppressed antidextran plaque-forming cells from CBA mice, but not from C57BL and *vice versa*. Thus, the autoantiidiotypic antibodies specifically recognized antidextran antibodies coded for by Igh-V genes in two different strains. Therefore, the Igh-V genes must be different in CBA and C57BL mice. It was formally established that the autoantiidiotypic antibodies from CBA mice did not suppress antidextran plaque-forming cells of CBA/Igh-1^b mice (Fig. 5). There were no autoantiidiotypic antibodies in dextran nonresponder strains after immunization with dextran, nor did dextran-tolerant mice of high-responder strains produce such antibodies.

TABLE II. Codominant Expression of Antiidiotypic Antibodies in F_1 Hybrids between CBA and C57BL Dextran High-Responder Mice[a]

Addition of serum	C57BL (%I)[b]	CBA (%I)[b]	(C57BL × CBA) F_1 (%I)[b]
C57BL	28	2	28
CBA	3	36	36
(C57BL × CBA) F_1	43	45	37

[a] *Sera were obtained 12 days after immunization with dextran and were absorbed with dextran before use. The sera were added to the agar in a final dilution of 1/1000. The spleen cells were obtained from the indicated strains 5 days after immunization with dextran.*

[b] *%I = inhibition of the number of plaque-forming cells by the autoantiidiotypic sera compared to untreated dishes.*

F_1 hybrids between CBA and C57BL mice produced autoantiidiotypic antibodies characteristic of each of the parental strains (Table II), indicating that F_1 hybrids express both Igh-V genes of the parents (presumably in different cells) and that the mice also synthesized two different autoantiidiotypic antibodies (13).

The strict relationship between heavy-chain allotype and the ability to respond to dextran did not hold when Baily recombinant strains were tested. These strains are derived from crosses between BALB/c and C57BL. In our hands BALB/c mice from Jackson and Bomholtgaard, Denmark, are nonresponders to dextran, whereas those from Dr. M. Cohn, La Jolla, are responders. We found that one $Igh\text{-}1^a$ recombinant strain responded to dextran. However, the antibodies did not possess the idiotype of C57BL or CBA mice. Instead, this strain produced its own autoantiidiotypic antibody, one that only suppressed antidextran antibodies produced by this strain.

IX. DICHOTOMY BETWEEN RESPONSE AND ALLOTYPE-LINKED IDIOTYPE

Two heavy-chain recombinant strains (CB.20 and BAB.14) were tested for their response to dextran (13). Both are recombinants between BALB/c and C57BL and contain heavy-chain genes from both strains. It was found that both strains responded to dextran (Table III). However, BAB.14 did not possess the idiotype of C57BL on the antidextran antibodies, whereas CB.20 did. Again BAB.14 produced its own autoanti-idiotypic antibody.

The relationship between response and allotype-linked idiotype is true for inbred mouse strains and strains that are coisogenic with regard to the entire heavy-chain locus, such as C57BL ($Igh\text{-}1^a$) and CBA ($Igh\text{-}1^b$), but not when recombinant inbred strains or heavy-chain recombinant strains were studied. In addition, there was a dichotomy between response and idiotype in BAB.14 mice. It is difficult to give a rational explanation for this finding, since it is not known whether or not the BALB/c strain used in the cross could respond to dextran. If it were a dextran responder, the finding would simply means that a recombination occurred in the heavy-chain locus so that the C57BL Igh-V gene coding for antibodies against dextran was lost and replaced by that of the BALB/c. However, if the BALB/c was a nonresponder to dextran the finding indicates that the Igh-V gene-determining response to dextran was different from an Igh-V gene-determining expression of the idiotype. Several other explanations are possible, however.

TABLE III. The Anti-α-1,6 Response of Strains BAB.14, CB.20, and C57BL Ig[a]

Strain	IgCH allotype	*H-2* type	V_H genes	PFC/spleen[1)a]
BAB.14	b	d	Partly BALB/c	4.37 ± 0.14(23442)
CB.20	b	d	C57BL	4.87 ± 0.12(74131)
C57BL/6($Ig-1^a$)	a	b	BALB/c	3.14 ± 0.50(1079)
CBA($Ig-1^b$)	b	k	C57BL	4.57 ± 0.06(37547)
DB-8 KN	b	d	Partly BALB/c	4.45 ± 0.30(33960)

[a] *The response is expressed as* log_{10} *mean ± SE (antilog of the mean).*

X. SUMMARY

The response to the α-1,6 epitope of dextran is determined by Igh-V genes linked to allotypes typical of CBA and C57BL strains. In addition, genes determining the expression of nonclonally distributed activation receptors (or cells carrying such receptors) for dextran are necessary for a response. High-responder strains produce IgM antibodies, but only C57BL mice or mice possessing an Igh-lb locus produce thymus-independent IgG antibodies to dextran. The inability of CBA mice to produce IgG antibodies to dextran is not due to suppressor cells or factors, but to properties of the B cell themselves that specifically lack the ability to make IgG antibodies to the α-1,6 epitope of dextran but can synthesize IgG to haptens coupled to dextran.

During the immune response to dextran autoantiidiotypic antibodies are spontaneously produced that specifically suppressed a subsequent response to dextran. CBA and C57BL mice make different autoantiidiotypic antibodies and F_1 hybrids between these strains make antidextran antibodies of both parental strains and also synthesize two different autoanti-idiotypic antibodies. In one heavy-chain recombinant inbred strain there was a dichotomy between the ability to respond to dextran and idiotype.

REFERENCES

1. Andersson, B. and Blomgren, B. T-cell dependency of the response to PVP is dependent on maturity of B cells. *In* "Immune Reactivity of Lymphocytes" (M. Feldman and A. Globerson, eds.), p. 283. Plenum, New York, 1976.

2. Coutinho, A., Möller, G., and Richter, W. Molecular basis of B cell activation. I. Mitogenicity of native and substituted dextrans. *Scand. J. Immunol. 3*, 321 (1974).

3. Fernandez, C., Hammarström, L., Möller, G., Primi, D., and Smith, C. I. E. Immunological tolerance only affects a subpopulation of the antigen-specific B lymphocytes. *Immunol. Rev. 43,* 3 (1979).

4. Fernandez, C., Lieberman, R., and Möller, G. The immune response to the α-1,6 epitope of dextran is determined by a gene linked to the IgCH locus. *Scand. J. Immunol. 10,* 77 (1979).

5. Fernandez, C. and Möller, G. The immune response against two epitopes on the same thymus-independent polysaccharide. I. Role of epitope density in carrier-dependent immunity and tolerance. *Immunology 33,* 59 (1977).

6. Fernandez, C. and Möller, G. The immune response against two epitopes on the same thymus-independent polysaccharide. II. Enhanced anti-hapten response by injection of unconjugated carrier. *Immunology 33,* 331 (1977).

7. Fernandez, C. and Möller, G. Immunological unresponsiveness to thymus-independent antigens. Two fundamentally different genetic mechanisms of B cell unresponsiveness to dextran. *J. Exp. Med. 146,* 1663 (1977).

8. Fernandez, C. and Möller, G. Irreversible immunological tolerance to thymus-independent antigens is restricted to the clone of B cells having both Ig and PBA receptors for the tolerogen. *Scand. J. Immunol. 7,* 137 (1978).

9. Fernandez, C. and Möller, G. Immunological unresponsiveness to native dextran B512 in young animals of dextran high responder strains in due to lack of Ig receptor expression. Evidence for a nonrandom expression of V genes. *J. Exp. Med. 147,* 645 (1978).

10. Fernandez, C. and Möller, G. A thymus-independent IgG response to the α-1,6 epitope of dextran is determined by a gene linked to the IgCH locus. *Scand. J. Immunol. 10,* 77 (1979).

11. Fernandez, C. and Möller, G. Antigen induced strain-specific autoantiidiotypic antibodies modulate the immune response to dextran B512. *Proc. Natl. Acad. Sci. U.S.A. 76,* 5944 (1979).

12. Fernandez, C. and Möller, G. A primary immune response to dextran B512 is followed by a period of antigen-specific immunosuppression caused by autoantiidiotypic antibodies. *Scand. J. Immunol. 11*, 53 (1980).

13. Fernandez, C., Mäkelä, O., and Möller, G. Genetics of the anti-dextran B512 and the autoantiidiotypic response: codominant expression in F_1 hybrids and dichotomy of response and allotype-linked idiotype. *Immunogenetics (N.Y.) 10*, 573 (1980).

14. Howard, J. G., Courtenay, B. M., and Hale, C. Lack of effect of thymectomy on spontaneous recovery from tolerance to levan. *Eur. J. Immunol. 6*, 837 (1976).

15. Howard, J. G., Vicari, G., and Courtenay, B. M. Influence of molecular structure on the tolerogenicity of bacterial dextrans. I. The α-1,6 linked epitope of dextran B512. *Immunology 29*, 585 (1975).

16. Möller, G. and Fernandez, C. Immunological tolerance to the thymus-independent antigen dextran can be abrogated by thymus-dependent dextran conjugation. Evidence against clonal deletion as the mechanism of tolerance induction. *Scand. J. Immunol. 8*, 29 (1978).

17. Moreno, C., Hale, C., and Ivanyi, L. The mitogenic and tolerogenic properties of dextrans and levans. Lack of correlation according to differences of molecular structure and size. *Immunology 33*, 261 (1977).

18. Mosier, D. E., Scher, I., Ruhl, H., Cohen, P. L., Zitran, I., and Paul, W. E. Activation of normal and defective B lymphocytes by thymus-independent antigen. *In* "Mitogens in Immunobiology" (J. J. Oppenheim and D. L. Rosenstreich, eds.), p. 313. Academic Press, New York, 1976.

19. Perlmutter, R. M., Nahm, M., Stein, K. E., Slack, J., Zitran, I., Paul, W. E., and Davie, J. M. Immunoglobulin in subclass specific immunodeficiency in mice with an X-linked B-lymphocyte defect. *J. Exp. Med. 149*, 993 (1979).

20. Sharon, R., McMaster, P. R. B., Kaks, A. M., Owen, J. D., and Paul, W. E. DNP-Lys-Ficoll: a T-independent antigen which elicits both IgM and IgG anti-DNP antibody secreting cells. *J. Immunol. 114*, 1585 (1975).

21. Vicari, G. and Courtenay, B. M. Restricted avidity of the IgM antibody response to dextran B512 in mice: Studies on inhibition of specific PFC by oligosaccharides. *Immunochemistry 14*, 253 (1977).

DISCUSSION[2]

DR. KLINMAN: How did you establish that CBA/N mice possess the Igh-V gene for dextran, since these mice do not respond to thymus-independent antigens of this type?

MÖLLER: We immunized (CBA/N × DNA) F_1 female mice with dextran and determined that the antidextran antibodies possessed the idiotype characteristic of CBA mice.

EICHMANN: Could the dichotomy between response and possession of idiotype be ascribed to different properties of V-J segments?

MÖLLER: Actually, one of the explanations we have offered for this dichotomy is that the ability to respond is determined by, e.g., a V segment, whereas the idiotype could be determined by the D or J segment. It is necessary to establish that the BALB/c mice used for the establishment of the BAB.14 strain is a nonresponder strain to dextran, before explanations of this type can be seriously considered.

EICHMANN: You showed that F_1 hybrids between responder and nonresponder strains gave about half the number of PFC, but in the figure on % inhibition of PFC by antiidiotypic sera, there was about equal suppression of PFC from parental and F_1 hybrids.

MÖLLER: To quantitate precisely inhibition of PFC by antiidiotypic antisera is difficult for several reasons. We do not know whether the antiidiotypic antisera from F_1 hybrids and the parental strain are equally strong nor do we obtain

[2] *Edited by Fernandez and Möller.*

complete suppression by parental antiidiotypic sera added to PFC from the same strain. Although we cannot formally show that the expression of idiotype is codominantly expressed, this is certainly the most plausible alternative.

Immunopathology: VIIIth International Symposium, 1980

MONOCLONAL-T CELL FACTORS: ANTIGENIC STRUCTURE, FUNCTIONS, AND GENETICS

Tomio Tada
Gen Suzuki
Keiichi Hiramatsu
Kyoko Hayakawa

Department of Immunology, Faculty of Medicine,
University of Tokyo,
Tokyo, Japan

Masaru Taniguchi

Laboratory for Immunology, School of Medicine,
Chiba University,
Chiba, Japan

I. INTRODUCTION

The recent development of hybridoma technology enabled us to make monoclonal antibodies specific for determinants of complex antigens, both soluble and membrane-associated forms (5). The same principle has been applied to make T-cell hybrids that secrete both antigen-specific and antigen-nonspecific mediators involved in T-cell-mediated immunological phenomena. It is especially pertinent to analyze antigen-specific

ISBN 0-12-218320-7

T-cell factors, which are apparently devices of T cells for recognizing antigen and interacting with other cells.

It is well known that these antigen-specific factors play substantial roles in the regulation of immune responses, yet their molecular basis remains obscure (9). They share certain immunological properties regardless of their diverse functions. The most important properties are that (a) they possess a specific affinity for antigen comparable to antibody molecules, (b) no immunoglobulin constant structures have been detected, and (c) they have antigenic determinants encoded in the I region of the major histocompatibility complex (MHC). Although there exist some discrepancies between the functionally defined Ia-bearing T-cell factors and biochemically extracted T-cell antigen receptors (2, 7, 9), these molecules lend clues to define the unknown antigen-recognition unit of T-cells. Biochemical analysis as well as critical comparisons between these two categories of antigen-specific molecules of T cells are hampered by the extremely low quantities of material obtained from normal antigen-primed T cells. Our laboratory has made an effort to establish T-cell hybridomas producing antigen-specific Ia-bearing T-cell factors and to characterize the material with respect to function and biochemistry. We will summarize some of the properties of the monoclonal products obtained from these hybridomas.

II. T-CELL HYBRIDOMAS WITH I-REGION DETERMINANTS

To make T-cell hybrids, we preselected antigen-binding T cells by a simple plating technique (13). Spleen cells from mice immunized with keyhole limpet hemocyanin (KLH) or a hapten, 4-hydroxy-3-nitrophenylacetyl (NP) coupled to nonimmunogenic carriers (gelatin and mouse immunoglobulin, MIg) were first incubated in petri dishes coated with anti-MIg to remove Ig-positive cells. The cells that did not adhere to the anti-MIg dishes were then applied to antigen (KLH or NP gelatin)-coated petri dishes at 37°C, and the nonadhering T cells were discarded. Cells bound to the dishes were eluted by washing with chilled medium (0°C). The fractions thus obtained were usually made up of more than 95% Thy-1 positive T cells, of which about 30% were Ia positive. This procedure also enriched Lyt-$1^{-}2^{+}3^{+}$ T cells. The recovery was 0.1 to 0.3% of original spleen cells.

Subregion specificities of Ia antigens on these antigen-binding T cells were determined by the cytotoxic test using anti-Ia directed at restricted subregions. In general, anti-I-J antisera killed these cells most effectively, except in the case of KLH-binding T cells from A/J mice. In this latter strain most Ia-positive T cells in the KLH-binding cell fraction were killed by anti-Ia directed at the I-A subregion, whereas I-J positive T cells were almost undetectable. This is consistent with our previous report that A/J mice were unable to produce I-J^{+} KLH-specific suppressor T cells (12). One further interesting fact is that 20-30% of antigen-binding T cells were found to carry immunoglobulin heavy-chain V region (V_H) determinants that were detectable by rabbit antibodies specific for the framework structure of V_H(11).

In the case of NP-binding, nearly 10% of the cells were stained with heterologous antiidiotypic antiserum raised against the major cross-reactive idiotype of anti-NP antibodies of strains with the Igh^{b} allotype (NP^{b}). A somewhat smaller percentage of cells was also stained with monoclonal antibody against the NP^{b} idiotype, which was kindly provided by Drs. Michael Reth and Klaus Rajewsky.

TABLE I. Heterogeneity of Ia-Bearing Hybridomas

Hybridoma	Parental T cell obtained from	Ia antigen coded by	Function*
9F18la	KLH-primed C57BL/6	$I\text{-}J^b$	Antigen-specific Ts, V_H^+
34S-11	KLH-primed C57BL/6	$I\text{-}J^b$	Antigen-specific Ts
34S-18	KLH-primed C57BL/6	$I\text{-}J^b$	Antigen-specific Ts, V_H^+
34S-704	KLH-primed C57BL/6	$I\text{-}J^b$	Antigen-specific Ts, V_H^+
8C-2	KLH-primed C57BL/6	$I\text{-}J^b$	Antigen-nonspecific Ts
8C-23	KLH-primed C57BL/6	$I\text{-}J^b$	Antigen-nonspecific Ts
34S-44	KLH-primed C57BL/6	$I\text{-}J^b$	Antigen-nonspecific Ts
34S-281	KLH-primed C57BL/6	$I\text{-}J^b$	No activity
8C-19	KLH-primed C57BL/6	$I\text{-}J^b$	No activity
4101FL10	KLH-primed A/J	$I\text{-}A^k$	Antigen-specific Ta, V_H^+
5108L1	KLH-primed A/J	$I\text{-}A^k$	Antigen-specific Ta, V_H^+
4704L2	KLH-primed A/J	$I\text{-}A^k$	Antigen-specific Ta
4318L14	KLH-primed A/J	$I\text{-}A^k$	Antigen-nonspecific Ta
5117L1	KLH-primed A/J	$I\text{-}A^k$	Antigen-nonspecific Ta
7C3	NP-primed B10.BR	$I\text{-}J^k$	Ts, NP-idiotype$^+$
7E7	NP-primed B10.BR	$I\text{-}J^k$	Ts? NP-idiotype$^+$
2D3	NP-primed B10.BR	$I\text{-}J^k$	No activity, NP-idiotype$^-$
4E12	NP-primed B10.BR	$I\text{-}J^k$	No activity, NP-idiotype$^-$

**Ts, suppressor activity in the extract. Ta, augmenting activity in the extract.*

Antigen-binding T cells thus obtained were fused with a thymoma cell line of AKR origin (BW5147) that lacks the enzyme hypoxanthine-guanine-phosphoribosyl transferase (HGPRT), by the method described by Taniguchi and Miller (14). After culturing in the medium containing hypoxanthine, aminopterin, and thymidine (HAT medium), the hybrid cells were first selected by Ia positivity with a fluorescence-activated cell sorter (FACS) followed by cloning with limiting dilution. The cell lines were occasionally recloned until they had stable expression of Ia, idiotype, or antigen-binding activity.

Table I lists our stock of hybridomas with Ia expression. The extracted material (TsF) from many of the $I\text{-}J^+$ hybridomas showed an antigen-specific or nonspecific suppressor activity when added to the cultured antigen-primed syngeneic spleen cells, whereas some others had no activities regardless of their I-J expression. The extracts from hybridomas with I-A subregion products had either antigen-specific or antigen-nonspecific augmenting activity in the *in vitro* secondary antibody response to DNP-KLH of A/J spleen cells.

III. SUPPRESSOR HYBRIDOMAS SPECIFIC FOR KLH AND NP

A number of suppressor hybridomas specific for KLH were established by Taniguchi and co-workers (15, 16). Many of them showed the KLH-specific suppressor activity in the secondary *in vitro* antibody response of syngeneic and semisyngeneic spleen cells against DNP-KLH, whereas others had an entirely nonspecific suppressor effect or no detectable activity even though all clones had been selected for the presence of I-J determinants.

The antigenic structures of the suppressor T-cell factor (TsF) were analyzed by absorption with various allo- and xeno-antibodies. It has been demonstrated that TsF activity was absorbed by columns composed of KLH, anti-H-2^b and anti-I-J^b, but not by anti-I-J^k and anti-MIg, thus indicating that the hybridoma-derived TsF has antigenic structures identical to those detected on TsF derived from normal primed suppressor T cells (16). The factor was also adsorbable by anti-V_H but not by anti-V_L (11); the results are shown in Fig. 1.

Some of the KLH-specific hybridomas were transplantable to F_1 animals of AKR × C57BL/6, since the original suppressor T cell for the fusion was derived from C57BL/6 mice (15). The cells can grow as a solid tumor when transplanted subcutaneously, and can produce a large quantity of ascites if

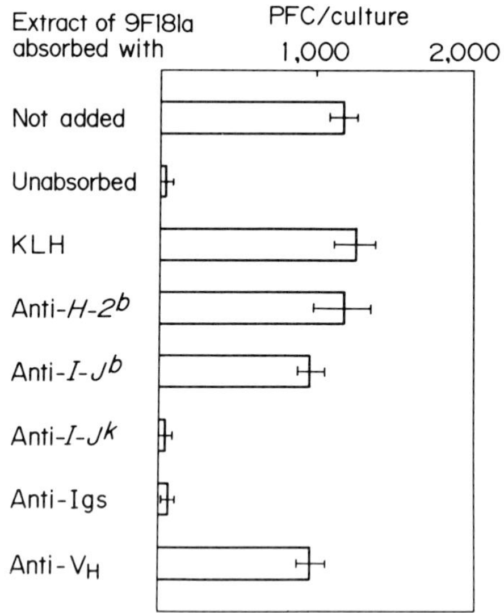

FIGURE 1. Characterization of a hybridoma(9F181a)-derived KLH-specific suppressor factor by absorption with antigen and antibodies. Note that the suppressor activity is removed by absorption with antigen (KLH), anti-H-2^b, anti-I-J^b, and anti-V_H but not with other antibody-coated columns. Absorption with anti-V_L column was ineffective (data not shown).

transplanted intraperitoneally. The ascitic fluid contained a strong antigen-specific suppressor activity which was also adsorbable with anti-I-J^b and KLH immunoadsorbent.

An interesting observation was made by Taniguchi *et al.* (17) indicating that the molecule consists of two discrete polypeptide chains. They absorbed the extracted TsF from one of the KLH-specific hybridomas (34S-704) either with KLH or an anti-I-J column. The adsorbed material had no suppressor activity after absorption by either column, whereas the 1:1 mixture of the ineffective filtrates reconstituted the strong suppressor activity. The same was true for the mixture of filtrates from anti-V_H and anti-I-J columns. These results indicate that the extracted material contains three different types of molecules: (1) a polypeptide chain with I-J determinant which can be adsorbed by anti-I-J, (2) a chain that carries V_H determinants responsible for the affinity for antigen, and (3) a molecule of the above two combined. The presence of the third molecule is indicated by the fact that the activity is fully recovered in the acid eluate from either the anti-I-J or the KLH column. The most feasible explanation for the reconstitution of the suppressor activity by the combination of ineffective filtrates is that the I-J coded and V_H-containing chains are recombined when they act on the target cells.

Such reconstitution of the suppressor activity by adsorbed materials was, however, not observed with ascitic fluid. Thus, it is suggested that I-J and V_H products are synthesized separately, but then combined to make an active molecule when they are secreted. In fact, a mild reduction of the secreted material with dithiothreitol separates these two determinants. Recent biochemical studies also indicate that the antigen-binding molecules from both suppressor and augmenting hybridomas are composed of heavy (MW 35,000-70,000) and light

(MW 25,000-30,000) chains detected by SDS gel electrophoresis under reducing conditions. The molecular weight of these chains has some inconsistency from one experiment to the other, perhaps due to proteolytic cleavage during the preparation or to the heterogeneity of the products themselves.

Similar observations had been made by Taussig and Holliman (19) with their sheep red blood cell-specific hybridoma. Although this hybridoma (A-1) had several features distinct from those described here, biochemical studies indicated that the internally labeled TsF from A-1 consists of two noncovalently linked polypeptide chains with MWs of about 85,000 and 25,000 and that the antigen-binding structure resides on the heavy chain whereas the H-2 coded structures are on the light chain. The subregion specificity of the light chains has not yet been determined, but it is encoded by the gene assigned to the right of I-J subregion of H-2 complex, most likely in the I-C subregion (20).

Another important point with the KLH-specific hybridoma-derived TsF is that there exists a strict genetic restriction with respect to the effect on the responding T cells (16). TsF derived from hybridomas with C57BL/6 parental T cells is capable of suppressing the responses mounted by syngeneic C57BL/6 and semisyngeneic (C3H × C57BL/6) F_1 spleen cells but not allogeneic C3H. This restriction is analogous to that observed with normal primed TsF in which restricting elements were mapped in the I-J subregion (8). This restriction is usually not observable with the antigen-nonspecific TsF from other hybridomas. We have recently established hybridomas with NP-binding activity. Since anti-NP antibodies have certain important characteristics, i.e., the possession of a major cross-reactive idiotype (NP^b) and heteroclicity (4, 6), NP-specific hybridomas are useful tools for studying the structure and genetic relations of the antigen-specific T cell factors. In fact, antigen receptor materials from NP-primed T cells have also been well documented (3).

The hybridomas were made by fusion with NP-binding splenic T cells of B10.BR mice (H-2^k, Igh-1^b) and BW5147. Some of the NP-binding hybrid clones expressed NP^b idiotype as detected by xenogeneic antiidiotype antibodies, although this was not the major cross-reactive one detectable by any of the monoclonals. However, the NP-specific receptor of the hybridomas clearly showed a heteroclicity in that the staining of the cell membrane with antiidiotype antibodies was inhibited by NIP better than by NP at the same concentrations. Furthermore, the culture supernatant as well as the receptor material bound to the NP-coupled nylon mesh from this hybridoma had an extremely high neutralizing activity for haptenated T_4 bacteriophages (Rajewsky, personal communication). The isolated material also showed a heteroclicity in which the affinity for NIP was 100 times higher than that for NP.

The extracted material could suppress the secondary anti-NP antibody response of H-2 *or* IgCH gene compatible strains. In IgCH gene compatible combinations, the expression of NP^b idiotype was also inhibited. This suggests that TsF is also involved in the idiotype regulation. Biochemical analysis of this idiotype-bearing suppressor molecule is now underway.

IV. KLH-SPECIFIC HYBRIDOMA WITH AUGMENTING ACTIVITY

We previously reported that there exists another antigen-specific T-cell factor that augments the antibody response (21). This factor, termed antigen-specific augmenting T-cell factor (TaF), was found in the extract of KLH-primed spleen cells of the A/J strain, which was found to be defective in the production of KLH-specific suppressor factors (12). This factor was not T-cell replacing, but was able to augment the specific antibody response against DNP-KLH in the presence of helper T cells. TaF was characterized by an Ia antigen coded for by the I-A subregion gene.

We have demonstrated that the Ia antigen on the KLH-specific TaF is different from those expressed on B cells and macrophages (21). This was further substantiated by a hybridoma cell line carrying Ia antigen encoded by the I-A subregion gene with an antigen-specific augmenting activity. The cell line 4101FL10 is a hybridoma made by fusion of the A/J derived KLH-binding T cell and BW5147 (3a). This cell line has both Thy-1.1 and Thy-1.2, I-A^k, Lyt-1, and V_H, but lacks the I-J expression. The extract of 4101FL10 had a definite enhancing activity in the *in vitro* secondary antibody response against DNP-KLH in syngeneic and I-region compatible combinations. The factor was adsorbable to KLH and anti-I-A columns and was successfully eluted from them by acid treatment. The factor is in all ways analogous to the previously described TaF, with respect to its inability to replace helper T cells and its enhancing activity in the presence of syngeneic, antigen-specific helper T cells.

Some important properties to be noted are that the hybridoma, in fact, carries an Ia antigen detectable by conventional anti-Ia (A.TH anti-A.TL) and that the subregion specificity of Ia antigen is clearly mapped in I-A subregion by cytotoxic killing with (gR × A.TFR 5) F_1 anti-A.TL (directed at I-A^k, I-B^k subregions). Despite that, none of the monoclonal anti-Ia antibodies with extremely high titers against private (Ia.2) and public (Ia.17) specificities of I-A^k were able to kill or stain the hybridoma cells. Moreover, after removal of the B-cell cytotoxicity by absorption with

T-cell-deprived spleen cells, the conventional anti-Ia (A.TH anti-A.TL) was equally effective in killing the hybridoma, whereas the antiserum absorbed with T cells was unable to kill this cell line even with the remaining strong cytotoxic activity against B cells. It was further noted that such anti-Ia antisera preabsorbed with B cells were able to absorb the KLH-specific TaF from normal as well as from I-A^+ hybridomas.

These results together with previous reports (1, 21) indicate that both I-J and I-A coded products detected on antigen-specific suppressor and helper T cells as well as on hybridoma counterparts, are a group of Ia molecules distinct from those detected on B cells and macrophages, and that there exist multiple T-cell Ia loci in the I region of the H-2 complex that are selectively expressed on functional subsets of T cells. It is further suggested that this unique family of Ia molecules in association with the antigen-bidning site on T cells is directly related to the functions born by T-cell subsets.

V. HETEROGENEITY OF Ia ANTIGENS ON HYBRIDOMAS

The results presented above suggest that the functional heterogeneity observed among I-J^+ hybridomas is due to structural differences in I-region-coded determinants. We have previously shown that I-J determinants expressed on suppressor and helper T cells are different (10). Taniguchi *et al.* (18) absorbed an anti-I-J^b antiserum with one of the hybridomas and tested its ability to kill other I-J^+ hybrids. It was found that after absorption with an antigen-nonspecific suppressor hybridoma, the antiserum was unable to kill either the homologous or other antigen-nonspecific hybrids, whereas the same antiserum was able to kill antigen-specific suppressor hybrids and nonfunctional ones. If the same antiserum was absorbed with an antigen-specific suppressor hybridoma, the resultant antiserum was still capable of killing both nonspecific and nonfunctional suppressor hybrids. Absorption with a nonfunctional hybridoma, however, abrogated the cytotoxic activity of the antiserum against both specific and nonspecific hybrids. These results indicate that conventional anti-I-J antiserum detected at least two different antigenic determinants that are expressed separately or together on functionally different hybridomas. If the I-J determinants on the Ia^+ helper T cell are also different, there should be at least three discrete loci that determine cell surface determinants expressed on functionally different T-cell subsets.

This was further supported by a recent experiment with $I\text{-}J^k$ positive hybridomas. A hybridoma derived from NP-primed B10.BR splenic T cells, 2D3, is a stable cell line continuously expressing a high density of I-J molecules on their surface. By screening a number of anti-$I\text{-}J^k$ (3R anti-5R) antisera with this hybridoma, we found that some anti-$I\text{-}J^k$ with high titers against 2D3 were unable to kill $H\text{-}2^k$ suppressor T cells. Other antisera with strong reactivity to KLH-specific suppressor T cells were incapable of killing 2D3. These latter antisera were able to kill another hybridoma (7C3) which had a NP-specific suppressor function. Absorption studies with these antisera by 2D3 or 7C3 indicated that these hybridomas carry distinct antigenic determinants. These results indicate that the I-J subregion accommodate more than two different loci which control distinct Ia specificities expressed on functionally different T cells and that monoclonal hybridomas are expressing one or more of these T cell Ia loci.

As already discussed, Ia antigen on the augmenting T-cell hybridoma is also different from B-cell Ia antigens, with respect to its antigenic specificities and cross-reactive patterns. Preliminary biochemical studies indicate that the basic structure of the molecule is entirely different from the prototype of B-cell Ia antigens, which are composed of α and β chains.

Future biochemical studies as well as molecular biological studies, which are now possible with these monoclonal hybrid cell lines, will clarify the structure of both I region-coded polypeptides and V_H-containing antigen-receptors of T cells. The second age of factorology has just now started.

V. SUMMARY

We were able to establish a number of T-cell hybridomas that produce monoclonal T-cell factors either suppressing or augmenting the specific antibody response. These T-cell factors carry I-region gene products in association with an IgV_H gene product. In certain cases, such as a NP-specific factor, an idiotypic determinant was detected, which was associated with a heteroclicity similar to that observed in the antibody molecule. Antigen-binding sites and Ia determinants are on separate polypeptide chains; the heavy chain contains a V_H structure and the light chain Ia. The exact molecular weight of the heavy chain has not been determined. Serological studies indicated that those Ia molecules on T cell hybrids are entirely different from B-cell Ia antigens. As yet there is no formal proof for the rearrangement of V_H and J genes in these hybridomas; they would provide important materials for the molecular biological studies on T-cell antigen receptors. In addition, these hybridoma-derived monoclonal T-cell factors can replace certain T-cell types in the regulatory circuit and are thus useful in elucidating the molecular basis of cell interactions.

REFERENCES

1. Asano, Y., Okumura, K., and Tada, T. Ia antigens on antigen-presenting cells do not carry the same Ia specificities as detected on suppressor and helper T cells. *Scand. J. Immunol. 13*, 353 (1981).

2. Binz, H. and Wigzell, H. Antigen-binding, idiotypic T-lymphocyte receptors. *Contemp. Top. Immunobiol. 7*, 113 (1977).

3. Cramer, M., Krawinkel, U., Hämmerling, G., Black, S. J., Berek, C., Eichmann, K., and Rajewsky, K. Antigen receptors on mouse T lymphocytes. *In* "Ir Genes and Ia Antigens" (H. O. McDevitt, ed.), p. 583. Academic Press, New York, 1978.

3a. Hiramatsu, K., Miyatani, S., Kim, M., Yamada, S., Okumura, K., and Tada, T. Unique T cell Ia antigen expressed on a hybrid cell line producing antigen-specific augmenting T cell factor. *J. Immunol. 127*, 1118 (1981).

4. Imanishi, T. and Mäkelä, O. Inheritance of antibody specificity. I. Anti-(4-hydroxy-3-nitrophenyl)-acetyl of the mouse primary response. *J. Exp. Med. 140*, 1498 (1974).

5. Köller, G. and Milstein, C. Derivation of specific antibody-producing tissue culture and tumor lines by cell fusion. *Eur. J. Immunol. 6*, 511 (1976).

6. Mäkelä, O. Single lymph node cells producing heteroclitic bacteriophage antibody. *J. Immunol. 95*, 378 (1965).

7. Rajewsky, K. and Eichmann, K. Antigen receptors of T helper cells. *Contemp. Top. Immunobiol. 7*, 69 (1977).

8. Tada, T., Taniguchi, M., and David, C. S. Suppressive and enhancing T-cell factors as I-region gene products: properties and the subregion assignment. *Cold Spring Harbor Symp. Quant. Biol. 41*, 119 (1977).

9. Tada, T. and Okumura, K. The role of antigen-specific T cell factors in the immune response. *Adv. Immunol. 28*, 1 (1979).

10. Tada, T., Nonaka, M., Okumura, K., Taniguchi, M., and Tokuhisa, T. Ia antigens on suppressor, amplifier and helper T cells. *In* "Cell Biology and Immunology of Leukocyte Function" (M. R. Quastel, ed.), p. 385. Academic Press, New York, 1979.

11. Tada, T., Hayakawa, K., and Taniguchi, M. Coexistence of variable region of immunoglobulin heavy chain and I region gene products on antigen-specific suppressor T cells and suppressor T cell factor — a minimal model of functional antigen receptor of T cells. *Mol. Immunol. 17*, 867 (1980).

12. Taniguchi, M., Tada, T., and Tokuhisa, T. Properties of the antigen-specific suppressive T-cell factor in the regulation of antibody response of the mouse. III. Dual gene control of the T-cell-mediated suppression of the antibody response. *J. Exp. Med. 114*, 20 (1976).

13. Taniguchi, M. and Miller, J. F. A. P. Enrichment of specific suppressor T cells and characterization of their surface markers. *J. Exp. Med. 146*, 1450 (1977).

14. Taniguchi, M. and Miller, J. F. A. P. Specific suppressive factors produced by hybridomas derived from the fusion of enriched suppressor T cells and a T lymphoma cell line. *J. Exp. Med. 148*, 373 (1978).

15. Taniguchi, M., Saito, T., and Tada, T. Antigen-specific suppressive factor produced by a transplantable I-J bearing T-cell hybridoma. *Nature (London) 283*, 227 (1979).

16. Taniguchi, M., Saito, T., Takei, I., and Tada, T. The establishment of T cell hybridomas with specific suppressive function. *In* "T and B Lymphocytes: Recognition and Function" (F. H. Bach, B. Bonavida, E. S. Vitetta, and C. F. Fox, eds.), p. 667. Academic Press, New York, 1979.

17. Taniguchi, M., Takei, I., and Tada, T. Functional and molecular organization of an antigen-specific suppressor factor derived from a T cell hybridoma. *Nature (London) 283*, 227 (1980).

18. Taniguchi, M., Takei, I., Saito, T., Haramatsu, K., and Tada, T. Functional organization of I-J subregion gene products on T cell hybridomas. *In* "Biochemical Characterization of Lymphokines" (A. L. de Weck, F. Kristensen, and M. Landy, eds.), p. 577. Academic Press, New York, 1980.

19. Taussig, M. J. and Holliman, A. Structure of an antigen-specific suppressor factor produced by a hybrid T-cell line. *Nature (London) 277*, 308 (1979).

20. Taussig, M. J. and Holliman, A. Antigen-specific suppressor factor for sheep erythrocytes and its B cell acceptor. Int. Congr. Immunol., *4th*, Abstr., 5.4.16.

21. Tokuhisa, T., Taniguchi, M., Okumura, K., and Tada, T. An antigen-specific I region gene product that augments the antibody response. *J. Immunol. 120*, 414 (1978).

Immunopathology: VIIIth International Symposium, 1980

A TUMOR MODEL OF IMMUNOREGULATION AND IMMUNOTHERAPY[1]

Jonathan W. Uhr
Keith Krolick
Peter Isakson
Ellen Puré
Ellen S. Vitetta

Department of Microbiology,
Southwestern Medical School,
University of Texas Health Science Center,
Dallas, Texas

I. INTRODUCTION

B-cell tumors in man account for approximately 75% of the non-Hodgkin's lymphomas and virtually all cases of chronic lymphocytic leukemia (CLL) (12). Present management of the B-cell lymphomas is in general unsatisfactory, particularly when compared with the results of treating Hodgkin's disease. In addition, there is a subset of patients with CLL who develop an aggressive form of the disease which responds poorly to chemotherapy (1, 5). For these reasons, there is an urgent need for the development of new therapeutic approaches.

[1]*Supported by Grants AI-12789, AI-11851, AI-13448, and CA-23115 from the National Institutes of Health.*

ISBN 0-12-218320-7

Through the pioneering work of Fu and colleagues (4), it is known that B-cell tumors in man are virtually always monoclonal and that the vast majority of tumor cells in individual patients bear surface immunoglobulin of a single idiotype. Hence, it is possible to utilize the idiotypic determinant(s) on surface immunoglobulin molecules of neoplastic B cells as tumor-specific antigens. We have chosen therefore to exploit the specificity of an antiidiotype response to a tumor immunoglobulin in order to develop more selective forms of immunotherapy. As a model system, we have used the BCL_1 tumor initially described by Slavin and Strober (20). This tumor resembles the prolymphocytic form of CLL in man (5). Our plan is to study in depth the biology of the tumor and the host response to it and subsequently to use such information and insights from these studies to eradicate the tumor. In addition, we want to use antiidiotypic antibody covalently coupled to cytotoxic agents as a means of delivering such agents selectively to the tumor cells.

In this chapter, we will summarize the biology of the BCL_1 tumor and then discuss two sets of experiments. One deals with the differentiative capacity of the BCL_1 cells *in vitro* and the other set of experiments with our attempts to kill BCL_1 cells selectively *in vitro* with antiidiotype antibody coupled to a toxic protein.

II. BIOLOGY OF THE BCL_1 TUMOR (10, 22)

Transfer of approximately 10^6 BCL_1 tumor cells to BALB/c mice results in enlargement of the spleen at approximately 3 weeks, and at 4 to 6 weeks leukemia appears. By 10 to 12 weeks after transfer of tumor cells, the spleen is massively enlarged (over 10^9 cells) and the leukemia has plateaued at approximately 10^8 cells per ml. About 80% of the cells in the spleen and over 90% of those in the blood are idiotype positive. The major cell type is a large lymphocyte that bears large amounts of IgM, trace amounts of IgD, and readily detectable I-A and I-E/C antigens. The mice live for 2-3 months after tumor inoculation in apparent good health. It is of interest that lymph nodes remain grossly normal and that tumor cells cannot be demonstrated in the thoracic duct lymph.

III. *IN VITRO* DIFFERENTIATION OF BCL_1 CELLS

We have observed two distinct pathways of differentiation of BCL_1 cells *in vitro*, depending upon the conditions of cultivation. If the cells are cultivated in the presence of fetal calf serum but without additional mitogens, the cells change their phenotype and functional characterisitics. Over a period of 2 to 4 days, BCL_1 cells acquire increased amounts of surface IgD (9), I-A and I-E/C antigens (7). Moreover, if freshly isolated cells are cultured with anti-Ig Sepharose beads, there is no increase in proliferation as judged by incorporation of $[^3H]$-thymidine. However, after four days of cultivation, a similar treatment results in a marked increase in $[^3H]$-thymidine incorporation (8). These changes in cell surface phenotype and the capacity to proliferate in response to treatment with anti-Igs are attributes of a mature B lymphocyte (24, 25). Immature B cells, like uncultured BCL_1 cells, express little surface IgD and do not proliferate in response to anti-Igs. Therefore, our tentative interpretation of these findings is that a relatively immature neoplastic B cell has matured *in vitro* into a more differentiated form that is now capable of responding to anti-Ig. We cannot formally exclude other possibilities, for example, BCL_1 cells might undergo other changes during culture that are unrelated to maturation but critical to activation by anti-Ig.

A second and distinct pathway occurs if lipopolysaccharide (LPS) is added to *either* freshly prepared or precultured cells. Three days later, secretion of pentameric IgM as detected by radioimmunoassay or by reverse-plaquing techniques can be readily demonstrated. Differentiation into Ig-secreting cells can also occur if T-cell helper factors (Con A or MLR supernatants) are added to BCL_1 cells that have been treated with Sepharose anti-Ig. Neither anti-Ig nor T-cell supernatants alone result in such differentiation (8). Thus, differentiation to Ig secretion requires two different signals: anti-Ig and T-cell help. Equivalent results are obtained if anti-δ or anti-μ are substituted for anti-Ig. Hence, either surface IgM or IgD is able to deliver a signal for replication and either surface isotype in conjunction with T-cell help can signal the cells to differentiate into Ig-secreting cells. These studies, therefore, confirm and extend in a clonal system the observations of Parker *et al.* (16) that support a two-signal model for B-cell stimulation.

It should be noted that Fu and co-workers first observed the differentiation of neoplastic lymphocytes to plasma cells both *in vivo* (4) and *in vitro* (2). More recent studies from this group (3), as well as from Saiki *et al.* (19), also demonstrated the ability of T-cell helper factors and/or mitogens to stimulate neoplastic human B cells to terminal differentiation. The new findings in the BCL_1 system include (a) the maturation from relatively immature to mature lymphocyte and (b) the ability to deliver one of the two signals needed for terminal differentiation with anti-Ig. Anti-Ig treatment of neoplastic human B cells has not been reported to deliver such signals, possibly because, like BCL_1, these cells must be incubated *in vitro* to develop into more mature and hence responsive B lymphocytes.

IV. USE OF TOXIN-ANTI-Id CONJUGATES TO KILL BCL_1 CELLS

The objective of the next series of experiments was to conjugate a toxin to antiidiotypic antibody and use such conjugates to kill neoplastic B cells bearing the idiotype in question. Since neoplastic B cells are monoclonal in origin, the idiotypic marker on such cells represents a tumor-specific antigen. We chose to use the highly poisonous toxin from castor beans, ricin, as the toxic material to be guided to the tumor cells by antibody. Ricin consists of an enzymatic polypeptide, the A-chain, which is responsible for inhibiting protein synthesis after gaining access to the cell cytoplasm, and the B chain, which is responsible for binding the protein to the surface of cells (15). Our plan was to cleave the disulfide bond between the A and B chains of ricin and covalently couple the A chain to specific antibody, thereby substituting the binding specificity of antibody for that of the B chain. In the first series of experiments we used antibody against immunoglobulin isotypes or allotypes to characterize the immunologic specificity and biologic activity of such complexes (11).

Conjugates were prepared with affinity purified anti-μ and the A chain of ricin. These conjugates were tested for antibody specificity and biological activity. By radioiodinating the A chain of ricin it could be shown that approximately one-half the input radioactivity could be bound to a Sepharose-IgM column but not to a Sepharose-ovalbumin immunoabsorbent. This observation suggested that at least half the conjugates formed retained antibody activity. These same conjugates were then tested for their biological effect on B lymphocytes. Since the mechanism of killing by ricin is inhibition of protein synthesis, it seemed reasonable to measure the toxic effect of ricin by determining its effect on LPS-stimulated protein synthesis in murine splenocytes. Since at least 90% of B cells in the spleen bear IgM these cells should be suitable targets for anti-μ A chain conjugates. Accordingly, splenocytes were admixed with such conjugates for 15 min at 4°C before addition of LPS. Protein synthesis was determined by incorporation of a pulse of [^{3}H]-leucine 72 hr later. The results of this experiment indicated that A chain conjugates were highly effective at inhibiting protein synthesis in splenocytes. Conjugates, 5-10 μg per ml of cells, virtually eliminated protein synthesis whereas the control conjugates of normal rabbit immunoglobulin and A chain had no effect on protein synthesis. Antibody by itself did not inhibit protein synthesis at these doses and under the conditions employed (15 min pulse at 4°C *before* addition of LPS). In the next series of experiments, we explored further the specificity of killing by anti-Ig A chain complexes using a hybridoma anti-δ allotype system. Thus, we prepared conjugates using monoclonal anti-δ directed against either of two IgD allotypes (a and b) and tested the effect of these conjugates on protein synthesis in spleen cells from strains bearing one or the other allotype (C57BL/6 bears the b allotype and BALB/c the a allotype). The results of this experiment were clear cut: protein synthesis was specifically inhibited only in spleen cells from mice bearing the appropriate δ allotype.

To evaluate the immunotherapeutic potential of a tumor-specific antibody conjugate, an affinity-purified rabbit anti-idiotype specific for the Ig on BCL_1 tumor cells (26) was coupled to the A chain and cultured with normal B cells or BCL_1 tumor cells (Fig. 1). The antiidiotype conjugate caused 70% inhibition of protein synthesis in LPS-stimulated spleen cells from mice bearing the BCL_1 tumor. As documented in previous experiments, an average of 77% of the splenic cells

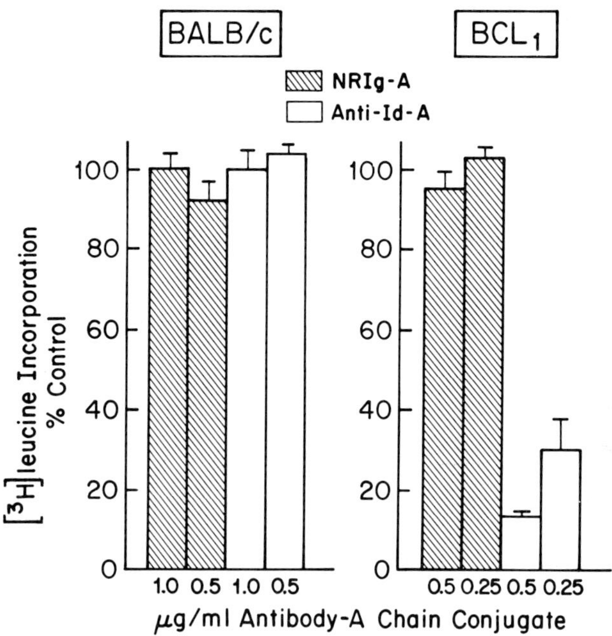

FIGURE 1. Inhibition of protein synthesis in BCL_1 tumor cells by affinity-purified antiidiotype-A chain. BALB/c spleen cells (2×10^5) were pulsed for 15-30 min with various concentrations of antiidiotype-A chain at 4°C, washed, and then cultured in triplicate for 2 days in the presence of LPS at 50 μg/ml. Cultures received 1 μCi of [^{3}H]-leucine, were incubated an additional 14-16 hr, and were then harvested and analyzed for incorporation of leucine into protein. Hatched bars, NRIg-A; open bars, antiidiotype-A. [From Krolick *et al.* (11).]

from mice injected with the BCL_1 tumor 7-10 weeks previously expressed the BCL_1 idiotype suggesting that virtually all BCL_1 cells were killed. The same conjugate caused only 5% inhibition of protein synthesis by normal BALB/c splenocytes. Neither NRIg coupled to A chain nor antibody alone had any effect on either normal or tumor cells.

The results presented in this study indicate that ricin A chain coupled to antibodies directed against either immunoglobulin isotypes or allotypes on normal B cells or to an idiotype on a B-cell tumor is specifically cytotoxic *in vitro*, as judged by inhibition of protein synthesis. The specificity of the cytotoxicity was demonstrated both by the inability of nonimmune Ig-A chain conjugates to kill any cells and the inability of the anti-Ig conjugates to kill cells lacking the corresponding Ig antigen. The specific binding of the antibody-A chain conjugates to their target cells was rapid, requiring only 15 min treatment to produce the subsequent inhibitory effect on protein synthesis. Moreover, the conjugates were effective at doses as low as 0.25-1 μg/ml. Unconjugated antibody was not cytotoxic under these conditions.

The immediate importance of these findings is that a purified antibody conjugate specific for the idiotype of the surface immunoglobulin on a particular B-cell tumor represents a specific toxin for that tumor. Thus, since a B-cell tumor expressing a particular idiotype is of monoclonal origin, all the tumor cells expressing that idiotype are potential targets for the cytotoxic agent. In contrast, only a negligible number of normal B cells express the same or cross-reacting idiotype and therefore the overwhelming majority escape the cytotoxic effect of the antiidiotypic conjugate. Fu *et al.* (4) and Stevenson and co-workers (21) have demonstrated the feasibility of preparing antiidiotype antibody to human B-cell tumors. Moreover, the above approach is theoretically applicable to any tumor to which a specific antibody can be generated. Therefore, with the development of hybridoma antibody technology, it is likely that antibodies that are highly specific to tumor-associated surface antigens can be generated to other types of tumors and used in a similar manner. Indeed there are numerous reports concerning the use of antitumor antibodies conjugated to toxins that selectively kill tumor cells (6, 13, 14, 17, 18, 23, 27).

Obviously, eradication of a tumor *in vivo* by the approach we have described above will depend on whether the tumor cells all bear the antigen in question, whether the tumor cells can all be killed by the conjugates, and the nonspecific toxicity of the conjugates. In addition, it will be important to determine whether such antigens are released by tumor cells *in vivo* since circulating antigen would decrease the effectiveness of such conjugates. In any case, it is likely that this approach will be most useful in eliminating a small number of residual tumor cells after nonspecific cytoreductive therapy.

REFERENCES

1. Bearman, R. M., Gerassimos, P. A., and Rappaport, H. Prolymphocytic leukemia. Clinical, histopathological, and autochemical observations. *Cancer (Philadelphia) 42*, 2360 (1978).

2. Fu, S. M., Chiorazzi, N., Kunkel, H. G., Halper, J. P., and Harris, S. R. Induction of *in vitro* differentiation and immunoglobulin synthesis of human leukemic B lymphocytes. *J. Exp. Med. 148*, 1570 (1978).

3. Fu, S. M., Chiorazzi, N., and Kunkel, H. G. Differentiation capacity and other properties of the leukemic cells of chronic lymphocytic leukemia. *Immunol. Rev. 48*, 23 (1979).

4. Fu, S. M., Winchester, R. J., Feizi, T., Walzer, P. D., and Kunkel, H. G. Idiotypic specificity of surface immunoglobulin and the maturation of leukemic bone-marrow-derived lymphocytes. *Proc. Natl. Acad. Sci. U.S.A. 71*, 4487 (1974).

5. Galton, D. A. G., Goldman, J. M., Wiltshaw, E., Catovsky, D., Henry, K., and Goldenberg, G. J. Prolymphocytic leukemia. *Br. J. Haematol. 27*, 7 (1974).

6. Gilliland, D. G., Steplewski, Z., Collier, R. J., Mitchell, K. F., Chang, T. H., and Koprowski, H. Antibody-directed cytotoxic agents: Use of monoclonal antibody to direct the action of toxin A chains to colorectal carcinoma cells. *Proc. Natl. Acad. Sci. U.S.A. 77*, 4539 (1980).

7. Isakson, P. C., Cook, R. G., Uhr, J. W., and Vitetta, E. S. Ia antigens on the murine B cell leukemia, BCL_1: Increase in surface expression of I-A and I-E/C antigens during differentiation *in vitro*, 1981.

8. Isakson, P. C., Puré, E., Uhr, J. W., and Vitetta, E. S. Induction of proliferation and differentiation of neoplastic B cells by anti-immunoglobulin and T cell factors. *Proc. Natl. Acad. Sci. U.S.A. 78*, 2507 (1981).

9. Isakson, P. C., Uhr, J. W., Krolick, K. A., Finkelman, F., and Vitetta, E. S. Acquisition of cell surface IgD after *in vitro* culture of neoplastic B cells from the murine tumor BCL_1. *J. Exp. Med. 151*, 749 (1980).

10. Krolick, K. A., Isakson, P. C., Uhr, J. W., and Vitetta, E. S. BCL_1, a murine model for chronic lymphocytic leukemia: Use of the surface immunoglobulin idiotype for the detection and treatment of tumor. *Immunol. Rev. 48*, 81 (1979).

11. Krolick, K. A., Villemez, C., Isakson, P., Uhr, J. W., and Vitetta, E. S. Selective killing of normal or neoplastic B cells by antibodies coupled to the A chain of ricin. *Proc. Natl. Acad. Sci. U.S.A. 77*, 5419 (1980).

12. Lennert, K. and Mohri, N. Histopathology and diagnosis of non-Hodgkins lymphomas. *In* "Malignant Lymphomas" (K. Lennert, ed.), pp. 111-136. 1978.

13. Masuho, Y., Hara, T., and Noguchi, T. Preparation of a hybrid of fragment Fab' of antibody and fragment A of diphtheria toxin and its cytotoxicity. *Biochem. Biophys. Res. Commun. 90*, 320 (1979).

14. Moolten, F. L., Capparell, N. J., Zajdel, S. H., and Cooperband, S. R. Antitumor effects of antibody diphtheria toxin conjugates. II. Immunotherapy with conjugates directed against tumor antigens induced by Simian virus 40. *J. Natl. Cancer Inst. 55*, 473 (1975).

15. Olsnes, S. and Pihl, A. Abrin, ricin and their associated agglutinins. *In* "Receptors and Recognition" (P. Cuatrecasas, ed.), Vol. 1, Halsted Press, London. pp. 130-173, 1976.

16. Parker, D. L., Fothergill, J. J., and Wadsworth, D. C. B lymphocyte activation by insoluble anti-immunoglobulin: Induction of immunoglobulin secretion by a T cell-dependent soluble factor. *J. Immunol. 123*, 931 (1979).

17. Raso, V. and Griffin, T. Specific cytotoxicity of a human immunoglobulin-directed Fab'-ricin A chain conjugate. *J. Immunol. 125*, 2610 (1980).

18. Ross, W. C. J., Thorpe, P. E., Cumber, A. J., Edwards, D. C., Hinson, C. A., and Davies, A. J. S. Increased toxicity of diphtheria toxin for human lymphoblastoid cells following covalent linkage to anti-human lymphocyte globulin or its $F(ab')_2$ fragment. *Eur. J. Biochem. 104*, 381 (1980).

19. Saiki, O., Kishimoto, T., Kuritani, T., Muraguchi, A., and Yamamura, Y. *In vitro* induction of IgM secretion and switching to IgG production in human B leukemic cells with the help of T cells. *J. Immunol. 124*, 2609 (1980).

20. Slavin, S. and Strober, S. Spontaneous murine B cell leukemia. *Nature (London) 272*, 624 (1977).

21. Stevenson, F. K., Hamblin, T. J., Stevenson, G. T., and Tutt, A. L. Extracellular idiotypic immunoglobulin arising from human B lymphocytes. *J. Exp. Med. 152*, 1484 (1980).

22. Strober, S., Gronowicz, E. S., Knapp, M. R., Slavin, S., Vitetta, E. S., Warnke, R. A., Kotzin, B., and Schröder, J. Immunobiology of a spontaneous murine B cell leukemia (BCL_1). *Immunol. Rev. 48*, 169 (1979).

23. Thorpe, P. E., Cumber, A. J., Williams, N., Edwards, D. C., Ross, W. C. J., and Davies, A. J. S. Abrogation of the non-specific toxicity of abrin conjugated to anti-lymphocyte globulin. *Clin. Exp. Immunol. 43*, 195 (1981).

24. Vitetta, E. S., Pure, E., Isakson, P., Buck, L., and Uhr, J. W. The activation of murine B cells: The role of surface immunoglobulins. *Immunol. Rev. 52*, 211 (1980).

25. Vitetta, E. S. and Uhr, J. W. IgD and B cell differentiation. *Immunol. Rev. 37*, 51 (1977).

26. Vitetta, E. S., Yuan, D., Krolick, K., Isakson, P., Knapp, M., Slavin, S., and Strober, S. Characterization of a spontaneous murine B cell leukemia (BCL_1). III. Evidence for monoclonality using anti-idiotypic antibody. *J. Immunol. 122*, 1649 (1979).

27. Youle, R. J. and Neville, D. M. Anti-Thy 1.2 monoclonal antibody linked to ricin is a potent cell-type-specific toxin. *Proc. Natl. Acad. Sci. U.S.A. 77*, 5483 (1980).

DISCUSSION

Dr. Seligmann pointed out that B cell neoplasms may arise from stem cells which would not carry the surface idiotype. Dr. Uhr replied that there are two distinct issues; the first is whether changes take place at the stem cell level that are necessary but possibly insufficient for malignancy. There is considerable evidence for this concept. The second issue is whether tumorigenic cells bear immunoglobulin. Dr. Uhr believes that this second and critical question cannot be answered at this time. The question can be approached by cell transfer studies in the BCL_1 system and by cloning human B cell tumors and determining whether clonable cells can be killed by ricin anti-Ig conjugates. Dr. Kunkel mentioned that Stevenson and co-workers have shown that the majority of patients with chronic lymphocytic leukemia have Ig in their serum that bears the idiotype of their tumor cell Ig. Such serum Ig would inhibit treatment of patients with antiidiotype-ricin conjugates. Dr. Uhr answered that the presence of a large amount of idiotype in the serum would clearly complicate the conjugate approach in such patients. A small amount of idiotype might not be a problem since the conjugates probably need only to bind to lymphocytes for a very short time to kill the cells. In BCL_1 bearing-animals, Ig bearing idiotype of the tumor cell Ig has not been detected in the serum. Dr. Lachman asked if the effects of Ig-ricin conjugates on macrophages are known. Dr. Uhr answered that no studies have been performed as yet of the potential untoward effects of such conjugates.

Immunopathology: VIIIth International Symposium, 1980

THE ROLE OF THE TOLERANCE TRIGGER IN THE EXPRESSION OF THE B-CELL REPERTOIRE[1]

Norman R. Klinman
Judy M. Teale

Department of Immunopathology,
Scripps Clinic and Research Foundation,
La Jolla, California

In order to facilitate conceptual approaches to the understanding of the expression of both T- and B-cell repertoires, we will put forward an old theory but with new data. The thesis is that the potential repertoire is vast, yet at the same time, largely genetically determined (15), and that "old mechanisms" such as clonal abortion (4, 19, 23) are extremely important in shaping that expressed repertoire in a highly specific and reproducible fashion. Furthermore, because one has both a very large inherited repertoire from which to choose and mechanisms that are highly reproducible and very specific to shape that repertoire, it is conceivable that there is no need to invoke a role for random mechanisms to derive the bulk of repertoire expression.

[1]*This work was supported by United States Public Health Service Grants AI-15797 and AI-06038.*

ISBN 0-12-218320-7

MECHANISMS THAT GOVERN REPERTOIRE EXPRESSION

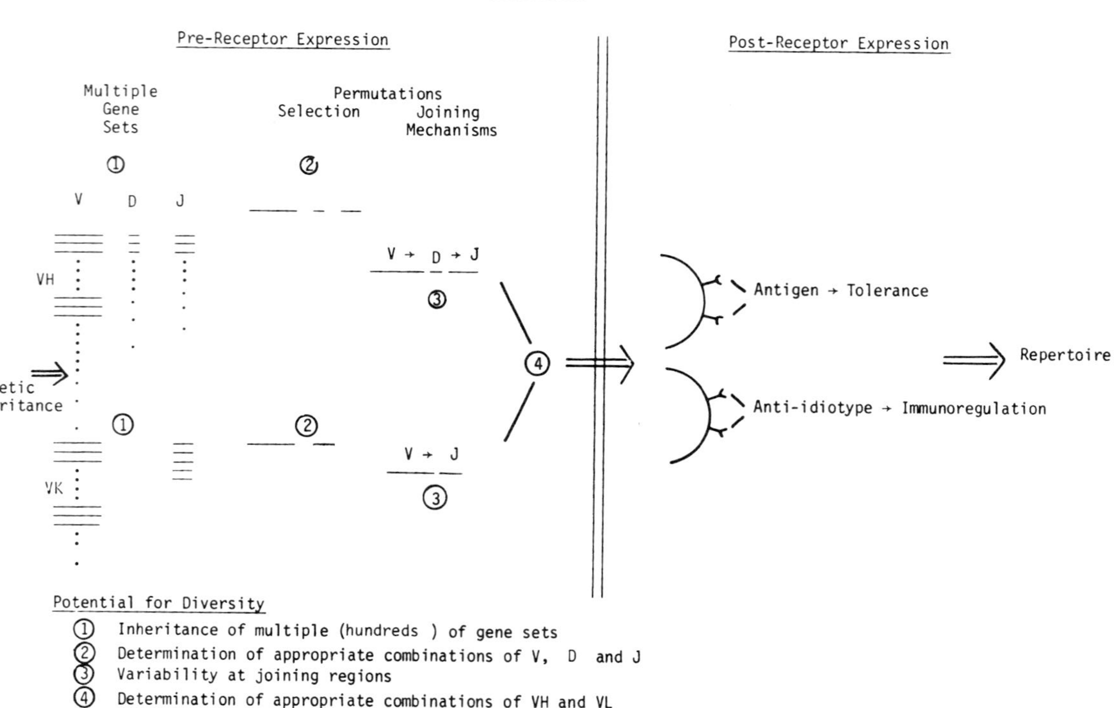

FIGURE 1

Figure 1 presents a general overview of what we currently believe to be the factors that account for the ultimate repertoire expression of primary B cells. We have divided, artificially, the mechanisms into two parts whose relative contribution is yet to be determined. The first pertains to the strictly molecular mechanisms that can give rise to a diverse repertoire and the second are those environmental mechanisms that might shape that repertoire. We know from the elegant molecular studies of a large number of laboratories that there are a fair number of inherited variable region genes both for the heavy and light chain; and more important, there are ways in which these genes can be selectively combined with other small gene pieces to amount to an extremely large repertoire (2, 3, 9, 24). Thus, for light chain one has a large set of mouse kappa-variable-region gene families. These combine, presumably in a fairly selective way, with a set of four or five J regions to yield, by combinatorial association, a repertoire of perhaps thousands of kappa chain sequences. In addition, there is variability at the joining region itself, which looks like "sloppiness" but may be relatively constrained since only selected amino acids, those encoded by deletion products of the V and J terminal sequences, can be substituted. With this added junctional diversity, a mouse could conceivably generate at least 10^4 light-chain sequences. Similar mechanisms obtain for heavy chain, with the addition of the D insert and junctional diversity on both sides of its combination with V and J. Thus, heavy chains might, in fact, express 10^5 or 10^6 sequences. Combinatorial association of heavy and light chains may multiply diversity so that the expressed repertoire prior to any extrinsic influence could easily include 10^9 or 10^{10} potential clonotypes without imposing somatic mutations within these variable region pieces. It should be stated, however, that such mutations apparently do occur (3) although their role in the expression of the functional repertoire is yet to be established. Thus, even without random mutations an individual could generate an extraordinarily large repertoire that may or may not be fully programmed. Certainly enzymatic events could account for each of the selective and joining processes which could render repertoire expression almost totally predetermined (15). On the other hand, random and stochastic mechanisms may play a role; but to what extent, if any, they actually do play a role is not known due to insufficient data. At the present time available data (see below) implies that repertoire expression is not random. In any case, as implied in Fig. 1, this entire diversification process and the expression of a vast repertoire could occur at a stage in development of B-cell clones which precedes the expression of immunoglobulin receptors and consequently precedes interaction with the antigenic environment.

At the time B-cell clones have sufficiently matured to express their immunoglobulin receptors and interact with the environment, the first part of the proposed mechanistic construct would end and the second part (to the right of the double line in Fig. 1) would ensue. Although the environment could presumably affect the expressed B-cell repertoire in many ways, two mechanisms are currently understood which might have a profound effect on the ultimate expression of the B-cell repertoire. The first is antiidiotypic immunoregulatory processes which have already been demonstrated to be capable of prohibiting the expression of given B-cell clonotypes within the mature repertoire (1, 10). The second, the subject that will occupy the major portion of this presentation, is the elimination of B cells from the repertoire by virtue of their recognition of self-antigenic determinants or tolerance induction (4, 19, 21, 23). If indeed all genetically identical individuals can express, by the aforementioned molecular mechanisms, the same vast B-cell repertoire, and, since genetically identical individuals should express most of the same self antigenic determinants, the combined effect of these two processes, network immunoregulation and tolerance induction, should reproducibly result in an extremely diverse but highly selected B-cell repertoire.

In recent years, a central role for processes such as tolerance induction in shaping the repertoire have been questioned because of several assumptions (22). First, it has appeared to some investigators that the repertoire is highly redundant, thus the selective elimination of a certain few specificities would have little or no affect on the overall capability of the repertoire to recognize either foreign or self determinants. Second, stimulation, at least by certain mechanisms, appears to be relatively nonspecific, so that if tolerance were to eliminate specifically a few clonotypes, many others with similar reactivity could presumably remain and be stimulated. Third, tolerance itself has seemed relatively nonspecific (30), so that if tolerance were to play a valid role and eliminate reactivity to all self antigens as well as those cross-reactive with self antigens, it would more than likely eliminate the total B-cell repertoire. Finally, certain experimental protocols have revealed self-reactive cells in mature individuals, and antigen-reactive cells in individuals that were presumably tolerant (22).

In an effort to address the controversial points listed above, we will present data obtained by studies of the repertoire which indicate that the repertoire, in terms of recognition of specific protein antigenic determinants, is not at all redundant. We will also show that the repertoire as expressed in F_1 individuals may reflect enormous deletions by virtue of contact with self antigens. And finally, we will demonstrate that both tolerance and antigenic stimulation are exquistely specific phenomena such that the elimination of clones that are specifically reactive to self determinants could be readily accomplished without diminishing the effectiveness of the repertoire as a whole in its recognition of foreign antigens.

What can studies of the repertoire itself reveal with respect to those processes responsible for the generation and shaping of the expressed repertoire? Studies over the past several years by many laboratories using a number of different approaches have all concluded that the clonotype repertoire of an inbred murine strain is extraordinarily diverse, probably exceeding 10^7 unique specificities (8, 17, 18, 26). Initially, such a large number of clonotypes appeared to be inconsistent with proposed genetic and somatic mechanisms for repertoire diversification. However, our current understanding of the molecular combinatorial process mentioned above and depicted in Fig. 1 place such estimates well within reasonable predictions for the molecular events leading to repertoire diversity.

High estimates of repertoire diversity have come from studies of antibody responses to many different antigens including small chemically defined moieties. Thus, studies of haptenic determinants such as 2,4-dinitrophenyl (DNP), 2,4,6-trinitrophenyl (TNP), and 4-hydroxy-5-iodo-3-nitrophenacetyl (NIP) have revealed that several thousand distinct clonotypes are available for response to such determinants. Since the frequency of B cells responsive to such determinants is in the range of 1 in 5,000 - 10,000 of the total B-cell population, it was concluded that the frequency of any given clonotype could not represent, on the average, more than 1 in 10^7 of the total B-cell pool. Recently, other frequency estimates have been derived from studies of responsiveness to the α-1,3-dextran and phosphorylcholine (PC) determinants. Here, as with the haptenic determinant *p*-azophenylarsonate (ARS), a much lower frequency of B cells is responsive, on the order of

1 in 20,000-50,000 (26). Whereas such responses were previously assumed to be highly restricted, it now appears that these responses involve primarily closely related families of clonotypes which are, themselves, extremely diverse (9, 26). Nonetheless, whereas all of these studies have implied an extremely diverse repertoire, they have also given the impression that because so many clonotypes recognize any given antigenic determinant, the repertoire is extraordinarily redundant. Thus, it was hard to imagine how a process such as tolerance, which might eliminate a few clonotypes against a given determinant, could markedly affect the overall responsiveness to such a determinant.

Another approach to repertoire estimation, however, has been carried out using complex protein antigen determinants such as the hemagglutinin molecule of the PR8 influenza virus (PR8-HA) (8) or β-galactosidase (17). Using these antigen systems, studies at the monoclonal response level have also revealed an extremely diverse repertoire with each clonotype representative of fewer than 1 in 10^7 B cells. In this case, however, the repertoire is clearly recognizing a multiplicity of distinct determinants expressed on the same antigenic moiety with few clonotypes available for the recognition of any one of these moieties. Thus, in the case of protein antigens, where recognized determinants may differ from self by small nuances, any individual may have few, if any, clonotypes recognizing available and potentially important determinants. For such potentially important physiologic recognition, therefore, repertoire redundancy is not apparent and tolerance of any given clonotype may be crucial to the capacity of the individual in recognizing that particular determinant.

A second important set of conclusions concerning control of repertoire expression comes from a series of studies of the B-cell repertoire as expressed in neonates. Several years ago, we observed that the repertoire of neonates during their first week of life was extremely restricted and at birth represented approximately 10^4 specificities which were present in all neonates of a given strain (13). In addition, the acquisition of new specificities during the first week of neonatal life appeared to be highly regular and reproducible in all genetically identical individuals (25, 26). Recently, these studies have been extended to a careful analysis of the B cells responsive to PR8-HA in two-week-old mice (7). Initial studies in the BALB/c strain demonstrated that, as opposed to adults which express hundreds of clonotypes specific for determinants of the PR8-HA molecule, two-week-old BALB/c neonates expressed fewer than 10 clonotypes recognizing these determinants, and all individuals at 2 weeks of age appeared to express the same set of clonotypes. Since each of these clonotypes on the average represent approximately 1 in 10^6 of all B cells, it can be concluded that at a time when the repertoire has diversified 100-fold subsequent to birth, all genetically identical individuals express essentially the same 10^6 specificities. Thus, when developing individuals are first encountering the environment, the repertoire is not terribly diverse. Moreover, many of the neonatal clonotypes screened recognized determinants different from those recognized by adult clonotypes, further arguing against redundancy as a major factor in B-cell repertoire function.

Studies using a second murine strain, B10.D2, confirmed the conclusions from the studies of BALB/c that all two-week-old genetically identical individuals express the same limited repertoire (6). However, many of the clonotypes expressed by B10.D2 neonates were not the same as those expressed by the BALB/c strain, providing evidence, at the level of total neonatal repertoire expression, of polymorphism in the expression of the B-cell clonotypes. By extending these studies to an analysis of the repertoire of F_1 hybrid individuals constructed between BALB/c and B10.D2 mice, several important facts were revealed (6). Similar to the parental strains, the F_1 neonates expressed a highly restricted repertoire, but this F_1 repertoire differed markedly from that of either parent with at least four of the eight observed clonotypes different from that seen in either parent at the neonatal stage. The reproducibility of clonotypes in early neonates within a strain and in F_1 hybrids is compelling evidence for overall genetic determination of repertoire expression. The finding that F_1 neonates express clonotypes not found in the neonates of either parental strain and lack clonotypes of both parental strains could be explained at either of the two levels depicted in Fig. 1. First, it is possible that the selective and molecular combinatorial events involved in variable region expression could be influenced by the presence of genes from two parental strains rather than a single parental strain. More pertinent to the present discussion, however, is the possibility that the set of self-antigens which constitute the tolerance gauntlet for developing B cells is very different in F_1 individuals than in either parental strain. In any case, the finding that the F_1 repertoire differs so markedly from the repertoire of either parent, raises the possibility that tolerance to self antigens has a profound effect in shaping the expressed repertoire.

The remainder of this presentation will discuss whether, in fact, a mechanism such as tolerance might be important in shaping the vast inherited repertoire. Figure 2 depicts a classical conceptualization of the relationship between the proportion of antibodies or B-cell receptors that can bind a determinant and the affinity of such binding. It can be seen that the lower the affinity of binding, the greater the number of cells that are capable of binding at that affinity.

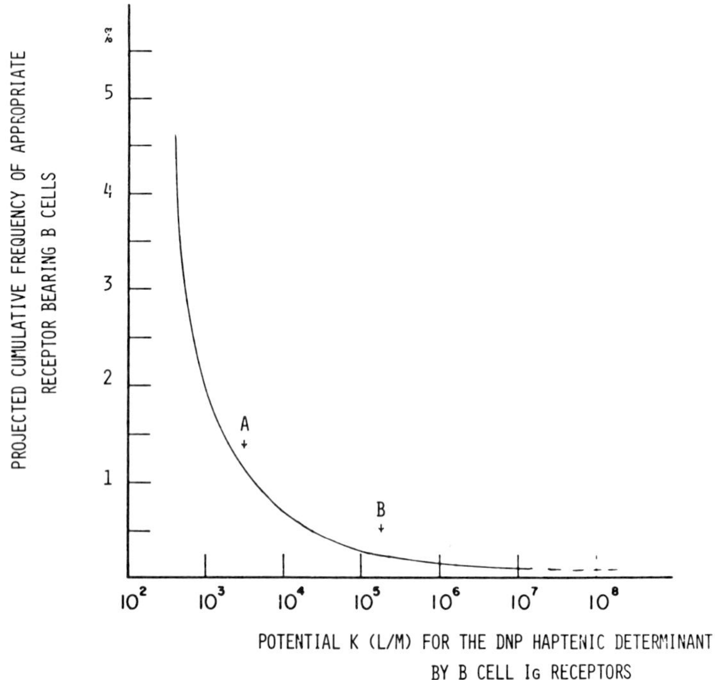

FIGURE 2

Accordingly, there would be very few cells with high affinity for any given antigen. If the threshold for stimulation or tolerance occurs at affinities depicted by arrow A, then for every antigen there would be an enormous number of cells responsive; and, conversely, if you were to tolerize to millions of self antigens using this affinity threshold, one could easily see eliminating the entire repertoire many times over. On the other hand, if stimulation and tolerance induction occur at affinities depicted by arrow B then they would be extremely specific and affect only a tiny portion of the repertoire. Providing stimulation is equally specific, such selective tolerance could have a profound impact but, at the same time, could preserve a considerable proportion of the initial repertoire for reactivity to foreign antigens.

Several years ago, we carried out experiments to test whether stimulation was, in fact, more specific than antigen binding *per se* (11, 12). The findings are summarized in Table I. Consistent with the results reported by several laboratories, as the concentration of antigen is increased the proportion of antigen-binding cells (ABC) is increased such that up to 4% of the B cells can specifically bind an antigen like DNP when presented polyvalently. In contrast, with increasing antigen concentrations, the number of cells that are stimulated in a T-dependent fashion increases only so far and then plateaus over a fairly wide range of antigen concentrations. Thus, a 10- to 100-fold increase in antigen-binding cells occurring over this concentration range results in no increase in cells recruited into the response (11). This would imply that, although antigen binding is important for antigenic stimulation, there is an apparent affinity requisite for stimulation that goes beyond simply binding the antigen to the cell. This is confirmed by the finding that, within the plateau region, with an increase in antigen concentration, there is no lowering of the affinity of the clones that respond (11). Affinity selection is only valid at very very low antigen concentrations.

In addition, we were able to document the exquisite specificity of stimulation by showing that whereas DNP and TNP are closely related, i.e., 90% of the antibodies cross-react; when you stimulate with both DNP and TNP, you stimulate the sum of the cells that you would stimulate with either alone (14). Therefore, although the antibody products are highly cross-reactive, DNP can stimulate very few, if any, TNP specific cells and *vice versa*. This was the evidence as it stood several years ago, leading us to believe that at least stimulation was exquisitely specific.

TABLE I. Evidence for Affinity Dependence of the Stimulation Trigger

Antigen determinant concentration (DNP on DNP-Hy)	Number of clones/10^6 transferred spleen cells	K_0 7°C ($\times 10^6$ l/m)	ABC/10^6 spleen cells (estimated)
10^{-5}	2.3	1.8	4×10^4 (4%)
10^{-6}	3.8	2.0	2×10^4 (2%)
5×10^{-7}	4.1	1.8	1×10^4 (1%)
10^{-7}	2.9	3.0	2×10^3 (0.2%)
10^{-9}	1.9	7.2	$<1 \times 10^3$ (<0.1%)
10^{-11}	1.3	10.1	

A few years ago, several laboratories demonstrated that it was possible to tolerize immature B cells passing through a very narrow window in their development, i.e., just when they are acquiring their receptors either as neonatal B cells or in the bone marrow of mature animals (5, 20, 21, 27, 28). This tolerance induction was found to be highly specific, could be induced with very low concentrations of antigen (as low as 10^{-9} *M* for the DNP determinant) and did not affect mature B cells, even at very high antigen concentrations (21, 28). Importantly, this tolerance was found to be totally carrier-independent in that good tolerogens as well as obligate immunogens such as DNP-ovalbumin (DNP-OVA) could tolerize very well. The only requirement was the multivalent presentation of DNP as evidenced by the fact that DNP lysine or DNP-S-papain, which are monovalent, did not tolerize (21).

Recently, we have extended this series of experiments and have demonstrated that the induction of tolerance in immature B cells apparently represents a bonafide triggering event since it could be abrogated by inhibiting either energy metabolism or protein biosynthesis (29). Figure 3 shows that DNP_{10}-OVA induces the tolerance trigger in about 70% of the neonatal B cells, but that this tolerance induction can be almost totally inhibited by the addition of 10^{-5} *M* DNP-L-lysine. This demonstrates that while DNP-L-lysine can bind to the receptors of DNP specific neonatal B cells and block tolerance induction, it, in itself, cannot induce tolerance. This suggests that tolerance induction requires multivalence as well as antigen binding (29). Additionally, even relatively low concentrations of DNP-L-lysine are effective in inhibiting tolerance induction. If one uses TNP-L-lysine, a cross-reacting antigen, to determine its capacity to inhibit the tolerance induction of DNP-specific B cells with DNP-OVA, it can be seen that at very high concentrations TNP-L-lysine is a very effective

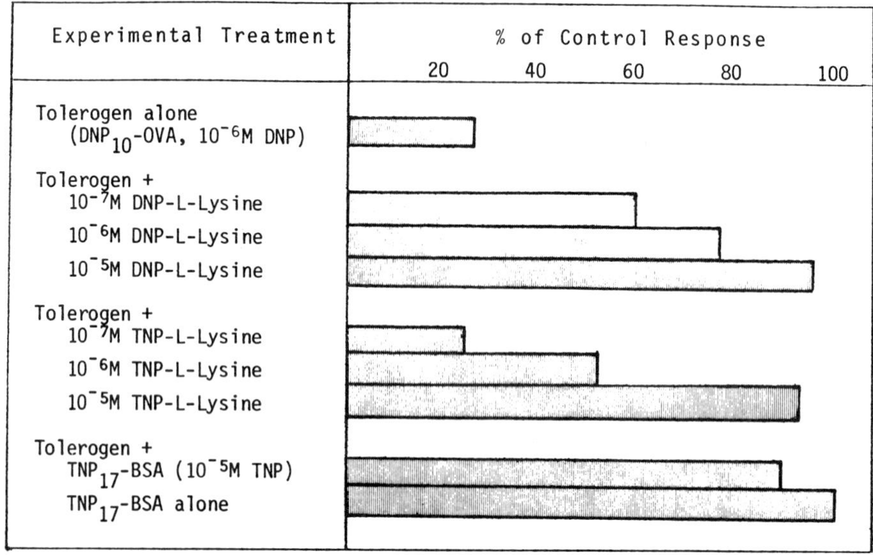

FIGURE 3. Data abstracted from Teale and Klinman (29).

inhibitor. At lower concentrations, however, it is not as effective as DNP-L-lysine. Thus, there is a measurable affinity difference in the binding interactions between the receptors of DNP-responsive B cells when DNP is compared with TNP, with TNP binding at a lower affinity. Nevertheless, TNP-L-lysine can bind the receptors and inhibit tolerance induced by DNP-OVA even though TNP cannot trigger these cells. Finally, in order to show that the tolerance trigger not only requires multivalent binding, but is exquisitely specific and affinity dependent, we assessed the ability of TNP bovine serum albumin (BSA) to block tolerance induction by DNP-OVA. TNP-BSA alone does not tolerize DNP-specific B cells although it tolerizes TNP-specific B cells very well. The important finding is that TNP-BSA can bind to the receptors of the DNP-specific B cells in such a way as to block tolerance induction by DNP-OVA. This demonstrates that the receptors of DNP specific neonatal B cells can be occupied by TNP-BSA but that these cells are not triggered to tolerance induction by that binding, presumably because the affinity is too low.

As depicted in Fig. 4, 1 out of 5000 B cells can be triggered by DNP in a highly specific, affinity dependent fashion. Cross-reacting antigens that bind the receptors have no real affect on these cells. Thus, in a sense, we have defined tolerance induction as an exquisitely specific phenomenon as it pertains to developing B cells and as such it could have a meaningful function in establishing the repertoire. Recently, with Dr. David Katz, we have carried out an experiment to see if any of this obtains for B cells *in vivo* (13). *In vivo* it has been possible with several antigens, including

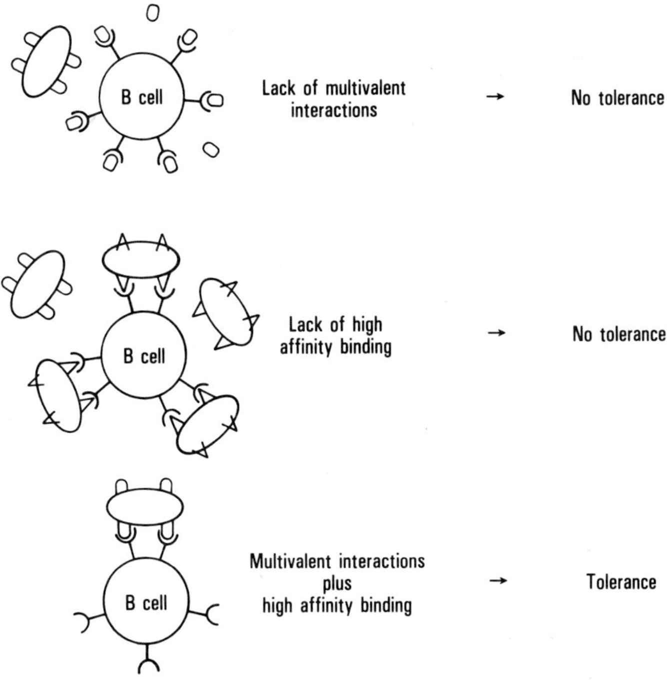

FIGURE 4

DNP coupled to the amino acid copolymer of D-glutamic acid and D-lysine (DGL), to tolerize not only immature cells, but B cells of mature mice. No evidence had heretofore been obtained that the highly specific mode of tolerance induction described above was playing any role whatsoever in the *in vivo* situation.

Recently, we tolerized a series of mice with very high doses of DNP-DGL. The animals were profoundly nonresponsive to both DNP and TNP within a few days after treatment as determined by serum antibody responses. However, when their splenic B cells were washed extensively, at least 80% remained fully functional after a week and a 60 to 70% diminution in frequency was observed only after a month. During this entire course, TNP specific precursors were essentially unaffected. Thus, after *in vivo* tolerance induction, the frequency of cells capable of responding to DNP is reduced very slowly with kinetics similar to that which would be expected if these cells were dying by their normal rate of attrition, i.e., their half-life being about one week to two weeks. Consequently, it appears that the DNP-responsive B cells are being lost from the mature cell pool due to normal turnover and the true effect of the tolerogen is to prohibit new cells from developing out of the bone marrow and replenishing the population. Consistent with this notion is the fact that B cells are eliminated from within the bone marrow more rapidly. Interestingly, the frequency of bone marrow B cells of the least mature pool, i.e., those which have not as yet expressed their Ig receptors, remains normal and, therefore, has not been affected by the "environmental" tolerogen.

Thus, it appears that, *in vivo* as well as *in vitro*, one can see an exquisite susceptibility of developing B cells to an extremely specific tolerance mechanism. This would indicate that such a tolerance phenomenon may play a physiologically crucial role during repertoire establishment. So, in summary, there are a series of extremely complex molecular events leading to a diverse repertoire. However, what eventually emerges in the mature repertoire is representative of many influences, not the least of which are the environmental antigens which probably serve an extremely important role in shaping repertoire expression.

REFERENCES

1. Accolla, R. S., Gearhart, P. J., Sigal, N. H., Cancro, M. P., and Klinman, N. R. Idiotype-specific neonatal suppression of phosphorylcholine-responsive B cells. *Eur. J. Immunol. 7*, 876 (1977).

2. Adams, J. M. The organization and expression of immunoglobulin genes. *Immunol. Today 1*, 10 (1980).

3. Brack, C., Hiramon, M., Lenhard-Schuller, R., and Tonegawa, S. A complete immunoglobulin gene is created by somatic recombination. *Cell 15*, 1 (1978).

4. Burnet, F. M. "The Clonal Selection Theory of Acquired Immunity." Cambridge Univ. Press, London and New York, 1959.

5. Cambier, J. C., Kettman, J. R., Vitteta, E. S., and Uhr, J. W. Differential susceptibility of neonatal and adult murine spleen cells to *in vitro* induction of B cell tolerance. *J. Exp. Med. 144*, 293 (1976).

6. Cancro, M. P. and Klinman, N. R. B cell repertoire ontogeny: Heritable but dissimilar development of parental and F_1 repertoires. *J. Immunol. 126*, 1160 (1981).

7. Cancro, M. P., Wylie, D. W., Gerhard, W., and Klinman, N. R. Patterned acquisition of the antibody repertoire: Diversity of the hemagglutinin specific B cell repertoire in neonatal BALB/c mice. *Proc. Natl. Acad. Sci. U.S.A. 76*, 6577 (1979).

8. Cancro, M. P., Gerhard, W., and Klinman, N. R. Diversity of the primary influenza specific B cell repertoire in BALB/c mice. *J. Exp. Med. 147*, 776 (1978).

9. Hood, L. and Early, P. Organization and rearrangements of heavy chain variable region genes. *In* "Immunoglobulin Genes and B Cell Differentiation" (J. R. Battisto and K. Knight, eds.), p. 7. Elsevier/North-Holland, Amsterdam, 1980.

10. Jerne, N. Towards a network theory of the immune system. *Ann. Immunol. (Paris) 125*, 373 (1971).

11. Klinman, N. R. The mechanism of antigenic stimulation of primary and secondary clonal precursor cells. *J. Exp. Med. 136*, 241 (1972).

12. Klinman, N. R., Pickard, A. R., Sigal, N. H., Gearhart, P. J., Metcalf, E. S., and Pierce, S. K. Assessing B cell diversification by antigen receptor and precursor cell analysis. *Ann. Immunol. (Paris) 127*, 489 (1976).

13. Klinman, N. R. and Press, J. L. The characterization of the B cell repertoire specific for the DNP and TNP determinants in neonatal BALB/c mice. *J. Exp. Med. 141*, 1133 (1975).

14. Klinman, N. R., Press, J. L., and Segal, G. Overlap stimulation of primary and secondary B cells by cross reacting determinants. *J. Exp. Med. 138*, 1276 (1973).

15. Klinman, N. R., Press, J. L., Sigal, N. H., and Gearhart, P. J. The acquisition of the B cell specificity repertoire: The germ line theory of predetermined permutation of genetic information. *In* "The Generation of Diversity: A New Look" (A. J. Cunningham, ed.), p. 127. Academic Press, New York.

16. Klinman, N. R., Schrater, A. F., and Katz, D. H. Immature B cells as the target for *in vivo* tolerance. *J. Immunol. 126*, 1970 (1981).

17. Kohler, G. Frequency of precursor cells against the enzyme β-galactosidase. An estimate of the BALB/c strain antibody repertoire. *Eur. J. Immunol. 6*, 340 (1976).

18. Kreth, H. W. and Williamson, A. R. The extent of diversity of anti-hapten antibodies in inbred mice: (4-Hydroxy-5-iodo-3-nitro-phenacetyl) antibodies in CBA/H mice. *Eur. J. Immunol. 3*, 141 (1973).

19. Lederberg, J. Genes and antibodies: Do antigens bear instructions for antibody specificity or do they select cell lines that arise by mutation? *Science 129*, 1649 (1959).

20. Metcalf, E. S. and Klinman, N. R. *In vitro* tolerance of bone marrow cells: A marker for B cell maturation. *J. Immunol. 118*, 2111 (1977).

21. Metcalf, E. S. and Klinman, N. R. *In vitro* tolerance induction of neonatal murine B cells. *J. Exp. Med. 143*, 1327 (1976).

22. Moller, G., Gonowicz, E., Persson, U., Coutinho, A., Moller, E., Hammerstron, L., and Smith, E. Spleen cells from animals tolerant to thymus-dependent antigen can be activated by lipopolysaccharide to synthesize antibodies to the tolerogen. *J. Exp. Med. 143*, 1429 (1976).

23. Nossal, G. J. V. and Pike, B. L. Evidence for the clonal abortion theory of B lymphocyte tolerance. *J. Exp. Med. 141*, 904 (1975).

24. Seidman, J. G., Max, E. E., Norman, B., Nau, M., and Leder, P. The source of kappa light chain diversity: A review. *In* "Immunoglobulin Genes and B Cell Differentiation" (J. R. Battisto and K. Knight, eds.), p. 35. Elsevier/North-Holland, Amsterdam, 1980.

25. Sigal, N. H., Gearhart, P. J., Press, J. L., and Klinman, N. R. Late acquisition of a germline specificity. *Nature (London) 259*, 51 (1976).

26. Sigal, N. H. and Klinman, N. R. The B cell clonotype repertoire. *Adv. Immunol. 26*, 255 (1978).

27. Stocker, J. W. Tolerance induction in maturing B cells. *Immunology 32*, 282 (1977).

28. Teale, J. M., Howard, M. C., and Nossal, G. J. V. B lymphocyte subpopulations separated by velocity sedimentation. II. Characterization of tolerance susceptibility. *J. Immunol. 121*, 2561 (1978).

29. Teale, J. M. and Klinman, N. R. Tolerance as an active process. *Nature (London) 288*, 385 (1980).

30. Weigle, W. O., Chiller, J. M., and Louis, J. A. Tolerance: Central unresponsiveness or peripheral inhibition. *Prog. Immunol., Proc. Int. Congr. Immunol., 2nd, Brighton, Engl. 3*, 187 (1974).

DISCUSSION

DR. ROIT: Do I understand you correctly to say that monovalent antigens like serum albumin would not tolerize neonatal cells?

DR. KLINMAN: Yes. As opposed to most other concepts of tolerance, where one would predict tolerance of your own albumin etc., it would seem that a prediction derived from our findings is that you would likely be tolerant mainly of cell surface antigens which would be in the bone marrow in a multivalent form and certain protein antigens, but you should not be tolerant of some of your own serum proteins, other monovalent antigens, and antigens which do not enter the bone marrow. My guess is that when the final story of this is all worked out, that will in fact be the case, and that the B cells are there but quiescent to self antigens.

DR. ROIT: How do these findings fit with those of Dr. Howard and others that neonatal cells do not readily reexpress their immunoglobulin receptors?

DR. KLINMAN: Whether or not that is relevant to this phenomenon is hard to know. Also, whether or not, for example, patching and capping are relevant to this phenomena is not known. As I said, I suspect that the TNP would cause such surface redistribution of DNP specific cells but does not tolerize them. On the other hand, concentrations of homologous antigens that are so low that there is no chance that they would patch or cap can tolerize. The parallels between these various phenomena and tolerance are as yet unclear.

DR. CLAMAN: Is it possible that some of what you observe is due to macrophages or other non B cells? Could you ask this question in a system where all populations could be defined?

DR. KLINMAN: In this particular instance, the technique requires that the B cells be in fragment cultures at the time you are tolerizing. The fragment culture technique has all kinds of disadvantages and all kinds of advantages. One of the advantages is that it does permit the cells to be stimulated; I think it is the only system, other than the mitogenic stimulation, which would permit such immature cells to be stimulated. So, we pay the price of not having the isolated cell populations.

DR. ROCKLIN: Is there any chance the *in vivo* experiments may involve a suppressor cell phenomenon?

DR. KLINMAN: This probably does not involve suppressor cells since Drs. Katz and Benacerraf showed several years ago, that DGL induced tolerance does not seem to evoke a suppressor cell phenomenon. In addition, Dr. Katz and I tried to find antiidiotypic suppression in these mice and there doesn't seem to be any.

Immunopathology: VIIIth International Symposium, 1980

ROLE OF T AND B CELLS IN AUTOIMMUNITY[1]

M. H. DeBaets
W. O. Weigle

Department of Immunopathology,
Scripps Clinic and Research Foundation,
La Jolla, California

J. M. Lindstrom

The Receptor Biology Laboratory,
The Salk Institute for Biological Studies,
San Diego, California

I. INTRODUCTION

Autoimmunity can best be defined as an apparent termination of a natural unresponsiveness to one's own body constituents. Although autoimmune diseases may involve abnormalities

[1]*Publication No. 2548 from the Department of Immunopathology, Scripps Clinic and Research Foundation. Dr. DeBaets was supported by a Fogarty Fellowship Award 1F05 TW02846-01 and a NATO Fellowship. Dr. Weigle was supported by United States Public Health Service Grant AI-07007 and a Biomedical Research Support Grant RR0-5514. Dr. Lindstrom was supported by grants from NIH (NS 11323), Muscular Dystrophy Association, and the Los Angeles Chapter of the MG Foundation.*

ISBN 0-12-218320-7

any place in the complex network of regulatory systems involved in the control of immune responses once they are induced, the events involved in the initiation of autoimmune responses are probably dictated by the manner in which self-antigen is presented to the immune system and the immune status of T and B cells to that autoantigen. A model can be constructed which is based on three assumptions.

First, tolerance to self is the result of a central unresponsiveness in which competent T and/or B cells specific for a given antigen are absent. Specific binding cells are not detected and no antibody-secreting cells appear even transiently. Although suppressor cells are at times associated with the tolerant state, they are not required for either the induction or maintenance of tolerance (1). Antigen blockade is not involved, and lymphocytes transferred from the tolerant donor to a neutral host remain unresponsive. Central unresponsiveness can be induced in adult animals with either a nonimmunogenic form of the antigen such as deaggregated IgG (2) or after a temporary inhibition of the immune system, but it is more easily and effectively induced before the immune system matures.

Second, there is a dramatic difference in the dose of tolerogen required for the induction of tolerance in T and B cells. The amount of tolerogen such as deaggregated human IgG required to induce tolerance in adult thymus cells is 100-1000 times less than that required to induce tolerance in adult bone marrow cells (3). Thus, when low doses of the tolerogen are used, B cells remain competent whereas T cells become tolerant. Similarly, one could expect that tolerance to self-antigens present in low concentrations in the extracellular fluids (e.g., thyroglobulin, certain classes of Ig, or growth hormone) would occur only in T cells and not in B cells, whereas tolerance to self-antigens in high concentration (e.g., serum albumin) would occur in both T and B cells. For still other antigens present in extremely low concentrations (basic protein, cytochrome C, idiotypic determinants and acetylcholine receptor) both T and B cells may be competent (Fig. 1). In order to maintain tolerance in the intact animal only T cells need be tolerant. Although tolerance induced by a single injection of deaggregated IgG is finite in either T or B cells, periodic injections of this tolerogen should perpetuate the tolerant state indefinitely, mimicking the life-long tolerance to self.

Third, the degree of tolerance in both the T and B cell compartments is dependent on the concentration of the self-antigen in the microenvironment.

In order to explore this hypothesis, we will review some of the cellular events that may be involved in experimental autoimmune thyroiditis (EAT). Some new data on experimental

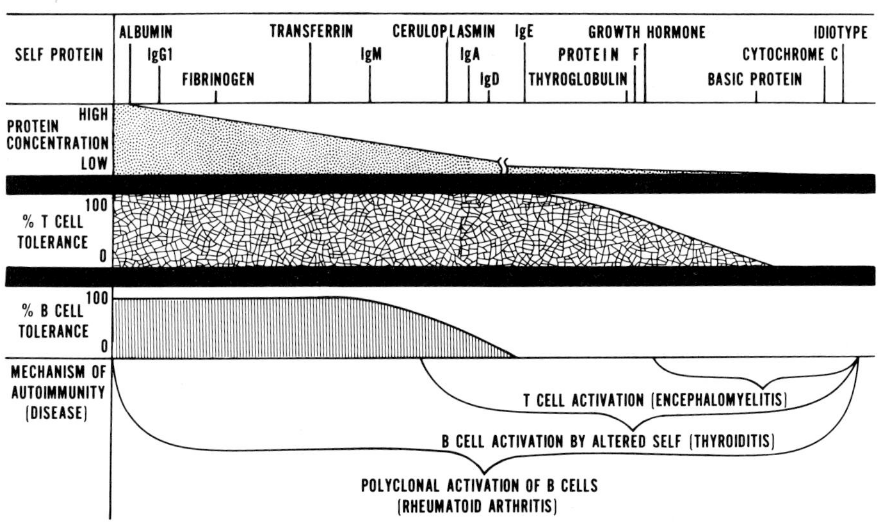

FIGURE 1. Relationship between levels of self-proteins in body fluids, immune status of T cells and B cells to self-proteins, and autoimmunity.

autoimmune myasthenia gravis (EAMG) will be summarized in the last section.

II. EXPERIMENTAL AUTOIMMUNE THYROIDITIS (EAT) AND EXPERIMENTAL ALLERGIC ENCEPHALOMYELITIS (EAE)

A. *Thyroiditis*

EAT can be induced in animals by injection of autologous thyroglobulin incorporated in complete Freund's adjuvant (4). The lesions brought about in these animals resemble those of Hashimoto's thyroiditis in the human. As mentioned previously, serum proteins such as thyroglobulin circulating in low concentration in the extracellular fluid maintain an unresponsive state in T cells but not in B cells. Injection of aqueous preparations of either heterologous or chemically altered autologous thyroglobulin in rabbits results in the termination of the self-tolerant state (5). Such immunized rabbits produce circulatory antibody reactive with autologous thyroglobulin, accompanied by inflammatory lesions in the thyroid gland. Thus non-self-determinants present in altered-self thyroglobulin or cross-reacting Tg activate T helper cells specific for these nonself-determinants resulting in differentiation of the competent B cells to autoantibody production (Fig. 2A). The absence of activation of T cells specific for syngeneic thyroglobulin is further supported by the fact that no proliferative responses were obtained by addition of rabbit thyroglobulin to the cultures of spleen cells of rats immunized with autologous Tg incorporated in CFA (6). These results are consistent with the existence of tolerance to autologous thyroglobulin at the T cell level, which, by appropriate immunization, can be bypassed to trigger competent B cells.

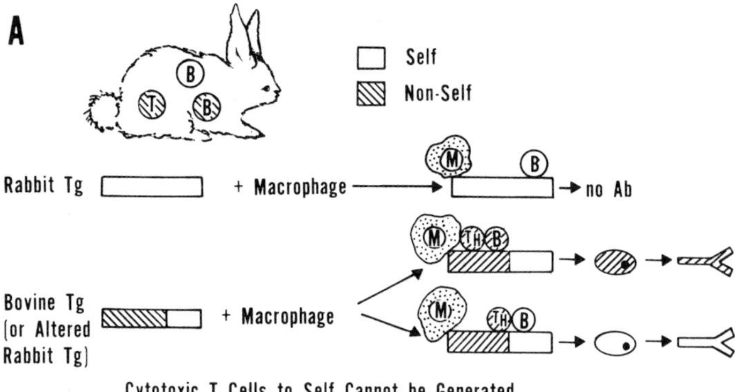

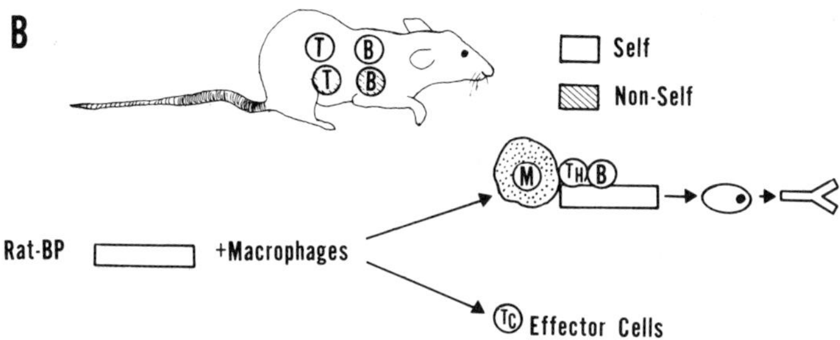

FIGURE 2. (A) Cellular events following injection of rabbits with homologous and heterologous thyroglobulin. (B) Role of effector T cells in rats with experimental allergic encephalitis (EAE).

Further studies in mice revealed that it was possible to inhibit both autoantibody production and development of thyroid lesions by prior incubation of bone marrow cells with syngeneic thyroglobulin heavily labeled with ^{125}I (7). The elimination of specific immunoreactive B cells by local inactivation then prevents the development of EAT. Moreover, the absence of significant numbers of antigen-binding cells in the thymus of normal A/J mice is compatible with the hypothesis that T cells are tolerant, whereas B-cells which specifically react with syngeneic thyroglobulin are fully immunocompetent.

As has been suggested in the rabbit model (5), immunization of mice with heterologous Tg apparently bypassed the specificity of T cells, and T cells activated by heterologous Tg supply a second signal needed for differentiation of competent B cells that have reacted with self-related determinants of heterologous Tg. In support of this mechanism is the nature of histological lesions that develop in the thyroid of mice immunized with aqueous preparations of heterologous Tg. The *in situ* formation of interstitial immune complexes in the gland with granular deposition along the follicular basement membrane is preceded by the appearance of neutrophils. These events are similar to those occurring in the Arthus reaction and are indicative of an antibody-mediated lesion.

B. Experimental Allergic Encephalomyelitis (EAE)

EAE can be produced by immunization with either central nervous tissue basic protein of myelin (BP) or peptides isolated from myelin or synthetically prepared and incorporated in CFA (8). It is characterized by acute vasculitis and perivascular demyelination of the central nervous system. In contrast to EAT, EAE is a cell-mediated disease because it is readily transferred by lymphocytes and not by serum (9). It further differs from EAT by the absence of tolerance in both T and B cells; moreover, both cell types are capable of specifically binding BP (10). The T cells, however, play the central role as effector cells, as shown by adoptive transfer studies. When thymectomized, irradiated Lewis rats were injected with lymphocytes obtained from syngeneic animals immunized 9 days previously with BP-CFA, they developed typical clinical and pathological symptoms. On the other hand, when the sensitized cells were first depleted of T cells by treatment with anti-rat-brain antiserum and complement, no disease occurred. The sera of these animals, however, had antibody titers similar to the sera from the recipients receiving a cell suspension not depleted of T cells (11). Thus, it appears that lymphocytes transferred 9 days after immunization were already committed to the production of antibodies to BP and needed no further T cell help. Also, it is clear from this experiment that the induction of EAE is dependent on effector T cells or mediators released from these cells rather than on serum antibodies to BP (Fig. 2B).

The role of T and B cells in the induction of EAE was further defined by antigen-suicide experiments where antigen-binding cells for BP with either T or B cell functions were specifically eliminated by treatment with BP heavily labeled with ^{125}I (10). No clinical symptoms, histological lesions, or antibody to BP were observed in thymectomized, irradiated recipients reconstituted with normal B cells along with T cells treated with [^{125}I]BP and subsequently immunized with BP-CFA. On the other hand, both clinical symptoms and histological lesions, but not antibody to BP, were observed in the recipient rats reconstituted with normal T cells along with B cells treated with [^{125}I]BP and subsequently immunized with BP-CFA. These observations clearly demonstrate that effector T cells and not antibody is responsible for the induction of EAE.

III. EXPERIMENTAL AUTOIMMUNE MYASTHENIA GRAVIS

Myasthenia gravis (MG) and its animal model (EAMG) are diseases characterized by rapid fatigability and progressive weakness of certain muscles on repetitive use. Impaired neuromuscular transmission is caused by antibodies against acetylcholine receptor (AChR) acting primarily by causing loss of AChR through complement-mediated focal lysis of the postsynaptic membrane (12-16) and an increased rate of AChR destruction (17-20). EAMG can be induced in a variety of species by the injection of AChR in CFA [reviewed in Lindstrom (21)]. The antigen used in most studies is affinity-purified AChR from *Torpedo californica* or *Electrophorus electricus*; however, the disease can be induced by AChR from mammalian muscle (22, 23). Syngeneic AChR has been successfully used to induce EAMG (24); extensive studies, however, have not been performed due to the limited amounts available. It is well established that EAMG is an antibody-mediated autoimmune disease, since disease can be passively transferred to normal rats by means of serum containing as little as 1×10^{-11} mol anti-rat AChR (25) or by monoclonal antibody (26, 27). Chronic high doses of IgG from MG patients can passively transfer MG to mice (28). Passive EAMG results in an infiltration of the muscle by macrophages, similar to that seen in acute EAMG which occurs 8-10 days after injecting AChR in CFA along with *Bordetella pertussis*. The cellular invasion of passively transferred acute EAMG is produced subsequent to C3 activation (29). The role of C3 is evident from studies of rats rendered temporarily resistent to acute EAMG by complement depletion (30). In chronic EAMG and MG, immune complexes containing C3, IgG, and C9 are present on the postsynaptic membrane (13, 15, 31); however, cellular infiltration is not observed. Cross-linking of AChR by antibody increases AChR degradation in muscle cells, independent of complement (18). This mechanism, termed antigenic modulation, probably accounts for most of the AChR loss, and hence transmission impairment observed in EAMG (32). Neuromuscular transmission is probably only slightly impaired by competitive and allosteric effect of antibodies on AChR function [reviewed in Lindstrom (21)].

In order to study the specific cellular immune response in EAMG, studies were designed to investigate both the *in vitro* proliferative response of lymphocytes to AChR and *in vitro* production of antibodies to AChR stimulated by the addition of AChR *in vitro*, as well as the correlation of these responses with *in vivo* levels of serum antibody, antibody bound to AChRs in muscle, and muscle AChR content. The roles of macrophages, helper T cells, and B cells in these responses were at least partially defined. Animals immunized with both electric organ and muscle AChR were studied for their response to the immunogen and to the cross-reacting antigen (33).

1. *The Role of T Helper Cells in EAMG.* In order to determine the role of T cells and accessory cells in chronic EAMG, we adapted a proliferative assay system of T lymphocytes and redefined the tissue culture conditions necessary to arrive at optimal antigenic stimulation (34).

Lewis rats were immunized with 15 μg affinity-purified AChR (35) from the main electric organ of *Torpedo californica* emulsified in CFA, in the footpads and at the base of the tail. A single-cell suspension prepared from the draining lymph nodes was cultured in microwells at a cell concentration of 1×10^6 cells/ml for 5 days. The solubilized AChR was added to the cultures after dialysis against RPMI-1640 in order to remove the detergent (cholate). The cultures were pulsed with 1 μCi tritiated thymidine 24 hr before harvesting. The results are expressed as mean counts per minute (cpm) of triplicate cultures ± standard error. Peripheral blood lymphocytes were purified from heparinized (40 IU/ml) blood obtained by cardiac puncture according to the procedure of Perper *et al.* (36). The addition of AChR *in vitro* to AChR-primed lymphocytes induced a mitogenic response. The $[^3H]$thymidine incorporation increased linearly with the amount of AChR used

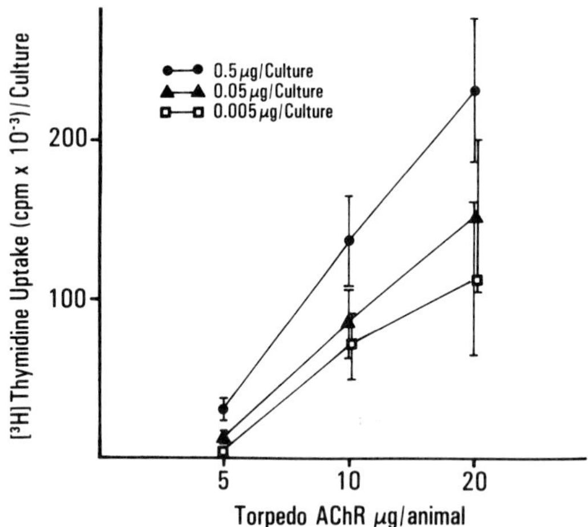

FIGURE 3. Proliferative response of lymph node cells *in vitro* after immunization with increasing amounts of Torpedo AChR. Each point is the average of five rats sacrificed 42 days after immunization. Lymph node cells were cultured with 3 different concentrations of Torpedo AChR (0.02, 0.2, 2 × 10^{-8} *M*) *in vitro* for 5 days.

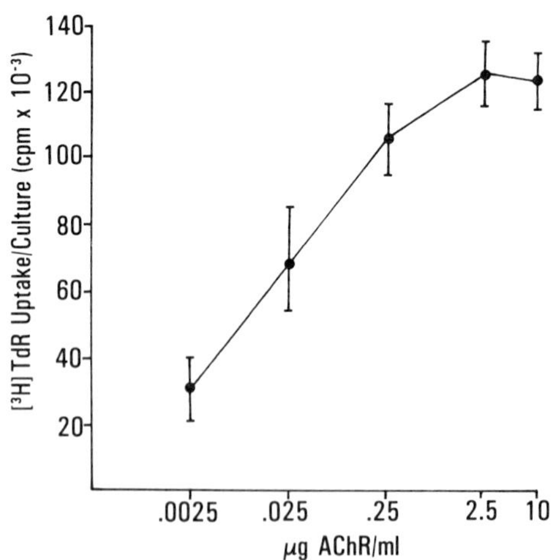

FIGURE 4. AChR concentration dependency of the proliferative response *in vitro*. 42 days after immunization with 15 μg of Torpedo AChR, lymph node cells were cultured in the presence of the indicated concentrations of Torpedo AChR (0.02 - 8 × 10^{-8} *M*) for 5 days.

for immunization over the range of 5-20 μg (Fig. 3). The proliferative response in lymphocyte cells of rats immunized with 15 μg AChR increased linearly with the log of the AChR concentration *in vitro*, starting at 0.0025 μg/ml to an AChR concentration of 0.25 μg/ml and reached a plateau at an AChR concentration of 0.25 μg/ml (Fig. 4). A culture period with AChR of 4 to 5 days was found to be optimal. Unlike the high proliferative response of lymph node cells, a much lower proliferative response was observed in peripheral blood lymphocytes (Fig. 5). This population presumably represents circulating lymphocytes that leave the draining lymph nodes. Thus, the responsiveness of peripheral blood lymphocytes in EAMG and possibly also in MG does not reflect the responsiveness in

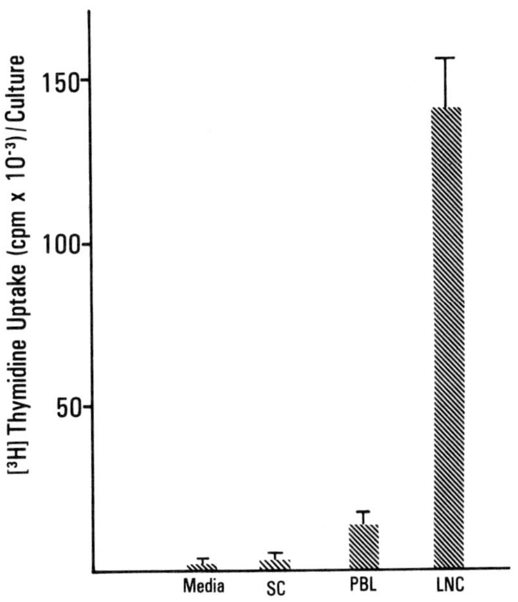

FIGURE 5. Comparison of the proliferative response to Torpedo AChR of peripheral blood lymphocytes (PBL), lymph node cells (LNC), and spleen cells (SC) in rats with EAMG. In each case, 2×10^{-5} cells were used per well.

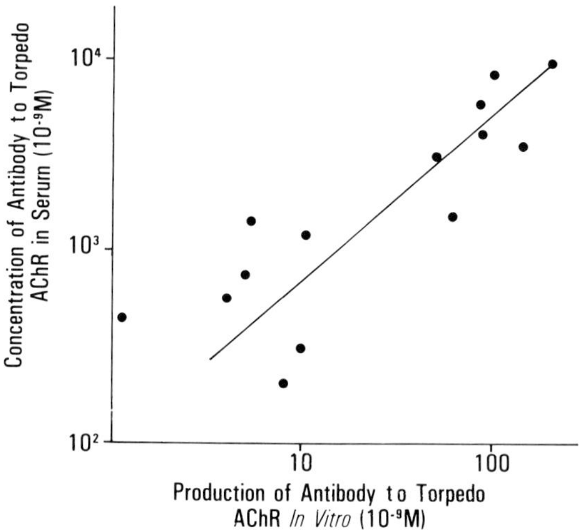

FIGURE 6. Production of antibody to AChR *in vitro* is directly proportional to the concentration of antibodies to AChR in the serum of rats from which the lymph node cells were removed. The lymph node cells were cultured in the presence of 25 ng AChR/ml (2×10^{-10} *M*). Rats (n = 14) receiving increasing doses of Torpedo AChR (5, 10, 20 μg) were used for this experiment.

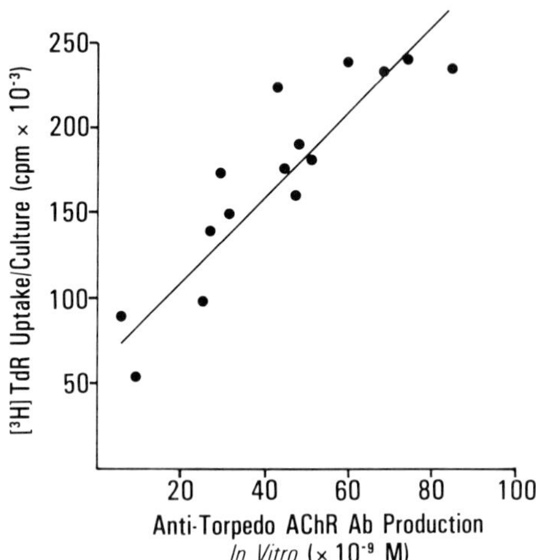

FIGURE 7. *In vitro*, the proliferative and antibody responses are directly proportional. Lymph node cells of 15 rats immunized with 15 μg Torpedo AChR with EAMG were cultured under optimal conditions for T proliferation (2.5 μg/ml) and for antibody production (25 ng/ml)

regional lymphoid tissue. Spleen cells cultured under identical conditions did not proliferate significantly (Fig. 5). Since only very low concentrations of the immunogen are used, most of the AChR preparation may be retained by macrophages in lymphocytes and therefore spleen cells may be unprimed. Alternatively, T or macrophage-like suppressor cells might be responsible for the inhibition of T proliferation in spleen cells, since suppressor cells preferentially "home" to this organ (37).

Since EAMG and MG are antibody-mediated diseases, the use of an *in vitro* system for anti-AChR antibody production could answer some of the questions concerning the immunoregulatory mechanisms operating in the experimental animal model. Immune lymph node cells (1×10^6 cells/ml) were cultured in triplicate wells in the presence of Torpedo AChR in 200 μl RPMI 1640 supplemented as described for the proliferative assay for 5 days. The cells were then washed in the microwells with cold HBSS to remove AChR that would interfere with the radioimmunoassay of anti-AChR antibody and 0.2 ml fresh medium was added, followed by an additional culture period of 24 hr. Aliquots of the tissue culture supernatants were assayed for anti-AChR antibody by indirect immunoprecipitation of [^{125}I]-α-bungarotoxin AChR (38).

In addition to proliferation, culture of immune lymphocytic cells in the presence of AChR resulted in the production of anti-AChR antibody. Moreover, antibody production *in vitro* was proportional to the serum titer of anti-torpedo AChR antibodies in the rats from which the lymphocytes were obtained (Fig. 6). Also, the amount of antibody generated *in vitro* was directly proportional to the proliferative response of the lymphocytic cells (Fig. 7). This observation suggested that the proliferating cells were T helper cells. More direct evidence for this concept was obtained by fluorescence-activated cell sorting of lymph node cells stained by indirect immunofluorescence with monoclonal antibody against the W3/25 antigen, a cell surface marker for T helper cells in the rat (39). Depletion of T cells with the W3/25 phenotype abolished both T proliferation and antibody production. The W3/25-positive lymphocytes were still capable of proliferating in the presence of AChR, but few antibody-producing cells were retained in this fraction. This *in vitro* system also allowed us to analyze the role of macrophages in antigen presentation. Lymphoid cells depleted of macrophages by filtration through Sephadex G-10 columns were reduced both in their proliferative and antibody-producing capacities. This probably reflects the requirement for antigen presentation to T cells in the context of major histocompatibility complex determinants (40) and more specifically the Ia molecule (I-A subregion) as shown for murine EAMG (41).

2. *Specificities of T and B Cell Responses for AChR.* Although the cross-reaction between antibodies raised against AChR from different species has been studied (22, 26, 42), the specificities of the T cells in EAMG have not been investigated thoroughly (43, 44). Immunization of rats with torpedo AChR (15 μg AChR in CFA, injected twice 1 month apart) elicits a strong specific antibody response ($5 \pm 0.75 \times 10^{-6}$ *M*, *n* = 11). Cross-reactive titers to fetal calf AChR were, respectively, 1.2 and 1.0% of the anti-torpedo antibody titer. Cross-reaction in the proliferative response appears considerably greater (25 ± 10%) (Fig. 8). Similar proliferative and serological cross-reactivities were observed with affinity-purified rat AChR, but because of the limited availability of rat AChR extensive studies were not possible. The discrepancy in cross-reactivity in the T and B cell response is compatible

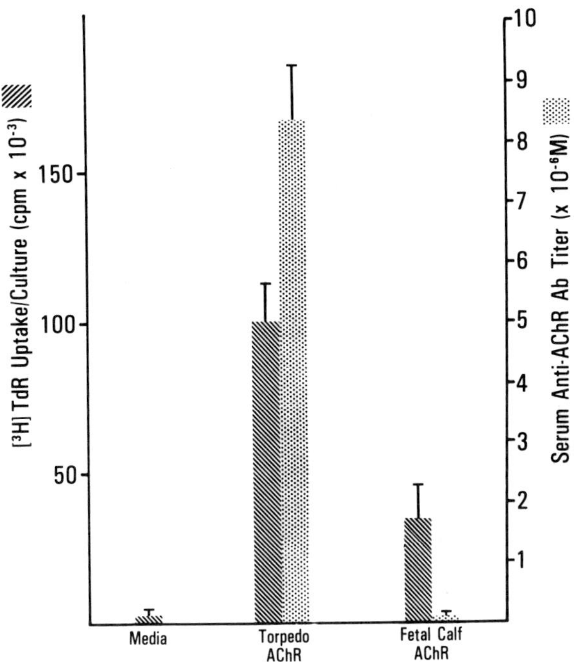

FIGURE 8. Cross-reaction of the proliferative response and serum anti-AChR of rats immunized with Torpedo AChR and stimulated with either Torpedo or fetal calf muscle AChR. Rats immunized and boosted with 15 μg of Torpedo AChR were sacrificed after 39 days for lymph node cells. Both the proliferative response and the serum titers were assayed with 2.5 μg/ml of Torpedo or fetal calf muscle AChR (2×10^{-8} *M*).

with different antigen specificities in T and B cells. In support of this theory, a high cross-reaction was also demonstrated between denatured subunits of torpedo AChR and native AChR, unlike the cross-reaction at the serum antibody level (<1%) (22). In several other studies it was suggested that T and B cells differ from one another in the way they recognize native and denatured forms of the antigens or serologically distinct viruses (45-48). However, antibody assays are direct binding determinations, whereas T proliferative responses are complex biological phenomena and need not be directly proportional to the interaction between T cell receptor and ligand.

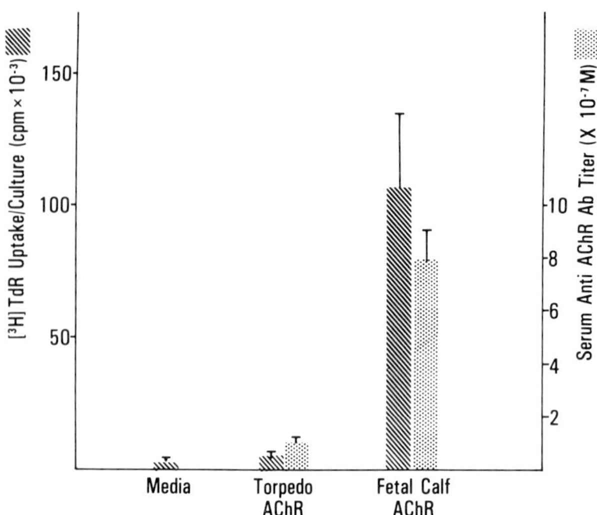

FIGURE 9. Cross-reaction of the proliferative response and serum anti-AChR antibody of rats immunized and boosted with 15 μg fetal calf muscle AChR and stimulated with either Torpedo or fetal calf muscle AChR. The proliferative response and the serum antibody concentrations were assayed with 2.5 μg/ml (2×10^{-8} *M*) Torpedo or fetal calf muscle AChR. Lymph node cells take 41 days after the initial immunization were cultured for 5 days.

Immunization of rats with fetal calf AChR induces severe EAMG. The titers of serum antibody to fetal calf AChR and to torpedo AChR were $7.9 \pm 1.1 \times 10^{-7}$ and $1.1 \pm 0.2 \times 10^{-7}$ *M*, respectively. The proliferative response to torpedo AChR of lymphocytic cells obtained from these animals was only 2.7% of the response to fetal calf AChR compared to 10% cross-reactivity at the serum antibody level (Fig. 9). Similar results were obtained in rats immunized with affinity-purified syngeneic AChR showing a cross-reaction of 32% in antibody specificity and 5% in the proliferative assay. These observations could be best explained by a restricted response to mammalian AChR in the rat, where antibody is produced to a limited number of epitopes on mammalian AChRs in comparison to a less restricted response to the more foreign torpedo AChR. Most of the cross-reactive epitopes between torpedo and mammalian AChR, as characterized by means of monoclonal antibodies, are localized on a region of the α subunit (49,50). The restrictions in the response to mammalian AChR are in agreement with other reports on the restrictions in the response to syngeneic thyroglobulin (51). Also, in patients with MG, the majority of autoantibodies are similarly restricted to a small region on the α subunit (52).

3. Relationship of the in Vitro *Assays and the Severity of EAMG.* A reasonable correlation was found between the *in vivo* anti-AChR responses, *in vitro* anti-AChR antibody production, and subsequent pathological effects. The log of the proliferative response *in vitro* is proportional to the loss of AChR from the muscles of rats with EAMG (Fig. 10) ($r = .85$, $p < .001$). This is in agreement with the concept that T helper activity is proportional to antibody production both *in vitro* (Fig. 7) and *in vivo* (Fig. 11) and that antibody levels *in vivo* are proportional to antibody production *in vitro* (Fig. 6) and that antibodies are responsible for AChR loss from muscle [reviewed in Parks and Weigle (1)]. Similar data were obtained in studies of murine EAMG, where it was shown that the proliferating cells express the lyt-1+2,3- phenotype of both helper T cells and cells mediating delayed-type hypersensitivity (53, 54). The proliferative response is proportional to the concentration of autoantibody to muscle AChR in serum and miniature endplate potential decrement in mouse strains with different sensitivities to EAMG. Our studies performed during the chronic phase of EAMG in the rat additionally demonstrate that the proliferative cell is not only phenotypically but also functionally a helper T cell (Fig. 11).

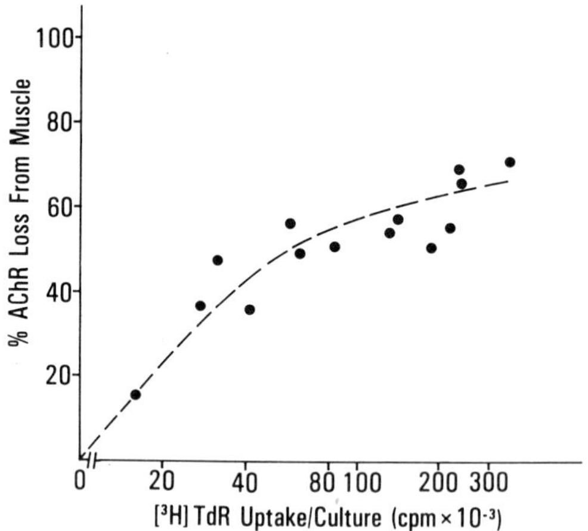

FIGURE 10. Correlation between the T proliferative response and disease severity. Rats immunized with 5, 10, and 20 μg of torpedo AChR were killed after 42 days. Loss of AChR from muscle was used as an index of severity of EAMG.

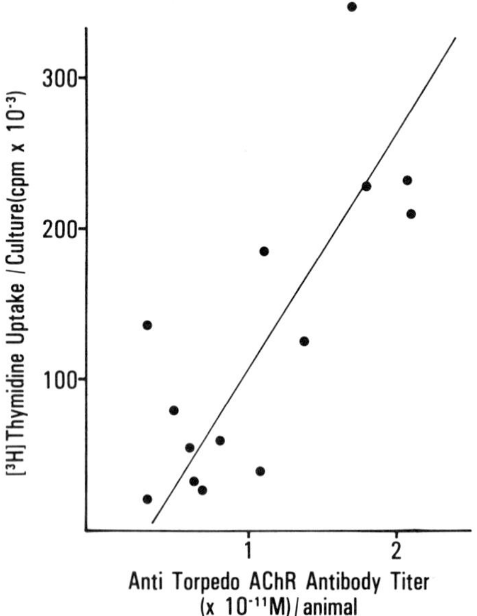

FIGURE 11. Comparison between the proliferative response and the amount of antibody bound to muscle AChR *in vivo*. The same rats were studied as in Fig. 10.

IV. CONCLUDING REMARKS

It is suggested that whether a given antigen is vulnerable to an autoimmune attack is dependent on the specific immune status of T cells and B cells to that antigen, which in turn is dependent on the concentration of self-antigen in the microenvironment. This suggestion and the observation that B cells require much higher concentrations of self-antigen than T cells for the maintenance of unresponsiveness are supported by data presented using an experimental model of acquired tolerance to serum proteins. Depending on the immune status of T and B cells for self antigens, three mechanisms were suggested for the initial events leading to autoimmunity. In the preceding sections, animal models illustrating each of these mechanisms were described. The mechanisms proposed for breaking tolerance and the model autoimmune diseases thought to illustrate it are listed below: (a) suppression of specifically tolerant T cells and activation of competent B cells (experimental autoimmune thyroiditis), (b) direct activation of competent T cells (experimental allergic encephalomyelitis), and (c) direct activation of competent T and B cells (experimental autoimmune myasthenia gravis).

ACKNOWLEDGMENTS

We thank A. Janssens, B. Einarson, and D. Finney for excellent technical assistance and J. Littrell for secretarial expertise.

REFERENCES

1. Parks, D. E. and Weigle, W. O. *Immunol. Rev. 43*, 217 (1979).

2. Weigle, W. O. *Adv. Immunol. 16*, 61 (1973).

3. Chiller, J. M., Habicht, G. S., and Weigle, W. O. *Science 171*, 813 (1971).

4. Rose, N. R. and Witebsky, E. *J. Immunol. 76*, 417 (1956).

5. Weigle, W. O. and Nakamura, R. M. *J. Immunol. 99*, 223 (1967).

6. Weigle, W. O. *Adv. Immunol. 30*, 159 (1980).

7. Clagett, J. and Weigle, W. O. *J. Exp. Med. 139*, 643 (1974).

8. Rauch, H. C. and Einstein, E. R. *Rev. Neurosci. 7*, 283 (1974).

9. Paterson, R. Y. *Adv. Immunol. 5*, 131 (1966).

10. Ortiz-Ortiz, L. and Weigle, W. O. *J. Exp. Med. 144*, 604 (1976).

11. Ortiz-Ortiz, L., Nakamura, R. M., and Weigle, W. O. *J. Immunol. 117*, 576 (1976).

12. Engel, A. G., Tsujihata, M., Lindstrom, J. M., and Lennon, V. *Ann. N.Y. Acad. Sci. 274*, 60 (1976).

13. Engel, A. G., Lindstrom, J. M., Lambert, E. H., and Lennon, V. A. *Neurology 27*, 307 (1977).

14. Engel, A. G., Lambert, E. H., and Howard, F. M. *Mayo Clin. Proc. 52*, 267 (1977).

15. Sahashi, K., Engel, A. G., Lindstrom, J. M., Lambert, E. H., and Lennon, V. A. *J. Neuropathol. Exp. Neurol. 37*, 212 (1978).

16. Engel, A. G., Sakakibara, H., Sahashi, K., Lindstrom, J. M., Lambert, E. H., and Lennon, V. A. *Neurology 29*, 179 (1979).

17. Kao, I. and Drachman, D. B. *Science 196*, 527 (1977).

18. Heinemann, S., Bevan, S., Kullber, R., Lindstrom, J. M., and Rice, J. *Proc. Natl. Acad. Sci. U.S.A. 74*, 3090 (1977).

19. Drachman, D. B., Angus, C. W., Adams, R. N., and Kao, I. *Proc. Natl. Acad. Sci. U.S.A. 75*, 3422 (1978).

20. Merlie, J. P., Changeux, J. P., and Gros, F. *J. Biol. Chem. 253*, 2882 (1978).

21. Lindstrom, J. *Adv. Immunol. 27*, 1 (1979).

22. Lindstrom, J. M., Walter (Nave), B., and Einarson, B. *Biochemistry 18*, 4470 (1979).

23. Fulpius, B. W., Zurn, A. D., Granato, D. A., and Leder, R. M. *Ann. N.Y. Acad. Sci. 274*, 116 (1976).

24. Lindstrom, J. M., Einarson, B. L., Lennon, V. A., and Seybold, M. E. *J. Exp. Med. 144*, 726 (1976).

25. Lindstrom, J. M., Engel, A. G., Seybold, M. E., Lennon, V. A., and Lambert, E. H. *J. Exp. Med. 144*, 739 (1976).

26. Tzartos, S. J. and Lindstrom, J. M. *Proc. Natl. Acad. Sci. U.S.A. 77*, 755 (1980).

27. Lennon, V. A. and Lambert, E. H. *Nature (London) 285*, 238 (1980).

28. Toyka, K. V., Drachman, D. B., Pestronk, A., and Kao, I. *Science 190*, 397 (1975).

29. Engel, A. G., Sakakibara, H., Sahashi, K., Lindstrom, J. M., Lambert, E. H., Lennon, V. A. *Neurology 29*, 179 (1979).

30. Lennon, V. A., Seybold, J., Lindstrom, J. M., Cochrane, C., and Yulevitch, R. *J. Exp. Med. 147*, 973 (1978).

31. Sahashi, K., Engel, A. G., Lambert, E. H., and Howard, F. M. *J. Neuropathol. Exp. Neurol. 39*, 160 (1980).

32. Lindstrom, J. and Einarson, B. *Muscle Nerve 2*, 173 (1979).

33. DeBaets, M. H., Einarson, B., Lindstrom, J. M., and Weigle, W. O. *J. Immunol.* (1982). In press.

34. Corradin, G., Etlinger, H. M., and Chiller, J. M. *J. Immunol.* *119*, 1048 (1977).

35. Lindstrom, J. M., Lennon, V., Seybold, M., and Whittingham, S. *Ann. N.Y. Acad. Sci.* *274*, 254 (1976).

36. Perper, R. J., Zee, T. W., and Mickelson, M. M. *J. Lab. Clin. Med.* *72*, 843 (1968).

37. Gershon, R. K. *Contemp. Top. Immunobiol.* *3*, 1 (1974).

38. Patrick, J., Lindstrom, J. M., Culp, B., and McMillan, J. *Proc. Natl. Acad. Sci. U.S.A.* *70*, 3334 (1973).

39. White, R. A. H., Mason, D. W., Williams, A. F., Galfre, G., and Milstein, C. *J. Exp. Med.* *148*, 664 (1978).

40. Yano, A., Schwartz, R. H., and Paul, W. E. *J. Exp. Med.* *146*, 828 (1977).

41. Christadoss, P., Lennon, V. A., and David, C. *J. Immunol.* *123*, 2540 (1979).

42. Lindstrom, J., Campbell, M., and Nave, B. *Muscle Nerve* *1*, (1978).

43. Noguchi, S. A., Drachman, D. B., Adams, R. N., and Hirsch, R. L. *Ann. Neurol.* *8*, 32 (1980).

44. Hohlfeld, R., Kalies, I., Heinz, F., Kalden, J. R., and Wekerle, H. *J. Immunol.* *126*, 1355 (1981).

45. Gell, P. G.H. and Benacerraf, B. *Immunology* *2*, 64 (1959).

46. Ishizaka, K., Okudaira, H., and King, T. P. *J. Immunol.* *114*, 110 (1975).

47. Chesnut, R. W., Endres, R. O., and Grey, H. M. *Clin. Immunol. Immunopathol.* *15*, 397 (1980).

48. Rosenthal, K. L. and Zinkernagel, R. M. *J. Immunol.* *124*, 2301 (1980).

49. Lindstrom, J. M., Einarson, B., and Merlie, J. *Proc. Natl. Acad. Sci. U.S.A.* *75*, 769 (1978).

50. Tzartos, S., Rand, D. E., Einarson, B. L., and Lindstrom, J. M. *J. Biol. Chem. 256*, 8635 (1981).

51. Nye, L., Pontes de Carvalno, L. C., and Roitt, L. M. *Clin. Exp. Immunol. 41*, 252 (1980).

52. Tzartos, S. J., Seybold, M. E., and Lindstrom, J. M. *Proc. Natl. Acad. Sci. U.S.A. 79*, 188 (1982).

53. Christadoss, P., Kroc, C. J., Lennon, V. A., and David, C. S. *J. Immunol. 126*, 1646 (1981).

54. Christadoss, P., Lennon, V. A., Kroc, C. J., Lambert, E. H., and David, C. S. *Ann. N.Y. Acad. Sci.* (1981).

CELLULAR ASPECTS OF MURINE SLE[1]

Argyrios N. Theofilopoulos
Frank J. Dixon

Department of Immunopathology,
Scripps Clinic and Research Foundation,
La Jolla, California

I. INTRODUCTION

New Zealand (NZ) strains of mice, particularly New Zealand Black (NZB) and New Zealand Black/White (NZB/W) F_1 hybrids, have been used for the last two decades as models for the study of systemic lupus erythematosus (SLE). Attempts to demonstrate abnormalities in the immune systems of these mice that might be responsible for their genetic susceptibility to and development of this autoimmune disorder have generated contradictory results concerning their immunocompetence

[1]*Supported by United States Public Health Service grants AI-07007, N01-CP-71078, CA-16600, CA-23322, and the Cecil H. and Ida M. Green Research Endowment. This is publication No. 2262 from the Department of Immunopathology, Scripps Clinic and Research Foundation, 10666 North Torrey Pines Road, La Jolla, California, 92037. Argyrios N. Theofilopoulos is supported by a Research Career Development Award, National Cancer Institute CA-00303.*

ISBN 0-12-218320-7

TABLE I. Derivation of SLE Mice and Genetic Markers

Strain	Derivation	*H-2*	Lymphocyte surface alloantigens	IgG allotype
NZB	Inbred for color from stock of undefined background	$H\text{-}2^d$	Thy-1.2, Ly-1.2, Ly-2.2, Ly-3.2, $Qa\text{-}1^a$, $M\ell s^a$, $T\ell a^a$	*e*
NZW		$H\text{-}2^z$	Thy-1.2	*e*
BXSB	Derived from (C57BL/6J × SB/Le) F_1	$H\text{-}2^b$	Thy-1.2, TL^-, Ly-1.2, Ly-2.2, Ly-3.2, $Qa\text{-}1^b$	*b*
MRL/ℓ	Genome = 75% LG, 13% AKR, 12% C3H, and 0.3% C57BL/6	$H\text{-}2^k$	Thy-1.2, TL^-, Ly-1.2, Ly-2.1, Ly-3.1, $Qa\text{-}1^b$	*a*

[reviewed in Talal (36), Theofilopoulos *et al.* (41), and Theofilopoulos and Dixon (40)]. Conspicuously missing from the voluminous research results on this subject is any common factor that points with certainty to a clear-cut cause-and-effect relationship between most of these animals' abnormalities and the etiology/pathogenesis of their autoimmune component.

Recently, Murphy and Roths (25) reported two genetically different murine strains, i.e., the MRL and BXSB strains, which develop typical lupus-like disorders. The availability of these two new strains allows us to look for pathogenetic and etiologic common denominators of the disease evolving on quite different genetic backgrounds. Below is a summarized description of our findings in NZ, BXSB and MRL mice.

II. DERIVATION OF SLE STRAINS

The derivations, major histocompatibility complexes, lymphocyte surface alloantigens and IgG allotypes of these new strains of autoimmune mice and of the NZ strains are described in Table I. It is evident that there is no association of murine SLE with any of these genetic markers. The MRL is notable because in its twelfth generation of inbreeding a spontaneous autosomal recessive mutation divided the stock into two substrains, one with *ℓpr* (lymphoproliferation) gene (MRL/ℓ substrain) and the other without (MRL/n substrain), leaving the two groups with at least 89% of their genomes in common. The *ℓpr* gene has been transferred to substrain MRL/n by five cycles of cross-intercross matings, reducing the estimated residual heterozygocity from 11 to 0.4% and producing the congenic inbred strains, MRL/Mp-*ℓpr*/*ℓpr* and +/+. The MRL/Mp-*ℓpr*/*ℓpr* substrain (MRL/ℓ) manifests early disease with 50% mortality in males and females at about 5 to 6 months of age, whereas the MRL/Mp-+/+ (MRL/n), which lacks the *lpr* gene, has delayed disease with 50% mortality at 17 to 23 months for female and male, respectively. Compared to the NZB/W (50% mortality at 8.5 months for females and 15 months for males), the male BXSB/Mp (BXSB) is affected much earlier than the female, with a 50% mortality for the males at around 6 months and for the females at 18 months.

III. HISTOIMMUNOPATHOLOGIC AND SEROLOGIC CHARACTERISTICS

Our findings on the histoimmunopathologic and serologic characteristics of the four kinds (NZB, NZB/W, MRL/*l*, BXSB) of autoimmune mice are summarized in Table II and detailed elsewhere (1, 2, 7-9, 17-19). Some characteristics are common to all these strains and some are strain specific. All these autoimmune mice develop immune complex glomerulonephritis and thymic atrophy. The degree of lymph node hyperplasia in older autoimmune mice varies considerably, being absent or minimal in NZ mice (2-3× the normal size), moderate in BXSB male mice (10-20× the normal size), and most prominent in older MRL/*l* mice (100× the normal size). Fifteen to thirty percent of mice in each SLE strain have acute and/or old myocardial infarcts and degenerative vascular disease due to immune complex deposits in heart vessels, although without accompanying cellular inflammation. Unique to their strain, over half MRL/*l* mice develop acute and/or necrotizing polyarteritis, and 25% of old, sick MRL/*l* mice have swollen joints of the hind feet and lower legs with associated articular destruction, joint effusions, and pannus formation, all resembling rheumatoid arthritis. Serologically, common characteristics of older autoimmune mice are hypergammaglobulinemia, antinuclear antibodies, anti-ds and ss DNA antibodies, antihapten antibodies,

TABLE II. Histoimmunopathologic and Serologic Characteristics of SLE Mice

		HISTOPATHOLOGIC FEATURES			
Strain	IC-GN*	Thymic atrophy	Lymphoid hyperplasia	Arteritis	Arthritis
NZB	+	+	+	0	0
NZBxW	+++	+	+	0	0
MRL/ℓ	+++	+	+++	+	+
BXSB	+++	+	++	0	0

SEROLOGIC FEATURES

Common =	Hyper-γ-globulinemia, antinuclear antibodies, anti-dsDNA, anti-ssDNA, antihapten antibodies, high levels of gp70, immune complexes, reduced complement levels (NZB is C5-deficient).
Uncommon =	Anti-Sm (MRL/n, MRL/ℓ), IgG + IgM rheumatoid factor (MRL/ℓ), anti-erythrocyte (NZB, NZBxW), NTA (NZB, NZBxW, BXSB).

IC-GN = immune complex glomerulonephritis.

significant levels of serum gp70, circulating immune complexes (composed of retroviral xenotropic gp70-anti-gp70 antibodies, rheumatoid factor-IgG and nuclear antigens-antibodies), and decreased hemolytic complement. Strain-specific serologic manifestations are antierythrocyte antibodies (high frequency in NZ mice but low in BXSB and MRL/ℓ), anti-Sm antibodies (exclusively in MRL/ℓ and MRL/n mice), rheumatoid factors of both the IgM and IgG classes (only in MRL/ℓ), and natural thymocytotoxic antibodies (NTA: high incidence and levels in NZ mice, intermediate in BXSB, and very low in MRL/ℓ mice). A primary role of NTAs in the development of murine SLE is questionable since we observed (8) that many immunologically normal strains of mice (RF, SN, NC, 129-GIX$^+$, 129-GIX$^-$) have similar incidences and titers of NTAs to those seen in NZ mice. Others have found that hereditarily asplenic (Dh/+) NZB mice develop autoimmune disease without NTAs (14) whereas recombinant NZB inbred strains express NTAs in the absence of other types of autoantibodies or, conversely, express anti-DNA and antierythrocyte autoantibodies without NTAs (29) (R. Riblet, personal communication). However, a secondary role of such NTAs in accelerating autoimmunity should still be considered.

IV. LYMPHOCYTE SURFACE CHARACTERISTICS

As indicated above, a multitude of studies have yielded only contradictory results in seeking altered phenotypic or functional characteristics of cells that participate and regulate immune responses of NZ mice and, consequently, foster their disease. To define better the nature of immunologic abnormalities associated with murine lupus, we have performed a thorough analysis of the phenotypic expression of various surface markers on lymphocytes from the lupus mice (38). Although we find that the lymphoid organs of each autoimmune strain vary somewhat from normals in cellular distributions, no two of the strains develop the same abnormality (Table III). For example, the number of T cells declines in older NZ animals, remains at normal levels in BXSB mice, and undergoes massive proliferation in older MRL/ℓ mice. The proliferating T cell in MRL/ℓ mice is Thy-1.2$^+$ and Ly "null" or weakly Ly-1$^+$. MRL/ℓ and BXSB mice have a numerically increased or normal content of I-J alloantigen-bearing T cells, respectively. Similarly, with regard to B cells, older NZ mice have low frequencies and absolute numbers, male BXSB mice have moderate proliferation, and MRL/ℓ mice have reduced frequencies but not

TABLE III. Lymphocyte Surface Markers in SLE Mice

Markers	NZB	NZB/W	MRL/ℓ	BXSB male
#Thy-1.2$^+$	↓	↓	↑	N*
I-J$^+$	-	-	↑	N
IgGFc	↓	↓	↓	↓
#sIg$^+$	↓	↓	N	↑
Capping sIg	N	N	N	N
Reexpression sIg	N	N	N	N
Isotype diversity	N	N	N	N
sIgM/sIgD	↑	↑	↓	↑
C3R^{+}**	↑	↑	↑	↑

*N = normal.

**C3R$^+$ = C3 receptor bearing B cells.

absolute numbers. As expected, B cells of older SLE mice are more mature than B cells of age-matched normal mice as evidenced by the formers' high frequency of complement receptor-bearing cells, loss of surface immunoglobulin (sIg), and high ratio of sIgM : sIgD-bearing cells. However, several surface characteristics of B cells from autoimmune mice are normal. For example, the developmental Ig-isotype diversity follows normal pathways with IgM present on spleen cells obtained immediately after birth and IgD appearing on spleen cells on the third day after birth. B cells from newborn BXSB and MRL/ℓ mice like B cells of normal strains do not reexpress sIg after modulation with $F(ab')_2$ anti-Ig; and the rates of sIg-anti-Ig complex endocytosis and of sIg capping in autoimmune mice are similar to those in normal strains.[2] However, splenocytes of newborn NZ mice, unlike those of normal mice, do reexpress sIg following modulation with $F(ab')_2$ anti-Ig. The relationship of this finding with the known resistance of NZ mice to tolerance induction remains to be determined.

V. B CELL FUNCTION

Immunologically, the most notable mark of the murine SLE syndrome is B lymphocyte hyperactivity, seen as hypergammaglobulinemia, spontaneous polyclonal antibody production, and secretion of various autoantibodies (41). We use three procedures in attempting to determine the functional and maturational state of the autoimmune animals' B cells. The results of these studies are summarized in Table IV. First, after assessing the numbers of Ig-secreting or -containing cells, we

TABLE IV. Functional Studies of B Cells from SLE Mice

Polyclonal B-cell activation	NZB	NZB/W	MRL/ℓ	BXSB male	C3H/St
Ig-secreting cells	6,000*	7,000	4,500	4,000	700
Ig-containing cells	66,000	72,000	61,000	21,000	12,000
Anti-TNP PFC	35	19	25	18	5
B-cell colonies**	9,480	5,200	5,640	5,040	920

**Numbers indicate the mean frequency of each cell type per 10^6 splenocytes.*

***In the absence of LPS.*

[2] *A. N. Theofilopoulos, R. S. Balderas, Y. Gozes, J. M. Fidler, F. T. Liu, A. Ahmed, F. J. Dixon. Surface and functional characteristics of B cells from lupus-prone murine strains.* Clinical Immunol. Immunopathol. *In press.*

find that all these SLE strains have many more mature, Ig-secreting cells in their spleens at one time or another than age-matched, immunologically normal strains (42). In NZB and NZB/W mice, the high frequency of splenic Ig-secreting cells is detectable as early as one month after birth and continues to increase somewhat. By contrast, in BXSB male and MRL/ℓ female mice, the high frequency of Ig-secreting cells first occurs only at or just preceding the clinical onset of disease. Spleen cells from mice of all autoimmune strains actively synthesize and secrete Ig, in young mice predominantly IgM, but with aging and the appearance of disease, IgG secretion predominates. The increased maturity of B cells in spleens of autoimmune mice is also shown by determining the number of cytoplasmic Ig-containing cells. Approximately 6 to 7% of the total spleen cells in the autoimmune mice versus 1% in normal mice stains positively for intracytoplasmic Ig. With advanced clinical disease, NZ mice have 5- to 10-fold and MRL/ℓ mice have 30-fold higher numbers of Ig-containing cells than younger, syngeneic animals.

Second, we assess the degree of polyclonal B cell activation by determining the number of antitrinitrophenyl (TNP) plaque-forming cells (PFC) in the spleens of these animals (17). All SLE strains contain significantly more PFC against TNP conjugated sheep red blood cells than normal mice (Table IV). The majority of NZB mice have significant elevations by two weeks of age, whereas the other three autoimmune strains (NZB/W, MRL/ℓ, BXSB) develp the increase at about four weeks of age. The increased polyclonal activation of B cells in spleens precedes the appearance of antihapten and anti-ssDNA antibodies in serum, but anti-ssDNA antibodies appear in serum at the same time as levels of antihapten antibodies increase.

Third, when we examine the generation of B-cell colonies in spleens of these mice, we find that the frequency of spontaneous B-cell colony-forming cells at one month of age is higher in spleens of all SLE strains compared to normals[2] (Table IV). All these results concerning Ig secretion, polyclonal antibody production, and B-cell colony formation strongly indicate to us and others (20, 23, 24, 26, 37) that generalized B cell hyperactivity is characteristic of mice with autoimmune syndromes.

VI. T CELL FUNCTION IN HUMORAL RESPONSES

The mechanisms responsible for the generalized B-cell hyperactivity and excessive production of autoantibodies in these mice are unknown. The cause may be one defect or a combination of defects such as primary or acquired B cell malfunction, endogenous or exogenous B-cell activators, lack of negative influence by suppressor T cells, an enhanced positive influence by helper T cells, defects in subsets of intra-T regulatory cells (i.e., Ly-123$^+$), and defects in other elements of the immune system such as macrophages. Some authors have claimed inadequacies of antigen-nonspecific suppressor T cells in NZ mice (3, 22), whereas others have failed to observe such a defect (14, 23, 28). Consequently, we have examined the functions of antigen-nonspecific and exogenous antigen-specific suppressor T cells, and of the antigen-nonspecific helper T cells during several phases of life and disease in the autoimmune murine strains with the results presented in the following paragraphs.

With regard to exogenous antigen-specific suppressor T cells (5), all the mice studied, autoimmune and normal, of all ages develop clear-cut ovalbumin (OVA)-specif.c suppressive activities that diminish IgG and IgE antibody production (exemplified in Fig. 1). In accord with the observations of Takatsu and Ishizaka (35), suppressor T cells were induced by injecting urea-denatured (UD)-OVA into OVA primed mice. Isolated T cells from UD-OVA treated autoimmune or normal donors, upon transfer to naive syngeneic recipients, efficiently suppress both IgG and IgE responses, confirming that T cells perpetrate the response we see.

Similarly, with regard to antigen nonspecific suppression (42), we find that concanavalin A (Con A) activated spleen cells not only from young and old normal mice but also from young and old autoimmune mice, including the NZ strains, effectively suppress lipopolysaccharide (LPS)-induced Ig synthesis by syngeneic cells (Fig. 2). Furthermore, contrary to a prior report (28), we find that LPS-responding B cells of young and old SLE mice are equally receptive to suppressor signals derived from Con A-activated syngeneic cells.

The above results taken together form the basis for our doubt that a *generalized* defect of suppressor T cells causes autoimmunity. However, it should be stressed that our experiments do not exclude the possible absence or abnormalities of specific subsets of suppressor T cells that control responses to autoantigens since Con A is an artificial inducer of antigen-nonspecific suppression, and immune responses to ordinary exogenous antigens may not depend on similar immunoregulatory mechanisms to those involved in responses to autoantigens. In addition, these experiments do not exclude the possible presence of subtle abnormalities of suppressor T cells or the development of late, secondary generalized suppressor T-cell abnormalities in these animals.

Ig hypersecretion and production of autoantibodies in SLE-prone mice may, at least in part, result from heightened T-helper activity. Therefore, we examined the degree of help provided by increasing numbers of isolated T cells from young

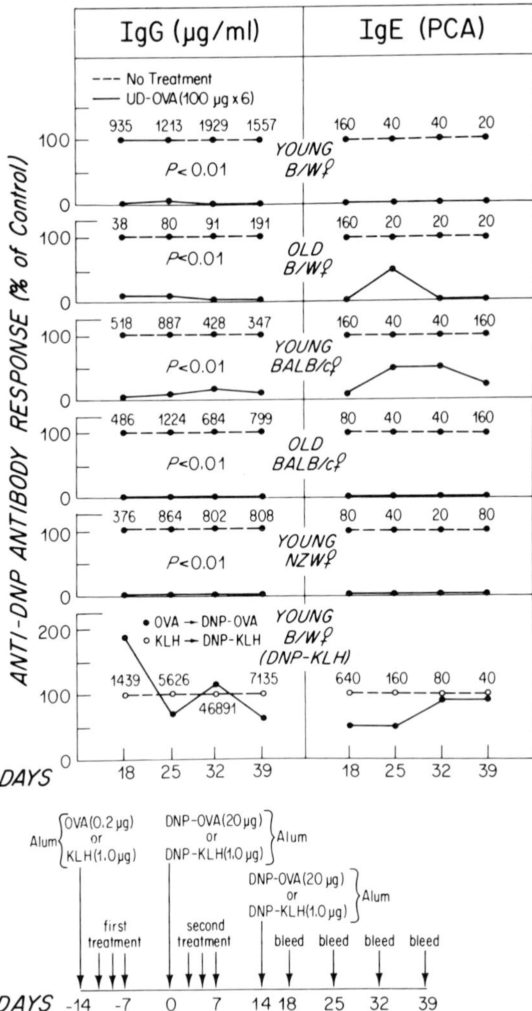

FIGURE 1. Induction of suppression in young and old $(NZB/W)F_1$ and BALB/c mice with UD-OVA [for details, see Creighton *et al.* (5)]. As summarized schematically at the bottom of the figure, groups of mice were immunized with 0.2 µg OVA (alum) or 1 µg DNP-KLH (alum) on day 14 and then given 100 µg UD-OVA iv on each of days -11, -9, -7, 3, 5, and 7. Primary and secondary immunization with 20 µg of DNP-OVA (alum) or DNP antibody responses were assayed on days 18, 25, 32, and 39. The IgE and IgG anti-DNP responses are presented as percentage of control responses with the control values given atop the corresponding point.

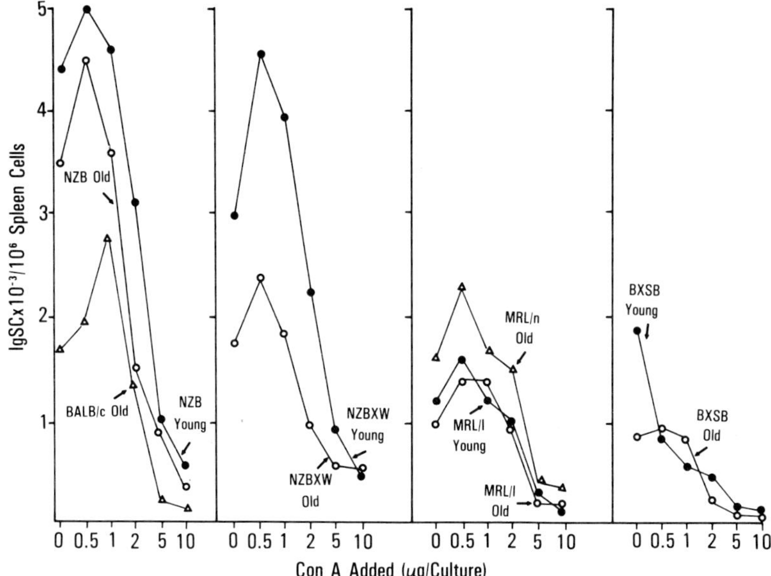

FIGURE 2. Direct suppression of LPS-induced Ig-secreting cells (IgSC) by Con A. Cells from the indicated strains were cultured in the presence of a standard amount of LPS (20 μg/ culture) and increasing concentrations of Con A. IgSC were assessed 3 days later.

and old animals to a standard number of mitogen-stimulated syngeneic and allogeneic but *H-2*-identical B cells isolated from spleens of young animals (Fig. 3) (42). Increments of T cells from young and old NZB and BXSB autoimmune mice added to a standard number of B cells from syngeneic young mice provide (at all doses and at both ages) equal help in enhancing the frequency of Ig-secreting cells after LPS stimulation. Moreover, the help provided by T cells from these two autoimmune strains to their own B cells is not significantly different from that provided by T cells from young and old normal mice of the same *H-2* haplotypes (BALB/c for NZB, C57BL/6 for BXSB). In the reverse situation, when T cells from young and old NZB and BXSB mice are added to B cells from young, normal counterparts, again the help is not significantly greater than that

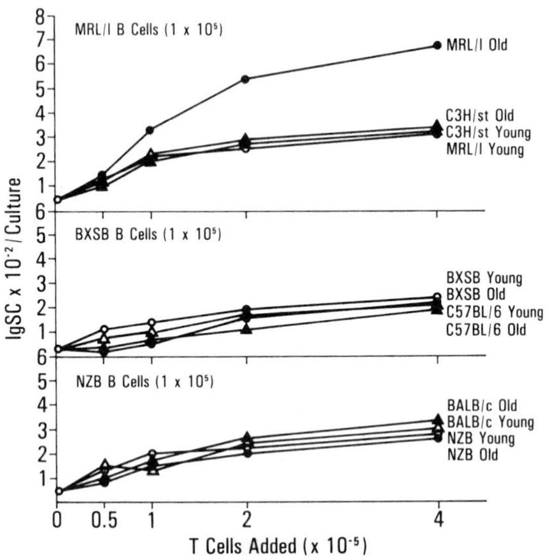

FIGURE 3. Antigen-nonspecific helper activity. Frequency of IgSC in B-cell enriched spleen cell populations obtained from 1-month-old SLE mice to which increments of isolated T cells from syngeneic and allogeneic but *H-2*-identical young (1-month-old) and old (4-7-months-old) animals were added together with LPS.

from T cells of the normal strains (data not shown). The only notable exception is the MRL/ℓ strain in which T cell-enriched populations from older animals (with clinically apparent lymph node hyperplasia) added at a 4:1 ratio to B cells from syngeneic young animals provide 2 to 3 times the help offered by equal numbers of T cells of young syngeneic animals or T cells from young and old normal mice of the same *H-2* haplotype (C3H/St). As we have demonstrated (38), the ratio of T to B cells in MRL/ℓ mice is significantly greater *in vivo* (10:1 in spleen and 30:1 in lymph nodes) than the maximal ratio employed in these experiments *in vitro*. Therefore, the helper activity seen *in vitro* should be far greater in the intact animal. Thus, these experiments and those of others (31) suggest that the advanced maturity of B cells from MRL/ℓ mice may be the result of a heightened helper T-cell activity exerted by the proliferating Ly-1$^+$ T cells.

VII. CELL-MEDIATED IMMUNITY

Several reports have described an age-dependent decline in certain T-cell functions of NZ mice such as allograft rejection, graft-versus-host reaction, *in vitro* responses to phytohemagglutinin, or Con A and killer cell activity against allogeneic tumor cells [reviewed by Zinkernagel and Dixon (45)]. Therefore, Zinkernagel and Dixon (45) and Creighton *et al.* (6) assessed the age-dependent capacities of autoimmune and various normal strains to generate T cell-mediated immune responses against alloantigens and virus-infected target cells as well as cell-mediated immune protection against *Listeria monocytogenes* after systemic infection. Their studies showed that, with the exception of older MRL/ℓ mice which are low responders, none of the remaining SLE-prone strains are particularly high or low responders when tested for the generation of cytotoxic T-cell responses against alloantigens in mixed lymphocyte cultures. Additionally, virus-specific cytolytic activity and recovery following *Listeria* infection are equivalent in all SLE strains to those in normal strains. Thus, the overall cell-mediated immunity of SLE-prone mice, as assessed in these models, is within normal limits.

Recently, Botzenhardt *et al.* (4) described the development of significant unidirectional, primary T cell-mediated lympholytic (CML) reactions by lymphoid cells of NZB mice against *H-2*-identical allogeneic cells. These investigators speculated that such CML reactions of NZB mice represent an abnormality that may be associated with the pathogenesis of their autoimmunity. Subsequently, our studies (39) and the work of

TABLE V. Primary *in Vitro* CML Reactions of SLE Mice against *H-2* Identical Allogeneic Cells

Effector	Stimulator	Target				% Specific release (Mean ± SD)
		Strain	*H-2*	*Qa-1*	*Mℓs*	
NZB ($H\text{-}2^d$, $Qa\text{-}1^a$, $M\ell s^a$)	BALB/c ($H\text{-}2^d$, $Qa\text{-}1^b$, $M\ell s^b$)	BALB/c	*d*	*b*	*b*	45.0 ± 5.6
↓	↓	DBA/2	*d*	*b*	*a*	49.2 ± 4.0
		B10.D2	*d*	*b*	*b*	46.8 ± 3.5
		DBA/1	*q*	*b*	*a*	55.5 ± 1.0
		AKR	*k*	*b*	*a*	46.9 ± 1.3
		ASW	*s*	*b*	*c*	55.6 ± 0.2
		C57BL/6	*b*	*b*	*b*	48.9 ± 5.9
NZB	BALB/c	B10.A	*k/d*	*a*	*c*	41.6 ± 3.2
↓	↓	SJL	*s*	*a*	*c*	27.7 ± 4.1
		B10.A(5R)	*b/d*	*a*	*b*	25.7 ± 10.0
		NZB	*d*	*a*	*a*	15.3 ± 2.2
		SWR	*q*	*a*	*	14.4 ± 12.4
		A/J	*a*	*a*	*c*	13.7 ± 10.8
MRL/ℓ ($H\text{-}2^k$, $Qa\text{-}1^b$)	AKR	AKR	*k*	*b*	*a*	-1.0 ± 4.8
MRL/ℓ ($H\text{-}2^k$, $Qa\text{-}1^b$)	C57BR	C57BR	*k*	*a*	*	7.7 ± 1.7
BXSB ($H\text{-}2^b$, $Qa\text{-}1^b$)	C57BL/6	C57BL/6	*b*	*b*	*b*	-2.4 ± 0.8
BXSB ($H\text{-}2^b$, $Qa\text{-}1^b$)	B6.Tla^a	B6.Tla^a	*b*	*a*	*	3.0 ± 2.0

* *Not known.*

Rich *et al.* (30) confirmed the above finding. Rich *et al.* (30) examined the cross-reactivity patterns of NZB anti-$H\text{-}2^d$ effector cells and concluded that such cells exhibit specificity for antigenic determinants associated with the murine $Qa\text{-}1^b$ genetic locus. We also attempted to determine whether such an activity is a general characteristic of all SLE-prone strains and to define the specificities of such reactions (43). The results summarized in Table V indicate the following: (a) NZB effector cells sensitized with BALB/c stimulators cross-react with target cells of varying *H-2* and *Mℓs* backgrounds; (b) Although such effector cells cause optimum lysis of targets bearing $Qa\text{-}1^b$ determinants, considerable degrees of specific lysis also occur with certain targets bearing $Qa\text{-}1^a$ antigenic determinants; (c) two other SLE-prone murine strains, BXSB and MRL/ℓ, do not display cytolytic activity against *H-2*-identical allogeneic cells irrespective of the *Qa-1* antigenic phenotype of the target cells; therefore, such CML reactions against *H-2*-identical allogeneic cells are not necessarily related to the development of murine SLE. As depicted in Fig. 4, significant inhibition of NZB anti-$H\text{-}2^d$ CML activity is observed when effector and stimulator cells are treated simultaneously, but not separately, with anti-Rauscher gp70 antibody. Curiously enough, independent treatment of the effector, stimulator, or target cells with anti-gp70 is without effect. As also shown in Fig. 4, this inhibition is specific, considering that $F(ab')_2$ anti-gp70 is as effective as whole IgG antibody; anti-gp70 adsorbed with Sepharose-bound gp70 is ineffective; nonimmune IgG, anti-p30, anti-Ig, anti-Thy-1.2 and a mixture of anti-Ig and anti-Thy-1.2 antibodies all are without effect. Anti-gp70 inhibits only primary and secondary NZB anti-$H\text{-}2^d$ responses, but not NZB responses against *H-2*-incompatible cells or secondary responses among $H\text{-}2^d$-compatible, immunologically normal strains of mice (Tables VI and VII).

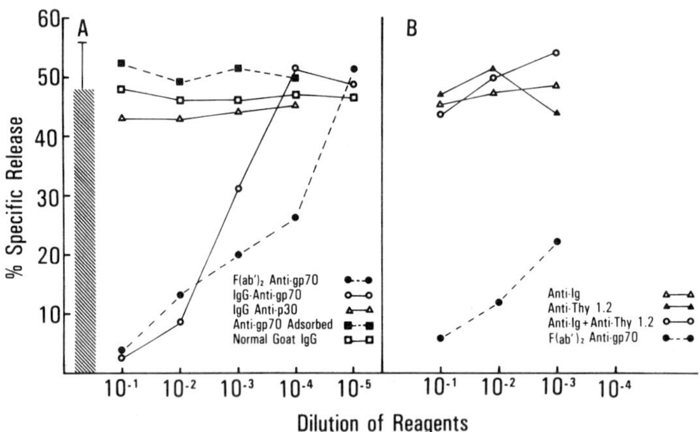

FIGURE 4. Specificity of anti-gp70 induced inhibition of NZB anti-*H-2*^{d} CML reactions. A mixture of NZB effector and BALB/c stimulator cells (6×10^6 each) were treated (30 min, 4°C) with 100 μl dilutions of the indicated reagents, washed once and then incubated for 5 days in triplicate cultures of 2×10^6 cells of each type. Untreated ^{51}Cr-labeled target cells (1×10^5) were added at the final 4 hr of incubation. Dashed column indicates degree of lysis in untreated controls.

Furthermore, anti-gp70 treatment of NZB effector and BALB/c stimulator cells inhibits the expression of NZB cytolytic cross-reactivity against both *Qa-1*^{b} and *Qa-1*^{a} bearing target cells and cross-reactivities not only against *H-2*-identical targets but also against *H-2*-incompatible, *Qa-1*^{b} target cells (data not shown).

Thus, it appears that generation of NZB effector cells depends on cognitive events occurring during incubation with BALB/c cells and subsequent expression of gp70 in the culture and not on histocompatibility or other alloantigens located on the target cells. NZB mice are known to express a unique form of virion-associated gp70 (12), and graft-versus-host reactions induce expressions of retroviral antigens (27). We may postulate that due to minor histocompatibility differences between NZB and BALB/c cells, retroviral gp70 is produced by NZB cells.

TABLE VI. Effect of Anti-gp70 on Primary and Secondary NZB Anti-BALB/c and on Secondary B10.D2 Anti-BALB/c and DBA/2 Anti-BALB/c CML Responses*

Type of response	Effector-stimulator	Target	Treatment of effectors and stimulators with:** Anti-gp70 % specific release (Mean ± SD)	Adsorbed anti-gp70 % specific release (Mean ± SD)
Primary *in vitro*	NZB-BALB/c	BALB/c	12.1	36.7
Secondary***	NZB-BALB/c	BALB/c	30.3	75.2
Secondary	B10.D2-BALB/c	BALB/c	51.8	45.4
Secondary	DBA/2-BALB/c	BALB/c	89.8	89.4

**Results of two experiments.*

***A mixture of effector and stimulator cells (6×10^6 of each) were treated (30 min, 4°C) with 100 μl (65 μl) IgG goat anti-Rauscher gp70 or anti-gp70 adsorbed with Sepharose-bound gp70 before being cultured for 5 days in triplicate cultures of 2×10^6 cells of each type.*

****NZB, B10.D2 and BDA/2 mice were first sensitized* in vivo *with BALB/c cells. Splenocytes were obtained at day 14 and incubated for 5 days* in vitro *with BALB/c irradiated stimulator cells. Five days later, BALB/c target cells were added.*

TABLE VII. Effect of Anti-gp70 on NZB CML Reactions against *H-2*-Compatible and -Incompatible Allogeneic Cells*

Effector	Stimulator-target		Treatment of effectors and stimulators with:**	
	Strain	*H-2*	Anti-gp70 % specific release (Mean ± SD)	Adsorbed anti-gp70 % specific release (Mean ± SD)
NZB ($H\text{-}2^d$) ↓	BALB/c	*d*	6.7	62.6
	B10.D2	*d*	3.9	50.9
	DBA/2	*d*	-4.8	34.8
	LG/J	*d*	11.4	44.8
NZB ($H\text{-}2^d$) ↓	C3H/St	*k*	76.7	76.9
	C57BL/6	*b*	78.6	86.8
	NZB	*z*	74.6	69.3
	MRL/ℓ	*k*	59.1	62.5
	129GIX$^+$	*bc*	50.7	46.7
	129GIX$^-$	*bc*	64.9	66.9
	SJL	*s*	61.9	63.8
	SWR	*q*	62.8	61.9
C57BL/6 ($H\text{-}2^b$)	BALB/c	*d*	92.9	90.3
SJL ($H\text{-}2^s$)	BALB/c	*d*	89.6	89.9
SWR	BALB/c	*d*	86.4	76.7

* *Results of three experiments.*

** *A mixture of effector and stimulator cells (6 × 10^6 of each) was treated (30 min, 4°C) with 100 µl (65 µg) IgG goat anti-Rauscher gp70 or anti-gp70 adsorbed on Sepharose-bound gp70, washed once and then incubated for 5 days in triplicate cultures of 2 × 10^6 cells of each type. Target cells were added at the final 4 hr of incubation.*

This in turn, induces secondary memory-type responses by the NZB effectors against stimulator cells that cross-react with various target cells. The accuracy of this interpretation is reinforced by our experiments,[3] in which Rauscher gp70 induced NZB spleen cells to become cytotoxic for BALB/c targets.

VIII. TOLERANCE SUSCEPTIBILITY

It has been demonstrated that six to eight-week-old NZB and NZB/W mice are relatively resistant to induction of tolerance by the T-dependent antigens, deaggregated bovine gamma globulin (BGG) and human gamma globulin (HGG), compared with many normal strains of mice (16, 33). This abnormality may be related to the pathogenesis of disease in these mice since the spontaneous development of autoantibody might result from resistance to, termination of, or breakdown of self-tolerance. In related experiments conducted in our laboratory by Izui *et al.*[4] not only NZB and NZB/W mice but also MRL/ℓ and BXSB mice exhibit resistance to the induction of tolerance to deaggregated HGG or even to biofiltered HGG (to ensure removal of any aggregates) at five weeks of age (Table VIII). Of interest, MRL/n and female BXSB, which are relatively normal immunologically compared with MRL/ℓ and male BXSB, are sensitive to the induction of tolerance. Therefore, this abnormal resistance to induction of tolerance to a T-dependent antigen seems to be a common feature of all autoimmune mice. Detailed studies in BXSB mice indicate that the defect in tolerance induction to HGG resides at the bone-marrow cell level. Of the

[3] *A. N. Theofilopoulos, D. L. Shawler, J. Elder, and F. J. Dixon. NZB anti-*H-2^{d} *CML responses induced by retroviral gp70. In preparation.*

[4] *S. Izui, L. M. Hang, L. Thor, and F. J. Dixon. Tolerance susceptibility in murine SLE strains. In preparation.*

TABLE VIII. Effect of DHGG on Induction of Tolerance to HGG

Strain*	Anti-HGG (μg/ml)** Control	DHGG	% of control
NZB	123 ± 20	79 ± 20	64
NZBxW	167 ± 45	123 ± 78	74
MRL/ℓ	35 ± 16	34 ± 14	97
BXSB male	196 ± 138	263 ± 118	134
MRL/n	110 ± 19	20 ± 8	18
BXSB female	24 ± 13	2 ± 1	8
NZW	71 ± 16	5 ± 2	7
BALB/c	36 ± 13	1 ± 2	3
C57BL/6	27 ± 13	2 ± 1	7
C3H/St	33 ± 12	2 ± 0.3	6
SJL	>400	>400	100

* *5 weeks old.*

** *3 mg DHGG (160,000 g, 150 min) were injected ip on day 0. 400 μg AHGG were injected iv on day 10 and anti-HGG activity in sera was determined on day 17 or 24 by RIA.*

strains that do not generally develop the lupus-like disease, only SJL mice are resistant to tolerance induction; but this strain is known for other immunologic abnormalities as well (13). Apart from abnormalities in tolerance induction to T-dependent antigens documented in the studies of Izui *et al.*,[4] others (15) have also demonstrated that splenic B cells derived from NZB/W mice are less susceptible than B cells from normal strains of mice to tolerance induction by a T-independent tolerogen (TNP-HGG) with low, but not high, epitope density. One can speculate that a similar loss of the susceptibility to tolerance induction to self-antigens at the B or T cell level might lead to autoantibody formation and disease.

IX. ROLE OF THYMUS

Several histologic and hormonally related defects of thymuses from NZB/W mice have been described [reviewed in Theofilopoulos and Dixon (40)]. Since the symptoms of autoimmune disease begin at different times in congenic MRL/ℓ and MRL/n mice and in male compared to female BSXB mice, we interchanged thymus grafts among these strains in attempting to learn how the actual thymus effect is related to the onset of SLE.[5] As depicted in Fig. 5, MRL/ℓ mice thymectomized when 1 day old and transplanted at 1 month of age with MRL/n thymuses retain the disease phenotype of the unmanipulated MRL/ℓ mice, including lymphoproliferation and a 50% mortality rate at 6 months of age. Similarly, 50% of thymectomized MRL/n mice transplanted with MRL/ℓ thymuses die by 17 months of age, as do the unmanipulated controls. In contrast, MRL/ℓ mice thymectomized when newborn but not given thymic transplants do not develop lymphoid hyperplasia and autoimmune disease, and 100% of them are alive by the 13th month of age (time of termination of the experiment), a point well beyond the 90% death rate of control unmanipulated mice (9 months of age). Serologically, the MRL/ℓ recipients of MRL/n thymuses behave like the unmanipulated MRL/ℓ animals with hypergammaglobulinemia and high levels of various autoantibodies.

In contrast, MRL/ℓ thymectomized but not transplanted mice have greatly reduced levels of serum IgG and background levels of anti-DNA antibodies (data not shown). We conclude that T-cell differentiation in the thymus is a necessary component in the MRL phenotype for development of lymphoproliferation and early autoimmune disease, but that the genotype of the thymic

[5] *A. N. Theofilopoulos, R. S. Balderas, D. L. Shawler, S. Lee, and F. J. Dixon. Role of the thymus in murine lupus.* J. Exp. Med. 153, *1405, 1981.*

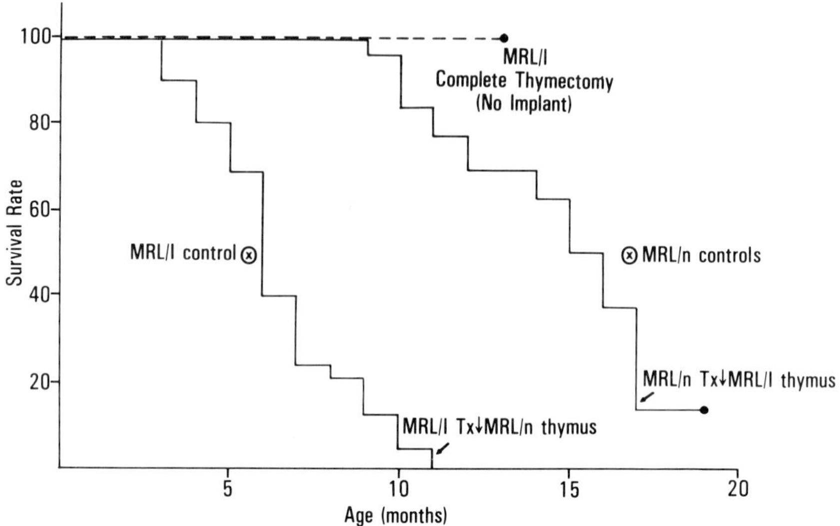

FIGURE 5. Survival rates of MRL/ℓ mice thymectomized when newborn but not transplanted, MRL/ℓ mice thymectomized and transplanted at 1 month of age with MRL/n thymus, and MRL/n mice thymectomized and transplanted at 1 month of age with MRL/ℓ thymus. The asterisk depicts the time of 50% survival for control unmanipulated mice.

microenvironment where differentiation occurs is irrelevant. Furthermore, the differentiation of MRL/n T cells in a thymic microenvironment that possesses the *ℓpr* genotype does not lead to abnormal T-cell differentiation or early autoimmunity. We do not know, as yet, whether the thymic effect in expression of lymphoproliferation and early disease in MRL/ℓ mice is exerted prethymically, intrathymically or postthymically, but these and other findings suggest that the defect associated with SLE in these mice lies at the stem cell level.

Preliminary experiments with BXSB mice indicate similarly that the genotype of the thymus is irrelevant in the development of autoimmunity since thymectomized BXSB males and females, when transplanted with thymuses from the opposite gender, sustain no alterations in the disease pattern typical for their strain. Additionally, our unpublished studies[6] and those of others (34) indicate that neonatal thymectomy enhances the disease of NZB/W mice, unlike that of MRL/ℓ mice, a finding that once again highlights the differences among the SLE-prone murine strains.

X. CELLULAR TRANSFER OF AUTOIMMUNE DISEASE

Transplantation of hematopoietic stem cells from bone marrow and spleen provides a biological approach to the question of the genetic and cellular basis for autoimmunity. Congenic inbred strains enable the researcher to perform cell-transfer studies without interference by background antigenic differences between graft and host. We recently transferred male and female bone marrow cells from 1-month-old BXSB mice into male and female lethally irradiated BXSB recipients of the same age, then watched for signs of disease (10). As shown in Fig. 6, the disease transfer is dependent not on the sex of the recipient but on the sex of the donor cells, with male bone marrow inducing early disease (glomerulonephritis and death) in both male and female recipients and female marrow inducing late disease in both male and female recipients. Similar results are obtained by transferring spleen cells from 4-month-old donors to 2-month-old lethally irradiated recipients. Once again the sex of the spleen cell donor and not the sex of the recipient determines the pace of disease development. Furthermore, the recipients express serologic markers similar to those of the donors. Based on these results, the male specific effect that accelerates autoimmune disease in the BXSB is not hormonally or environmentally

[6] *A. N. Theofilopoulos, R. S. Balderas, and F. J. Dixon. Transfer of autoimmune disease among MRL/ℓ and MRL/n mice.* Fed. Proceed. 40, *973, 1981 (abstract).*

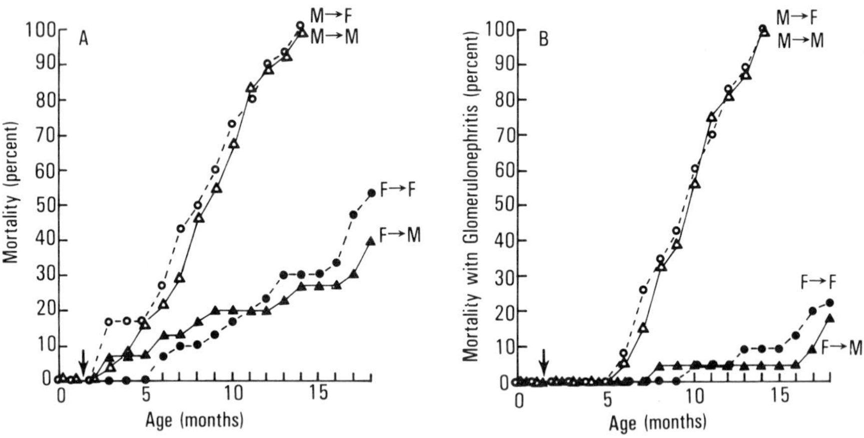

FIGURE 6. (A) Mortality from all causes in BXSB bone marrow chimaeras. Recipients were lethally irradiated (850R) and infused with donor bone marrow (5×10^7 cells) at six weeks of age, as shown by the arrow. Male recipients are depicted by triangles; females by circles. Male bone marrow is shown by open symbols; females by closed symbols. In summary, (△) M → M; (○) M → F; (▲) F → M; and (●) F → F. (B) Mortality from documented glomerulonephritis in BXSB bone marrow sex chimeras.

mediated, but rather is expressed in the hematopoietic/lymphoid stem-cell populations. Moreover, since spleen cells obtained from older male mice that previously manifested disease do not produce disease in the recipients any faster than bone marrow from premorbid mice, the active cells in these transfers seem to be stem cells, not differentiated autoantibody secreting B cells; and the development of BXSB disease does not appear to result from an accumulation of defects at the stem cell level, which are equally abnormal throughout the animal's life. Further experiments seem to indicate that the male dominant effect in BXSB mice is Y-chromosome associated, since the autoimmune phenotype is transmitted as a dominant trait to F_1 hybrids (25, 40) and since castration of male BXSB mice has no effect on disease development (11).

Similar bone marrow and spleen cell transfer experiments have been performed among the congenic MRL/ℓ and MRL/n mice. In each instance, 1-month-old lethally irradiated MRL/n mice that received bone marrow or spleen cells from 1-month-old MRL/ℓ mice, as well as those receiving MRL/ℓ fetal liver cells from 17-day-old fetuses, developed at 3 to 5 months post-transplantation a severe wasting syndrome without lymphadenopathy but, instead, severe depletion of lymph node and spleen cells (Table IX). The basis of this phenomenon, resembling an advanced graft-versus-host reaction, is unclear at this time, but further analysis may provide important clues on the etiopathogenesis of the MRL/ℓ disease. In contrast, the MRL/n → MRL/ℓ chimeras showed significantly prolonged survival (>10 months) as well as suppression of lymphadenopathy and splenomegaly, indicating again the irrelevance of the host's thymus and environment in disease development. Also serum IgG levels and autoantibodies were significantly lower than in MRL/ℓ → MRL/ℓ chimeras, which die within 5 to 6 months of birth. In MRL/ℓ recipients of spleen cell inocula derived from both MRL/ℓ and MRL/n mice, a prolongation of survival and inhibition of lymphoadenopathy was seen. If this type of chimera is shown to be composed of both cell types, then the results may suggest modulation of *ℓpr* gene expression by the MRL/n lymphoid cells.

To overcome the problem of the wasting syndrome in MRL/n recipients of MRL/ℓ cells, we intend to substitute irradiated MRL/ℓ mice as recipients. This approach stems from our observation (44) indicating amelioration of disease, lack of lymphoproliferation and long survival in 3-month-old MRL/ℓ mice exposed to total lymphoid irradiation (17 fractions of 200 rad each for a total of 3,400 rad) or a single dose of whole body irradiation (300 rad; Fig. 7). Considering the ameliorating effects of irradiation in MRL/ℓ mice, like those

TABLE IX. Effect of Cell Transfers on the *ℓpr* Phenotype

Donor	850r Recipient	50% Survival in days BM			Clinical signs
		BM	Spleen	Fet. liver	
+/+	+/+	344(11)*	>300(21)**	--	None
ℓpr	+/+	117(41)	140(16)	90(8)	Wasting-LN atrophy
+/+	*ℓpr*	>300(20)***	--	--	Slight LN enlargement
ℓpr	*ℓpr*	150(9)	186(9)	--	Lymphadenopathy
mixed****	*ℓpr*	--	203(11)	--	Slight LN enlargement

* *Numbers in parenthesis indicate the number of animals studied in each group.*

** *19 of 21 animals alive beyond 300 days.*

*** *11 of 20 dead (3 at 7 months, 6 at 9 months, 2 at 10 months). Nine alive beyond 300 days.*

**** *Equal number of splenocytes* (5×10^7) *from 1-month-old ℓpr and +/+ mice.*

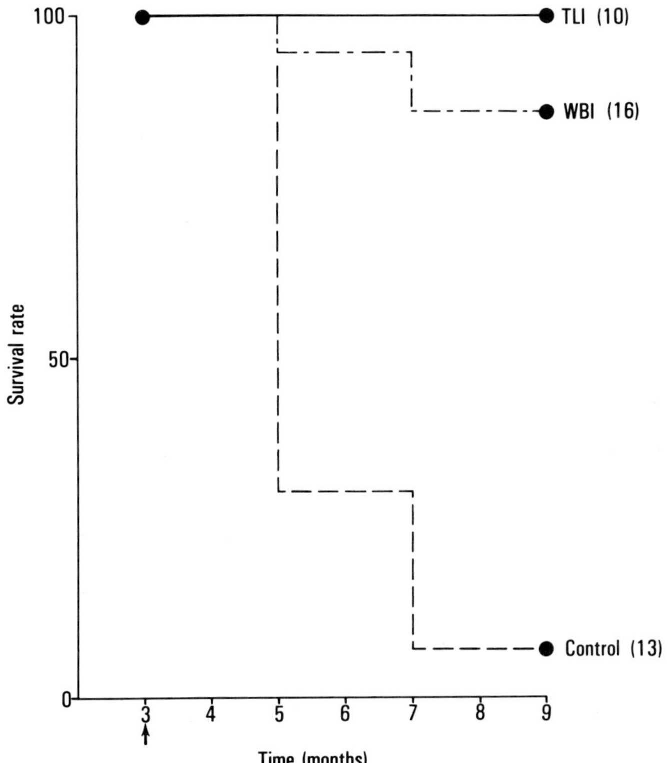

FIGURE 7. Survival rates of total lymphoid irradiation (TLI) or whole body irradiation (WBI) treated animals compared to controls. Numbers in parenthesis indicate the numbers of mice included in each group. The arrow indicates the time of irradiation.

previously reported in the NZB/W strain (21, 32) (A. N. Theofilopoulos, unpublished observations), irradiation may become a practical method for treating SLE and for defining more explicitly the humoral and cellular abnormalities involved.

XI. CONCLUSIONS

It is obvious from the foregoing discussion that the pathogenic mechanisms fundamental to murine SLE are highly complex, apparently well-programmed genetically but still ill-defined.

We now have identified many hallmarks of this disorder, put into proper perspective the role of certain autoantibodies in disease development, demonstrated that a *generalized* suppressor T cell defect is not a factor of murine SLE, and in general determined that different types of primary or secondary humoral and cellular abnormalities can underlie SLE as a syndrome. The variable and consistent immunopathologic features of the SLE-prone murine strains are summarized in Tables X, XI, and XII. If there is a common etiology for these defects of the several murine strains that develop SLE, it has not yet been defined.

TABLE X. Murine SLE Variable Immunopathologic Features

Immunopathologic features	MRL/ℓ	BXSB male	NZB/W female	NZB
NTA	±	+	+++	+++
Anti red blood cells	0	+	++	+++
Anti Sm	++	0	0	0
Rh Factor and arthritis	+	0	0	0
Vasculitis	+	0	0	0
Lymphoid hyperplasia	+++	++	+	+
Cell type	T↑	B↑	B&T↓	B&T↓
Sex	F&M	M	F	F
Sex hormone dependence	?	0	+	±

TABLE XI. Murine SLE-Consistent Immunopathologic Features

I.	Polyclonal B-cell hyperactivity (<1 mo)
	Hypergammaglobulinemia
	Early resistance to tolerance
	No associated generalized T-cell regulatory defect
II.	Multiple autoimmune responses
	Antinuclear (DNA) antibodies
	Antiretroviral gp70 antibodies
III.	Accelerating factors with early SLE
IV.	Immune complex pathogenesis
	Circulating immune complexes → C activation
	Fatal IC glomerulonephritis (DNA-gp70)
	Degenerative arterial lesions and myocardial infarcts
	Early thymic atrophy

Our analysis of F_2 offspring derived from crosses of SLE strains among themselves and with normal strains (40), as well as the studies of others (29) (R. Riblet, personal communication) on recombinant inbred strains derived from NZB crosses with normal strains further indicate that (a) murine SLE has a multifactorial genetic basis; (b) many of the individual SLE traits appear to be determined by single genes segregating quite independently from other disease-related genes; (c) in recombinant mice there is no association of any *H-2* phenotype with autoantibody production; (d) murine SLE can be associated with various constellations of such genetic abnormalities and some constellations predispose to late life SLE; and (e) a variety of different disease accelerating factors exist (viral, hormonal, Y-chromosome associated, *ℓpr* gene) which, when superimposed on the predisposition to late life disease, cause

TABLE XII. Murine SLE

Genetic background	
Various independent A-I traits	
Immunologic characteristics	
Stem cells	- Transfer disease, BXSB
B cells	- Hyperfunction, all strains
	- A-I responses, all strains
	- # ↑, BXSB
T cells	- Generalized Ts normal, all strains
	- Th ↑ MRL/ℓ
	- # ↑ MRL/ℓ
Thymus	- Essential for MRL disease
	- Not essential for NZ disease
Nonlymphoid tissues	- Noncontributory to disease, BXSB, MRL/ℓ
Accelerating factors	
Intrinsic	- Female hormones, NZBxW
	- Y linked, BXSB
	- *ℓpr* gene, MRL
Extrinsic	- LCM, all strains
Pathogenesis	
Auto-Abs-IC-C activation	
Glomerulonephritis	
Vascular disease, myocardial infarction	
Arthritis, MRL/ℓ	
Thymic atrophy	

an early, severe SLE. Our cell-transfer experiments in BXSB mice clearly indicate that the disease in this strain is associated with a lymphohemopoietic stem-cell defect, but it is not yet clear whether the defect is positive (i.e., the presence of an abnormal cell type) or negative (i.e., the absence of a normal cell type). Furthermore, thymectomy and irradiation experiments clearly indicate that the MRL/ℓ disease is due to the presence of an abnormal T-cell type that accelerates autoantibody formation. Future genetic and cell-transfer experiments with well-defined cell populations in this and the other autoimmune murine strains as well as study of immunoregulation of responses to autoantigens should provide further insights into the etiopathogenesis of murine and, it is hoped, human SLE.

REFERENCES

1. Accinni, L. and Dixon, F. J. Degenerative vascular disease and myocardial infarction in mice with lupus-like syndrome. *Am. J. Pathol. 96*, 477 (1979).

2. Andrews, B. S., Eisenberg, R. S., Theofilopoulos, A. N., Izui, S., Wilson, C. B., McConahey, P. J., Murphy, E. D., Roths, J. B., and Dixon, F. J. Spontaneous murine lupus-like syndromes. Clinical and immunopathological manifestations in several strains. *J. Exp. Med. 148*, 1198 (1978).

3. Barthold, D. R., Kysela, S., and Steinberg, A. D. Decline in suppressor T cell function with age in female NZB mice. *J. Immunol. 112*, 9 (1974).

4. Botzenhardt, V., Klein, J., and Ziff, M. Cytotoxic reactions of NZB spleen cells with lymphocytes of MHC identical strains. *J. Exp. Med. 147*, 1435 (1978).

5. Creighton, W. D., Katz, D. H., and Dixon, F. J. Antigen-specific immunocompetency, B cell function and regulatory helper and suppressor T cell activities in spontaneously autoimmune mice. *J. Immunol. 123*, 2627 (1979).

6. Creighton, W. D., Zinkernagel, R. M., and Dixon, F. J. T cell-mediated immune responses of lupus-prone BXSB mice and other murine strains. *Clin. Exp. Immunol. 37*, 181 (1979).

7. Eisenberg, R. A., Tan, E. M., and Dixon, F. J. Presence of anti-Sm reactivity in autoimmune mouse strains. *J. Exp. Med. 147*, 582 (1978).

8. Eisenberg, R. A., Theofilopoulos, A. N., Andrews, B. S., Peters, C. J., Thor, L. J., and Dixon, F. J. Natural thymocytotoxic autoantibodies in autoimmune and normal mice. *J. Immunol. 122*, 2272 (1979).

9. Eisenberg, R. A., Thor, L. J., and Dixon, F. J. Serum-serum interactions in autoimmune mice. *Arthritis Rheum. 22*, 1074 (1979).

10. Eisenberg, R. A., Izui, S., McConahey, P. J., Hang, L. M., Peters, C. J., Theofilopoulos, A. N., and Dixon, F. J. Male determined accelerated autoimmune disease in BXSB mice: transfer by bone marrow and spleen cells. *J. Immunol. 125*, 1032 (1980).

11. Eisenberg, R. A., Lee, S., and Dixon, F. J. Effect of castration on male-determined acceleration of autoimmune disease in BXSB mice. *J. Immunol. 125*, 1959 (1980).

12. Elder, J. H., Gautsch, J. W., Jensen, F. C., Lerner, R. A., Chused, T. M., Morse, H. C., Hartley, J. W., and Rowe, W. P. Differential expression of two distinct xenotropic viruses in NZB mice. *Clin. Immunol. Immunopathol. 15*, 258 (1980).

13. Fujiwara, M. and Cinader, N. Cellular aspects of tolerance. VI. The effect of age on responsiveness and tolerance inducibility of SJL mice. *Cell. Immunol. 12*, 205 (1974).

14. Gershwin, M. E., Castles, J. J., Ikeda, R. M., Erickson, K., and Montero, J. Studies of congenitally immunologic mutant New Zealand mice. I. Autoimmune features of hereditarily asplenic (Dh/+) NZB mice; reduction of naturally occurring thymocytotoxic antibody and normal suppressor function. *J. Immunol. 122*, 710 (1979).

15. Goldings, E. A., Cohen, P. L., McFadden, S. F., Ziff, M., and Vitetta, E. S. Defective B cell tolerance in adult (NZBxNZW)F_1 mice. *J. Exp. Med. 152*, 730 (1980).

16. Golub, E. S., and Weigle, W. O. Studies on the induction of immunologic unresponsiveness. III. Antigen form and mouse strain variation. *J. Immunol. 102*, 389 (1979).

17. Izui, S., McConahey, P. J., and Dixon, F. J. Increased spontaneous polyclonal activation of B lymphocytes in mice with spontaneous autoimmune disease. *J. Immunol. 121*, 2213 (1978).

18. Izui, S., McConahey, P. J., Theofilopoulos, A. N., and Dixon, F. J. Association of circulating retroviral gp70-anti-gp70 immune complexes with murine systemic lupus erythematosus. *J. Exp. Med. 149*, 1099 (1979).

19. Izui, S. and Eisenberg, R. A. Circulating anti-DNA-rheumatoid factor complexes in MRL/ℓ mice. *Clin. Immunol. Immunopathol. 15*, 536 (1980).

20. Kincade, P. W., Lee, G., Fernandes, G., Moore, M. A. S., Williams, N., and Good, R. A. Abnormalities in clonable B lymphocytes and myeloid progenitors in autoimmune NZB mice. *Proc. Natl. Acad. Sci. U.S.A. 76*, 3464 (1979).

21. Kotzin, B. L. and Strober, S. Reversal of NZB/NZW disease with total irradiation. *J. Exp. Med. 150*, 371 (1979).

22. Krakauer, R. S., Waldmann, T. A., and Strober, W. Loss of suppressor T cells in adult NZB/NZW mice. *J. Exp. Med. 144*, 662 (1976).

23. Manny, N., Datta, S. K., and Schwartz, R. S. Synthesis of IgM by cells of NZB and SWR mice and their crosses. *J. Immunol. 122*, 1220 (1979).

24. Moutsopoulos, H. M., Boehm-Truitt, M., Kassan, S. S., and Chused, T. N. Demonstration of activation of B lymphocytes in New Zealand black mice at birth by an immunoradiometric assay. *J. Immunol. 119*, 1639 (1977).

25. Murphy, E. D. and Roths, J. B. Autoimmunity and lymphoproliferation: induction by mutant gene *ℓpr*, and acceleration by a male-associated factor in strain BXSB mice. *In* "Genetic Control of Autoimmune Disease" (N. R. Rose, P. E. Bigazzi, and N. L. Warner, eds.), p. 207. Elsevier-North-Holland, Amsterdam, 1979.

26. Ohsugi, Y. and Gershwin, E. Studies of congenitally immunologic mutant New Zealand mice. III. Growth of B lymphocyte clones in congenitally athymic (nude) and hereditarily asplenic (Dh/+) NZB mice: A primary B cell defect. *J. Immunol. 123*, 1260 (1979).

27. Phillips, S. M., Hirsch, M. S., Andre-Schwartz, J., Solnik, C., Black, P., Schwartz, R. S., Merrill, J. P., and Carpenter, C. B. Cellular immunity in the mouse. V. Further studies on leukemia virus activation in allogeneic reaction mice: stimulating parameters. *Cell. Immunol. 15*, 169 (1975).

28. Primi, D., Hammarstrom, L., and Smith, C. I. E. Genetic control of lymphocyte suppression. I. Lack of suppression in aged NZB mice is due to a B cell defect. *J. Immunol. 121*, 2241 (1978).

29. Raveche, S., Brown, L. J., Novotny, E. A., Tjio, J. H., Shreffler, D. C., and Steinberg, A. D. Separable genetic traits in NZB mice. *Arthritis Rheum. 23*, 735 (1980). Abstr.

30. Rich, R. R., Sedberry, D. A., Kastner, D. L., and Chu, L. Primary *in vitro* cytotoxic response of NZB spleen cells to *Qa-1*^{b}-associated antigenic determinants. *J. Exp. Med. 150*, 1555 (1979).

31. Sawada, S. and Talal, N. Evidence for a helper cell promoting anti-DNA antibody production in murine lupus. *Arthritis Rheum. 22*, 655 (1979). Abstr.

32. Slavin, S. Successful treatment of autoimmune disease in (NZB/NZW) F_1 female mice by using fractionated total lymphoid irradiation. *Proc. Natl. Acad. Sci. U.S.A. 76*, 5274 (1979).

33. Staples, R. J. and Talal, N. Relative inability to induce tolerance in adult NZB and NZB/NZW F_1 mice. *J. Exp. Med. 129*, 123 (1969).

34. Steinberg, A. D., Roths, J. B., Murphy, E. D., Steinberg, R. T., and Raveche, E. S. Effects of thymectomy or androgen administration upon the autoimmune disease of MRL/Mp-*ℓpr/ℓpr* mice. *J. Immunol. 125*, 871 (1980).

35. Takatsu, K. and Ishizaka, K. Reaginic antibody formation in the mouse. VIII. Depression of the ongoing IgE antibody formation by suppressor T cells. *J. Immunol. 117*, 1211 (1976).

36. Talal, N. Disordered immunologic regulation and autoimmunity. *Transplant. Rev. 31*, 240 (1976).

37. Taurog, J. D., Moutsopoulos, H. M., Rosenberg, Y. J., Chused, T. M., and Steinberg, A. D. CBA/N X-linked B cell defect prevents NZB B cell hyperactivity in F_1 mice. *J. Exp. Med. 150*, 31 (1979).

38. Theofilopoulos, A. N., Eisenberg, R. A., Bourdon, M., Crowell, J. S., Jr., and Dixon, F. J. Distribution of lymphocytes identified by surface markers in murine strains with SLE-like syndromes. *J. Exp. Med. 149*, 516 (1979).

39. Theofilopoulos, A. N., Shawler, D. L., Katz, D. H., and Dixon, F. J. Patterns of immune reactivity in autoimmune murine strains. II. Cell-mediated immune responses induced by *H-2*-identical and *H-2* incompatible stimulator cells. *J. Immunol. 122*, 2319 (1979).

40. Theofilopoulos, A. N. and Dixon, F. J. Etiopathogenesis of murine SLE. *Immunol. Rev. 55*, 179 (1981).

41. Theofilopoulos, A. N., McConahey, P. J., Izui, S., Eisenberg, R. A., Pereira, A. B., and Creighton, W. D. A comparative immunologic analysis of several murine strains with autoimmune manifestations. *Clin. Immunol. Immunopathol. 15*, 258 (1980).

42. Theofilopoulos, A. N., Shawler, D. L., Eisenberg, R. A., and Dixon, F. J. Splenic immunoglobulin-secreting cells and their regulation in autoimmune mice. *J. Exp. Med. 151*, 446 (1980).

43. Theofilopoulos, A. N., Shawler, D. L., Balderas, R. S., Elder, J. H., Katz, D. H., and Dixon, F. J. Specificities of NZB anti-$H\text{-}2^d$ CML reactions: Role of *Qa-1* and retroviral gp70 antigens. *J. Immunol. 126*, 1154 (1981).

44. Theofilopoulos, A. N., Balderas, R. S., Shawler, D. L., Izui, S., Kotzin, B. L., Strober, S., and Dixon, F. J. Inhibition of T cell proliferation and SLE-like syndrome of MRL/ℓ mice by whole body or total lymphoid irradiation. *J. Immunol. 125*, 2137 (1980).

45. Zinkernagel, R. M. and Dixon, F. J. Comparison of T cell-mediated immune responsiveness of NZB, (NZBxNZW) F_1 hybrid mice and other murine strains. *Clin. Exp. Immunol.* *29*, 110 (1977).

Immunopathology: VIIIth International Symposium, 1980

RETROVIRAL GENE EXPRESSION AND MURINE SYSTEMIC LUPUS ERYTHEMATOSUS[1]

Shozo Izui
John E. Elder
Patricia J. McConahey
Frank J. Dixon

Department of Immunopathology,
Scripps Clinic and Research Foundation,
La Jolla, California

Vicki E. Kelley

Department of Medicine,
Brigham and Women's Hospital,
Boston, Massachusetts

Ikuo Hara

Okayama University Medical School
Okayama, Japan

I. INTRODUCTION

Mice of four strains, NZB, NZBxNZW F_1 hybrids (NZBxW), MRL/ℓ and BXSB, spontaneously develop a disease that closely resembles human systemic lupus erythematosus (SLE) (3, 19).

[1]*This is publication No. 2286 from the Immunology Departments, Scripps Clinic and Research Foundation, La Jolla, California. This work was supported in part by U.S.P.H.S. Grant AI-7007, N01-CP-71018, R01-CA-25533, CA-255803, CA-16600, the Cecil H. and Ida M. Green Research Endowment, the Department of Health Service Contract, Commonwealth of Pennsylvania, and the Health Research and Service Foundation of Pittsburgh.*

ISBN 0-12-218320-7

The adjunct immunologic abnormalities are formation of several types of autoantibodies and immune complex (IC) glomerulonephritis. The newly developed MRL/ℓ strain, which has the *ℓpr* (lympho-proliferation) gene, is characterized by massive proliferation of T lymphocytes and glomerulonephritis with high levels of anti-DNA antibodies; 50% of MRL/ℓ mice die by 5 months of age. BXSB is also a new strain, but only the males succumb to this early glomerulonephritis, and their levels of anti-DNA antibodies are low.

An important aspect of murine SLE is the involvement of endogenous retrovirus-related antigens. This relationship was first suggested when retroviral antigens and antibodies to them were found in the circulations of New Zealand mice (22). Subsequently, it was demonstrated that among the several viral proteins, the major envelope glycoprotein gp70 is preferentially expressed in sera of these mice and is also identifiable in IC deposits within their diseased glomeruli (30). This factor is consistent in all the four strains of SLE-prone mice (3). Furthermore, careful immunohistologic study indicates the apparent deposition of ICs containing gp70 in the walls of blood vessels associated with degenerative vascular disease and myocardial infarction, in the ovaries, particularly the zona pellucida surrounding developing ova, and along the basement membranes of epithelia of the genital tract, the gastrointestinal tract, and the female breast (1-3). Therefore, we have investigated endogenous retroviral gp70 as a participant in the pathogenesis of the immunologic disease, murine SLE.

II. EXPRESSION OF RETROVIRAL gp70 IN SERA OF MICE

It is now clear that a variety of immunologically and structurally related gp70s are expressed in every mouse, either in a form that is associated or not associated with viral particles (8) (Table I). The gp70s associated with endogenous retroviruses can be classified largely into three groups, according to the tropism of retroviruses, as follows: (a) ecotropic viruses, which grow in and infect only murine cells, (b) xenotropic viruses, which are produced by murine cells but infect only cells of other species, and (c) amphotropic viruses, which can infect both murine cells and cells of other species. Based on the analysis of tryptic peptide fingerprints of these retroviral gp70s, each group of retroviruses has structurally different molecules of gp70 on its envelope (8, 9). Of further note, even in a single group of viruses, individual retroviruses isolated from different strains of mice do not have identical gp70 molecules.

TABLE I. Classification of Virion- and Non-Virion-Associated gp70s

Virion-associated gp70s	Non-virion-associated gp70s
Xenotropic virus	
NZB type: NZB, NZBxW mice	Serum gp70
Non-NZB type: NIH Swiss, NZW, wild mice, etc.	Thymocyte gp70
Ecotropic virus: AKR, NZBxW, MRL/ℓ, NZW mice, etc.	Epididymal fluid gp70
Amphotropic virus: wild mice	

Besides these virion-associated gp70s, mice express several kinds of non-virion-associated gp70s (Table I). This virion-free gp70 circulates in the blood and is also evident in lymphatic and epithelial tissues (3, 8, 20, 30). The structure of gp70 found free in the serum of many laboratory and wild murine strains is relatively conserved and is closely related to that of gp70 on xenotropic virus isolated only from NZB and NZBxW mice but not from other strains of mice (8, 9). This suggests that the serum gp70 is probably a partial expression of a single provirus present in most murine strains but expressed as complete virus only in NZB and NZBxW mice. Additional studies show that gp70 expressed on surfaces of such lymphoid cells as thymocytes or spleen cells and gp70 found in the epididymis or seminal fluid of the genital tract differ in molecular characteristics from the serum gp70. Lymphoid cell-associated gp70 resembles gp70 of xenotropic viruses isolated from mice other than NZB and NZBxW, including those from NIH Swiss, NZW, and wild mice (9). The genital tract-associated gp70 is structurally similar to ecotropic viral gp70 (8).

Structural analysis of these several kinds of retroviral gp70s provides us with a number of important facts. First, the expression of serum gp70 does not require the production of complete virus particles, since most mice other than NZB and NZBxW have considerable amounts of NZB-type xenotropic viral gp70 in their sera but do not form an NZB-type xenotropic virus. Second, lymphoid cells do not seem to be a major source of serum gp70, because their gp70 is structurally different from serum gp70. Supporting evidence is that neither thymectomy nor exchange of hematopoietic tissues between $129GIX^{+}$ and $129GIX^{-}$ mice changes levels of serum gp70 in either strain (24). Third, the structural unrelatedness between serum gp70 and epididymal gp70 excludes the possible contribution of genital tract gp70 to the circulating pool, although male mice always have higher concentrations of gp70 in sera than females (3, 12). However, because castration of male mice reduces the level of serum gp70 to that of females, and since the higher level is fully restored by injecting testosterone (24), the main source of serum gp70 is apparently a tissue or organ common to males and females and directly or indirectly responsive to testosterone.

We have recently observed that a single intraperitoneal injection of bacterial lipopolysaccharides (LPS) increases the serum concentrations of gp70 5 to 15 times in several strains of mice. These increases begin hours after the injection of LPS, peak after 24 hr, and return to the preinjection levels 3 days after the injection (Fig. 1). Generally, this response occurs only in murine strains that have high concentrations of gp70 (>10 μg/ml) in their sera; strains such as C57BL/6, C3H/St, and BALB/c mice, whose gp70 levels are lower, have little or no response. Although LPS activates xenotropic virus

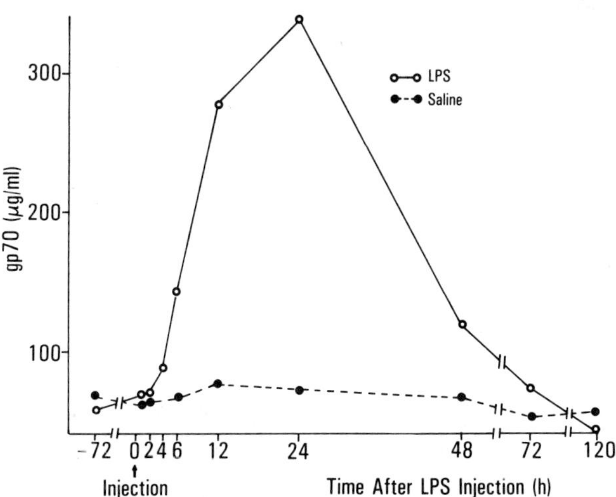

FIGURE 1. Serum gp70 response after a single intraperitoneal injection of 25 μg *E. coli* 0111:B4 LPS in 2-month-old NZB female mice. Each point represents the mean value of 7 mice.

in spleen cell cultures of BALB/c mice (23, 25), the serum gp70 response induced by LPS is independent of virus activation, based on the following experimental results. First, no xenotropic virus was detectable in MRL/ℓ or BXSB mice after the injection of LPS. Second, sucrose density gradient analysis showed that serum gp70 induced by LPS was not associated with viral particles. Third, there was no marked increase in serum concentrations of p30, which is the major structural protein of retrovirus.

The fact that LPS increases serum levels of gp70 in T cell-depleted mice as much as in control mice with normal numbers of T cells excludes the possible involvement of T lymphocytes. In addition, this response is not related to the activation of B lymphocytes by LPS. The irradiation of mice with a lethal dose (1000 rads) 2 days before the injection of LPS completely abolishes the activation of B lymphocytes by LPS, but has no effect on the serum gp70 response. These results are compatible with the hypothesis that lymphoid cells are not a major source of serum gp70. Moreover, the increase in serum levels of gp70 after LPS injection is not a by-product of cell death caused by LPS and subsequent release of gp70, since simultaneously injecting an inhibitor of protein synthesis greatly suppresses the gp70 response. This indicates, instead, that LPS stimulates the synthesis of serum gp70.

A most significant observation is that inducers of acute phase reactants (APR), such as turpentine or poly I-poly C, induce the production of gp70 as effectively as LPS (Table II). However, these APR inducers fail to activate B lymphocytes, ruling out possible contamination with LPS in these preparations. The kinetics of gp70 responses to LPS and to APR inducers are identical. Furthermore, these gp70 responses are kinetically similar to those of APR such as serum amyloid A

TABLE II. Induction of gp70 by Various APR Inducers in NZBxW Mice

Treatment	*gp70* (μg/ml)		*IgM* (μg/ml)	
	Pre	Day 1	Pre	Day 5
LPS*	62 ± 11	590 ± 69	730 ± 150	1670 ± 640
Turpentine**	59 ± 8	413 ± 38	610 ± 40	520 ± 50
Poly I-poly C***	60 ± 7	426 ± 58	460 ± 70	510 ± 90
Saline	52 ± 4	53 ± 7	640 ± 50	690 ± 100

* *25 μg LPS from* E. coli *0111:B4 were injected ip on day 0.*

** *0.05 ml turpentine oil.*

*** *200 μg polyriboinosinic-polyribocytidylic acid.*

protein or haptoglobin (17, 21). Apparently, the expression of gp70 in sera is controlled by a mechanism similar to that for APR.

If gp70 is indeed an APR, gp70 might be synthesized in the liver like most APR. The dependence of serum gp70 concentrations on sex hormone supports this possibility, since liver is a known source of several proteins whose serum concentrations are markedly dependent on sex (10). Additionally, our preliminary studies have demonstrated that the amounts of gp70 in liver homogenates of LPS-injected mice are about five times higher than in uninjected controls. There are no significant increases in other tissue homogenates of these injected animals, including lung, kidney, or spleen. Moreover, the injection of colchicine, which is a known inhibitor of protein release from hepatic cells (27), greatly suppresses the serum gp70 response. Accordingly, the amount of gp70 recoverable in liver homogenates from colchicine-treated mice increases, indicating the accumulation of newly synthesized gp70 in hepatic cells as colchicine inhibits its release. In all probability, hepatic cells are the major source of the NZB-type xenotropic viral gp70 that eventually enters the circulation.

III. IMMUNE RESPONSE TO SERUM gp70 IN MICE

It is clear that several strains of mice respond immunologically to their own retroviral gp70s by forming the corresponding antibodies. Free antibodies to some nonserum gp70s such as AKR ecotropic viral gp70 or Rauscher murine leukemia virus (MuLV) gp70 have been detected in sera of mice carrying the AKR viral genome (7, 12). Apparently, this anti-gp70 antibody is made in response to the AKR ecotropic viral gp70; therefore, this antigen-antibody system could theoretically be a potential source of pathogenic ICs, the importance of which would depend upon the amount of AKR gp70 formed. However, in view of the facts that (a) the serum titers of antibodies to AKR ecotropic viral gp70 do not correlate with the progression of autoimmune disease; (b) two SLE-prone strains of mice, NZB and BXSB, do not have detectable amounts of these antibodies; (c) several immunologically normal strains spontaneously develop these antibodies; and (d) these antibodies are not significantly concentrated in renal eluates of SLE mice (3, 7, 12), it appears that antibodies to AKR ecotropic viral gp70 do not play a significant role in murine SLE.

We have recently demonstrated that murine strains with SLE respond immunologically to serum xenotropic viral gp70 in addition to nonserum gp70s (12). Because of the great excess of xenotropic viral gp70 in sera from these strains, antibodies reacting with xenotropic viral gp70 are not detectable in a free form; nevertheless, one can find antibody-bound gp70 ICs

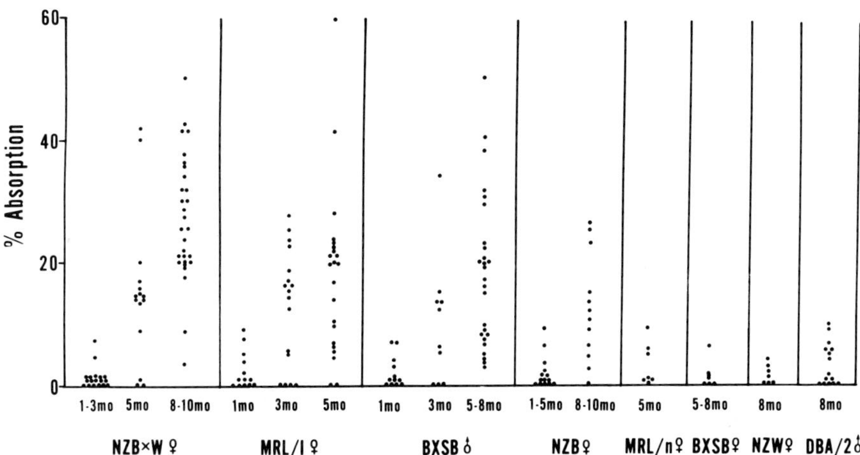

FIGURE 2. Quantitation of Ig-bound gp70 in sera from SLE-prone and normal mice at various ages. Concentrations of gp70 were determined before and after removal of serum Ig by rabbit antimurine IgG antibodies. Results are expressed as the percentage of serum gp70 absorbed with anti-IgG antibodies. [From Izui *et al.* (12).]

in sera from all the SLE-prone mice. In contrast, immunologically normal strains of mice do not develop significant amounts of antibody to serum gp70, at least during the first year of life. This conclusion followed our demonstration that one-fifth to one-half of the gp70 is removable from sera of SLE mice, but not other strains, through absorption by anti-IgG antibodies (Fig. 2). Clearly, the capacity to develop an immune response in this situation is not related to the serum concentrations of xenotropic viral gp70. Even though murine strains with SLE generally tend to have more gp70 than most normal strains, several immunologically normal strains equal or surpass the gp70 values of SLE mice (3, 12). Of course, one cannot exclude the possibility that SLE mice might produce a unique and as yet undiscovered form of retroviral gp70 that may be responsible for the formation of gp70 IC. However, our recent studies of tryptic peptide maps of gp70 isolated from the circulating ICs have shown its resemblance to gp70 from the NZB-type xenotropic virus expressed commonly in sera of all mice, but distinct from gp70s belonging to viruses with other tropisms.

Further immunochemical characterization by two different competitive radioimmunoassays that distinguish AKR ecotropic viral gp70 from xenotropic viral gp70 reveals that gp70 isolated from the circulating ICs does not carry the determinants specific for the AKR ecotropic viral gp70, ruling out the possible involvement of AKR ecotropic virus or a recombinant virus formed between ecotropic virus and xenotropic virus. Isolated antibodies to gp70 from the circulating ICs seem to be directed primarily to gp70 from NZB-type xenotropic virus and have a minimal cross-reactivity with other retroviral gp70s (Table III). This rules out the possibility that antibodies to AKR ecotropic virus or Rauscher MuLV gp70 occasionally found in sera of NZBxW and MRL/ℓ mice (12) participate in the formation of these circulating ICs.

TABLE III. Binding of Anti-gp70 Antibodies Isolated from Circulating ICs to gp70s from Serum and Various Retroviruses

gp70 from	% binding of gp70**
Serum*	66.5
NZB xenotrope virus	59.5
AKR xenotrope virus	25.4
AKR ecotrope virus	10.7
AKR recombinant virus	11.3
Amphotrope virus	<5.0

**Pool from 2-month-old NZBxW mice.*

***Binding of gp70 by anti-gp70 was determined by quantitating the amounts of gp70 absorbed specifically with protein A in the presence of anti-gp70. Without anti-gp70, protein A absorbed less than 5% of serum or retroviral gp70.*

Our observations that the gp70 involved in the formation of circulating ICs is identical to free gp70 commonly present in sera of virtually all murine strains, and that the anti-gp70 antibodies isolated from these ICs react preferentially with NZB-type xenotropic viral gp70, suggest that the abnormality of SLE mice manifested as production of antibodies to their own serum xenotropic viral gp70 and formation of ICs does not originate from their unusual type of gp70, but rather from their unique ability to make an antibody to their own NZB-type xenotropic viral gp70. Such an abnormal immune response may result from their well-known immunologic dysfunction, for example, lack of T cell regulatory function (6), loss of suppressor T cells (4, 18), and/or increased B cell activity (11).

IV. PATHOGENIC SIGNIFICANCE OF gp70 ICs IN MURINE SLE

Several lines of evidence suggest that gp70-anti-gp70 ICs (gp70 ICs) play a role in the pathogenesis of glomerulonephritis that accompanies murine SLE. These complexes increase not only in incidence but also in amount with the progression of renal disease in all the SLE strains (12). The appearance of gp70 ICs in circulating blood varies with age among the SLE susceptible strains, but parallels the onset of renal disease and persists throughout its course. For example, MRL/ℓ and male BXSB mice with the most rapidly progressive disease develop gp70 ICs in their sera earlier than the other SLE mice. However, a substrain of MRL/ℓ mice, MRL/n, and female BXSB mice, which develop glomerulonephritis in the second year of life with a 50% mortality after about 15 months, fail to develop any Ig-complexed gp70 during the first 8 months of life. The presence of the Ig-complexed gp70 in eluates from the diseased kidneys, but not in those from healthy mice, also indicates the involvement of these gp70 ICs in the renal lesions. In addition, renal eluates from these sick mice contain larger quantities of gp70 than those of young, healthy mice or those of old, but immunologically normal mice. However, amounts of the retroviral structural protein p30 are similar in both eluates.

These results strongly suggest, but do not prove, that circulating gp70 ICs are a potential source of renal injury in all mice with SLE. In fact, these mice produce a variety of antibodies reactive with native or altered autologous antigens (3). Such antibodies also seem to be involved in the pathogenesis of murine SLE by virtue of their combination with soluble tissue antigens released in circulating blood or in extravascular spaces to form ICs that eventually result in tissue damage. For example, the probable participation of DNA-anti-DNA ICs has been demonstrated by the significant concentration of anti-DNA antibodies found in eluates of diseased kidneys from these mice (3, 19). Furthermore, supporting these complexes' pathologic role, the induction of tolerance to DNA antigen in NZBxW mice prolongs survival and decreases nephritis as well as anti-DNA production (5). Therefore, it is important to determine how much of the immunologic injury in murine SLE is associated with complexes containing gp70 and how much with other complexes exemplified by those containing nuclear DNA antigen.

To examine the importance of gp70 ICs and anti-DNA antibodies in the renal disease of SLE-prone strains, we treat NZBxW and MRL/ℓ mice with pharmacologic quantities of prostaglandin E_1 (PGE) to analyze its effect on the development of renal disease and the appearance of gp70 ICs and anti-DNA antibodies. Injections of 200 μg PGE, twice daily beginning when the animals are 2 months old, effectively retard the

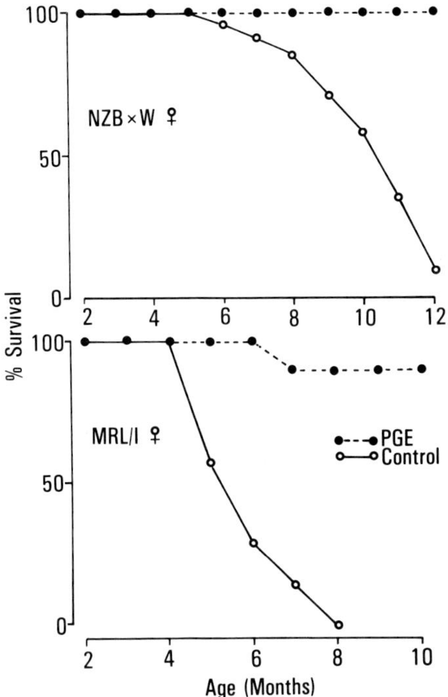

FIGURE 3. Survival rates of NZBxW and MRL/ℓ female mice treated with PGE beginning at 2 months of age.

development of SLE in both strains (14, 15, 31). The development of IC glomerulonephritis is dramatically suppressed, and survival is greatly prolonged (Fig. 3). PGE also prevents almost completely the development of generalized lymphadenopathy characterized by the massive proliferation of T lymphocytes that accompanies the SLE of MRL/ℓ mice.

Despite the beneficial effects of PGE in lessening renal pathology and lengthening life span in NZBxW and MRL/ℓ mice, production of anti-ssDNA and anti-dsDNA remains virtually unchanged throughout the experiment (Tables IV and V). Since the qualitative and quantitative aspects of the anti-DNA response in murine SLE may be equally important in provoking renal disease, PGE might function by suppressing the formation

TABLE IV. Effect of PGE Treatment in NZBxW Female Mice*

	PGE	Control
IgG (mg/ml)	11.0 ± 0.2	10.1 ± 0.2
Anti-dsDNA (%)**	17.2 ± 4.1	22.3 ± 2.7
Anti-ssDNA (%)**	44.3 ± 5.5	51.5 ± 4.2
Total gp70 (μg/ml)	50.2 ± 15.3	45.7 ± 16.9
Ig-bound gp70 (μg/ml)	5.9 ± 7.4	19.1 ± 10.8

*All values were determined at 10 months of age.

**% binding of 20 ng ^{125}I-DNA by 10 μl of serum.

of a specific subpopulation(s) of anti-DNA antibodies that is more pathogenic than others. However, we find no qualitative differences in the isotypes or avidities of serum anti-DNA antibodies in PGE-treated and untreated mice. Apparently, PGE achieves its therapeutic effect through mechanisms that do not

TABLE V. Effect of PGE Treatment in MRL/ℓ Female Mice*

	PGE	Control
IgG (mg/ml)		
IgG1	3.0 ± 2.2	6.4 ± 1.6
IgG2a	11.7 ± 3.0	13.8 ± 5.0
IgG2b	1.1 ± 0.4	1.6 ± 0.9
Anti-dsDNA (%)**	12.2 ± 7.5	14.5 ± 9.8
Anti-ssDNA (%)***	41.9 ± 20.4	49.1 ± 17.4
Total gp70 (μg/ml)	17.7 ± 9.3	21.0 ± 9.5
Ig-bound gp70 (μg/ml)	3.4 ± 5.0	10.0 ± 9.9

*All values were determined at 4 months of age.

**% binding of 20 ng ^{125}I-dsDNA by 10 μl of serum.

***% binding of 20 ng ^{125}I-ssDNA by 2 μl of serum.

directly involve the formation of anti-DNA antibodies. Other forms of therapy that can prolong survival in NZBxW mice also act without altering anti-DNA levels (26, 28).

In contrast to the negligible effect on anti-DNA production by PGE, the incidence and quantity of Ig-complexed gp70 are greatly reduced in the sera of NZBxW and MRL/ℓ mice treated with PGE compared with those of untreated mice (Tables IV and V). Over 90% of sera from 8- to 10-month-old untreated NZBxW female mice and 75% of sera from 4-month-old untreated MRL/ℓ female mice have significant amounts (>1/5) of gp70 complexed with IgG, whereas less than 25% of sera from PGE-treated 8- to 10-month-old NZBxW and 4-month-old MRL/ℓ mice contain significant amounts of Ig-bound gp70. Of course, the reduced amount of circulating complexed gp70 could result from accelerated clearance as well as from reduced formation. However, it is difficult to believe that gp70 ICs alone are cleared more rapidly from the circulation, since relatively large amounts of other ICs detectable by Raji cell test are present in sera from the PGE-treated mice.

Other data clearly show that the decreased quantities and incidences of circulating gp70 ICs in the PGE-treated mice correlate well with the reduced deposition of ICs of all kinds in glomeruli. In the kidneys of PGE-treated SLE mice, as in immunologically normal mice (20), gp70 is seen by direct immunofluorescence only in the tubules, but in untreated SLE mice glomeruli as well as tubules are involved. The amount of gp70 elutable from kidneys of one-year-old PGE-treated mice is only one-third that from the untreated mice, but similar to that from young healthy mice of the same strain and sex. This association of circulating gp70 ICs with renal disease strongly suggests the importance of such complexes in the fatal glomerulonephritis of mice susceptible to SLE.

The probability that PGE inhibits or modulates immune responsiveness to xenotropic viral gp70 in serum is exemplified by the relative absence of lymphoid hyperplasia in PGE-treated NZBxW and MRL/ℓ mice (16, 29). Moreover, PGE exerts its immunosuppressive effect in a somewhat selective manner, because only the production of IgG1 is suppressed in PGE-treated MRL/ℓ mice without affecting IgG2 production (Table V). Such selective suppression is compatible with the observation that serum levels of anti-DNA antibodies are unchanged by PGE treatment, since most of anti-DNA antibodies in MRL/ℓ mice belong to the IgG2a subclass (13). Considering that PGE seems to decrease anti-gp70 antibody formation, these antibodies might belong mainly to the IgG1 subclass in MRL/ℓ mice. If so, immune responsiveness to xenotropic viral gp70 must be regulated by a different mechanism than governs anti-DNA antibody production. Thereby, PGE could selectively prevent the formation of anti-xenotropic viral gp70 antibodies. Indeed, the separation of anti-DNA formation and gp70 IC formation in mice with SLE is supported by the evidence that MRL/ℓ mice infected with lactic dehydrogenase virus have approximately one-tenth the amount of anti-DNA antibodies as do uninfected control mice, but both have similar levels of gp70 ICs and develop early fatal glomerulonephritis.

Our recent genetic analysis of the F_2 generation of NZBxW mice underscores the significant association between the presence of circulating gp70 ICs and the development of fatal glomerulonephritis. However, no significant association is observed between the presence of anti-DNA antibodies and fatal glomerulonephritis. Although both NZB and NZW strains share high concentrations of gp70 in their sera, only NZB and NZBxW mice produce detectable amounts of gp70 ICs. Apparently, the NZB genes responsible for the appearance of gp70 ICs are the same genes that determine or regulate the production of anti-gp70 antibodies. The association of anti-gp70 antibody production, but not anti-DNA antibody production, with the development of renal disease strongly suggests that the genes responsible for the production of anti-gp70 antibodies may be one of the major genes for renal disease segregated in NZBxW F_2 generations.

In conclusion, endogenous retroviral gp70 complexed to antibody is prominantly involved in the renal disease of murine strains with genetic SLE-like disease. Not only SLE-prone mice but also many immunologically normal mice have relatively high concentrations of gp70 in their sera; however, only SLE mice develop antibodies directed against these serum xenotropic viral gp70. Subsequently, these antibodies combine with circulating gp70 and form ICs that deposit in the renal glomeruli where they produce glomerulonephritis. A significant association of circulating gp70 ICs with the development of glomerulonephritis has been demonstrated in SLE-prone mice under several experimental conditions such as treatment with PGE, chronic infection with lactic dehydrogenase virus, or genetic manipulation. These combined results strongly suggest that gp70 ICs play an important role in the pathogenesis of murine SLE.

ACKNOWLEDGMENTS

The expert technical assistance of Ms. Sharon Pascoe, Ms. Susan G. Hensley, Ms. Jeanne Godene, Ms. Christine Ethridge, Ms. Judith Shonnand, Ms. Ardith Ries, and Mr. John P. Clark, and the excellent secretarial and editorial assistance of Ms. Lisa A. Flores and Ms. Phyllis Minick are gratefully acknowledged.

REFERENCES

1. Accini, L. and Dixon, F. J. Degenerative vascular disease and myocardial infarction in mice with lupus-like syndrome. *Am. J. Pathol. 96*, 477 (1979).

2. Accini, L., Albini, B., Andres, G., and Dixon, F. J. Deposition of immune complexes in ovarian follicles of mice with lupus-like syndrome. *Am. J. Pathol. 99*, 589 (1980).

3. Andrews, B. S., Eisenberg, R. A., Theofilopoulos, A. N., Izui, S., Wilson, C. B., McConahey, P. J., Murphy, E. D., Roths, J. B., and Dixon, F. J. Spontaneous murine lupus-like syndrome. Clinical and immunopathological manifestations in several strains. *J. Exp. Med. 148*, 1198 (1978).

4. Barthold, D. R., Kysela, S., and Steinberg, A. D. Decline in suppressor T cell function with age in female NZB mice. *J. Immunol. 112*, 9 (1974).

5. Borel, Y., Lewis, R. M., and Stollar, B. D. Prevention of murine lupus nephritis by carrier dependent induction of immunologic tolerance to denatured DNA. *Science 182*, 76 (1973).

6. Cantor, H., McVay-Boudreau, L., Hugenberger, J., Naidorf, K., Shen, F. W., and Gershon, R. K. Immunoregulatory circuits among T cell sets. II. Physiologic role of feedback inhibition *in vivo*: absence in NZB mice. *J. Exp. Med. 147*, 1116 (1978).

7. Dixon, F. J., Jensen, F. C., McConahey, P. J., and Croker, B. P. Oncornaviruses and immunologic disease. *In* Proceedings of the VIIIth Symposium of *Immunopathology*, Bad Schachen, Germany (ed. by P. A. Miescher), p. 131. Schwabe & Co., Basel (1977).

8. Elder, J. H., Jensen, F. C., Bryant, M. L., and Lerner, R. A. Polymorphism of the major envelope glycoprotein (gp70) of murine C-type viruses: virion associated and differential antigens encoded by a multigene family. *Nature (London) 267*, 23 (1977).

9. Elder, H. H., Gautsch, J. W., Jensen, F. C., Lerner, R. A., Chused, T. M., Morse, H. C., Hartley, J. W., and Rowe, W. P. Differential expression of two distinct xenotropic viruses in NZB mice. *Clin. Immunol. Immunopathol. 15*, 493 (1980).

10. Gustafasson, J. A., Eneroth, P., Pousette, A., Skett, P., Sonnenschein, C., Steinberg, A., and Ahlén, A. Programming and differentiation of rat liver enzymes. *J. Steroid Biochem. 8*, 429 (1977).

11. Izui, S., McConahey, P. J., and Dixon, F. J. Increased spontaneous activation of B lymphocytes in mice with spontaneous autoimmune disease. *J. Immunol. 121*, 2213 (1978).

12. Izui, S., McConahey, P. J., Theofilopoulos, A. N., and Dixon, F. J. Association of circulating retroviral gp70-anti-gp70 immune complexes with murine systemic lupus erythematosus. *J. Exp. Med. 149*, 1099 (1979).

13. Izui, S. and Eisenberg, R. A. Circulating anti-DNA-rheumatoid factor complexes in MRL/ℓ mice. *Clin. Immunol. Immunopathol. 15*, 436 (1980).

14. Izui, S., Kelley, V. E., McConahey, P. J., and Dixon, F. J. Selective suppression of retroviral gp70-anti-gp70 immune complex formation by prostaglandin E_1 in murine systemic lupus erythematosus. *J. Exp. Med. 152*, 1645 (1980).

15. Kelley, V. E., Winkelstein, A., and Izui, S. Effect of prostaglandin E on immune complex nephritis in NZB/W mice. *Lab. Invest. 41*, 531 (1979).

16. Kelley, V. and Winkelstein, A. PGE_1 prevents lymphoproliferation and renal disease in MRL/ℓ mice. *Fed. Proc. 39*, 471 (1980).

17. Koj, A. Acute-phase reactants. *In* "Structure and Function of Plasma Proteins" (A. C. Allison, ed.), Vol. 1, p. 73. Plenum, New York, 1974.

18. Krakauer, R. S., Waldmann, T. A., and Strober, W. Loss of suppressor T cells in adult NZB/NZW mice. *J. Exp. Med. 144*, 662 (1976).

19. Lambert, P. H. and Dixon, F. J. Pathogenesis of glomerulonephritis of NZB/W mice. *J. Exp. Med. 127*, 507 (1968).

20. Lerner, R. A., Wilson, C. B., Del Villano, B. C., McConahey, P. J., and Dixon, F. J. Endogenous oncornaviral gene expression in adult and fetal mice: Quantitative, histologic and physiologic studies of the major viral glycoprotein, gp70. *J. Exp. Med. 143*, 151 (1976).

21. McAdam, K. P. W. J. and Sipe, J. D. Murine model for human secondary amyloidosis: Genetic variability of the acute-phase serum protein SAA response to endotoxins and casein. *J. Exp. Med. 144*, 1121 (1976).

22. Mellors, R. C., Aoki, T., and Huebner, R. J. Further implications of murine leukemia-like virus in the disorder of NZB mice. *J. Exp. Med. 129*, 1045 (1969).

23. Moroni, C. and Schumann, G. Lipopolysaccharide induced C-type virus in short term cultures of BALB/c spleen cells. *Nature (London) 254*, 60 (1975).

24. Obata, Y., Stockert, E., Yamaguchi, M., and Boyse, E. A. Source and hormone-dependence of G_{IX}-gp70 in mouse serum. *J. Exp. Med. 148*, 793 (1978).

25. Phillips, S. M., Stephenson, J. R., Greenberger, J. S., Lane, P. E., and Aaronson, S. A. Release of xenotropic type-C RNA virus in response to lipopolysaccharide: activity of lipid A protein upon B lymphocytes. *J. Immunol. 116*, 1123 (1976).

26. Roubinian, J. R., Talal, N., Greenspan, J. S., Goodman, J. R., and Suteri, P. K. Delayed androgen treatment prolongs survival in murine lupus. *J. Clin. Invest. 63*, 902 (1979).

27. Stein, O., Sanger, L., and Stein, Y. Colchicine-induced inhibition of lipoprotein and protein secretion into the serum and lack of interference with secretion of biliary phospholipids and cholesterol by rat liver *in vivo*. *J Cell Biol. 62*, 90 (1974).

28. Walker, S. E., Anver, M. R., Schecter, S. L., and Bole, G. G. Prolonged lifespan and high incidence of neoplasma in NZB/NZW mice treated with hydrocortisone sodium succinate. *Kidney Int. 14*, 151 (1978).

29. Winkelstein, A. and Kelley, V. E. The effects of PGE_1 on lymphocytes in NZB/W mice. *Clin. Immunol. Immunopathol. 17*, 212 (1980).

30. Yoshiki, T., Mellors, R. C., Strand, M., and August, J. T. The viral envelope glycoprotein of murine leukemia virus and pathogenesis of immune complex glomerulonephritis of New Zealand mice. *J. Exp. Med. 140*, 1011 (1974).

31. Zurier, R. B., Damjanov, I., Miller, P. L., and Biewer, B. F. Prostaglandin E_1 treatment prevents progression of nephritis in murine lupus erythematosus. *J. Clin. Lab. Immunol. 1*, 95 (1978).

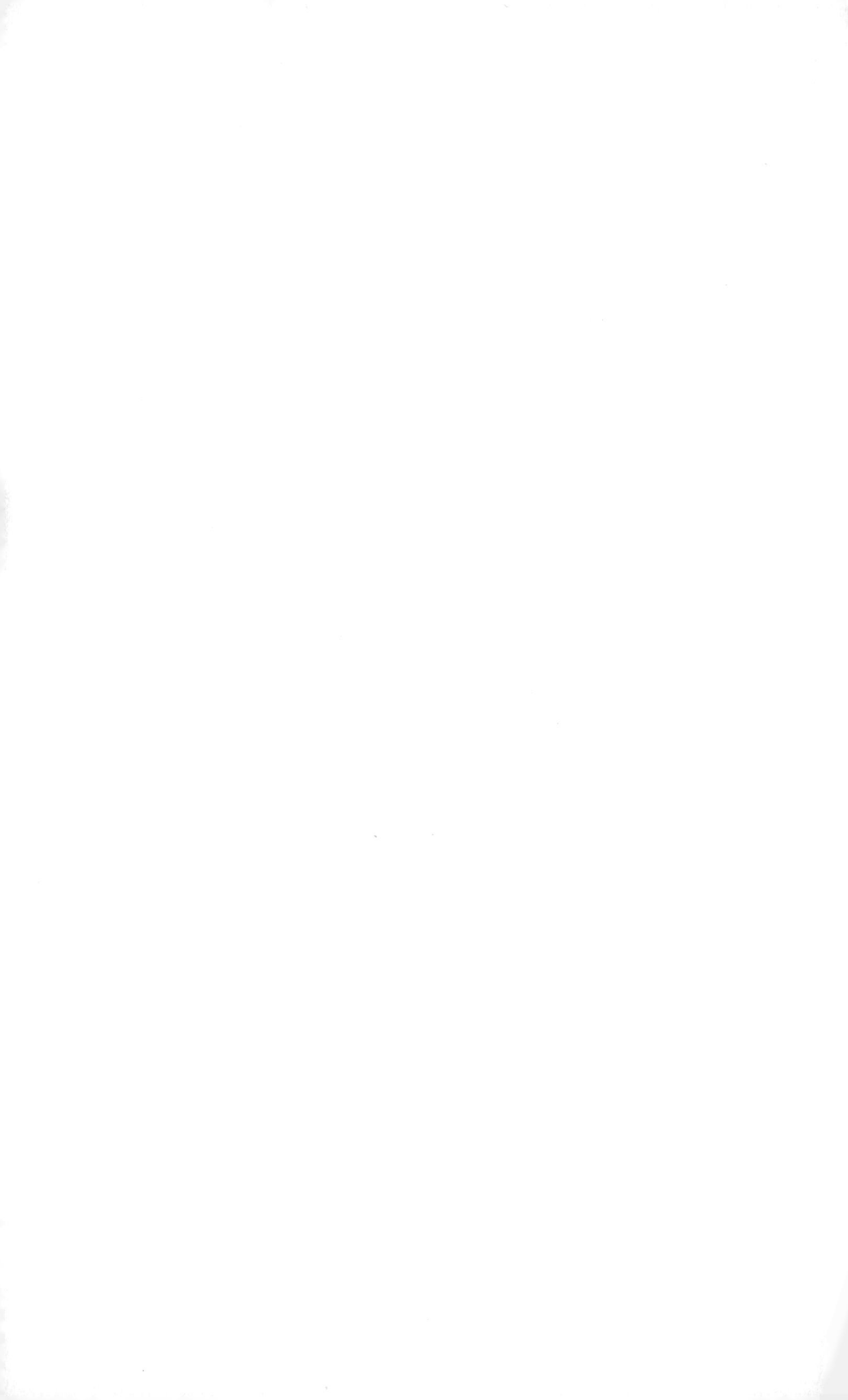

Immunopathology: VIIIth International Symposium, 1980

MONOCLONAL LUPUS AUTOANTIBODIES[1]

Joyce Rauch
Chester Andrzejewski, Jr.
Robert S. Schwartz

Department of Medicine,
Tufts University School of Medicine,
Boston, Massachusetts

Eileen Lafer
B. David Stollar

Department of Biochemistry and Pharmacology,
Tufts University School of Medicine
Boston, Massachusetts

SLE stands out from most other autoimmune diseases because of the unusual diversity of its clinical and serological manifestations. Some of the clinical aspects of SLE can be accounted for by the deposition in tissues of soluble immune complexes that circulate in the blood (9). This mechanism cannot explain other clinical aspects of SLE, however. The hematological complications, for instance, are not due to circulating immune complexes, but to autoantibodies that bind directly to the target cell (5). The mechanism of central nervous system lesions remains enigmatic and evidence that

[1]*Supported by NIH Grants AM-27232 and AI-14534.*

ISBN 0-12-218320-7

immune complexes can enter and damage the brain is elusive (8). The pathogenesis of membranous lupus nephropathy, a common lesion of the disease, is also unclear and may not be due to glomerular deposition of immune complexes, as previously thought (7).

The serological manifestations of SLE match the complexities of its clinical findings. A tendency to form antibodies that react with numerous components of the normal cell, from nuclear DNA to antigens on the membrane, is characteristic (Table I). To be sure, not every patient with SLE forms all of the antibodies listed in Table I, but in the aggregate lupus patients manifest an unparalleled array of serological abnormalities. This situation contrasts sharply with that in most

TABLE I. Autoantibodies in SLE

Nucleoprotein
Nuclear glycoprotein
Double-stranded DNA
Single-stranded DNA
Double-stranded RNA
Single-stranded RNA
Sm antigen
Polynucleotides
Ribosomes
Lysosomes
Ro antigen
La antigen
Red cells
Platelets
Granulocytes
Lymphocytes

"organ-specific" autoimmune diseases. In those conditions the serological abnormalities are far more restricted than in SLE, and they usually focus on a single antibody-antigen system.

An understanding of the diversity of lupus autoantibodies is therefore essential for an understanding of this disease. Detailed knowledge of the properties of lupus autoantibodies could explain not only the varied clinical aspects of SLE, but also its genetic (4) and immunologic (6) disturbances.

We have embarked upon a program to address some of these issues by the application of hybridoma technology to lupus autoantibodies. Monoclonal antibodies produced by hybridomas have an obvious advantage over complex mixtures of serum antibodies for analyses of immunochemical specificities. Moreover, the search for serological, structural, and genetic relationships among antibodies by analysis of idiotypes is greatly enhanced with monoclonal antibodies as reagents.

Our studies were initiated with hybridomas prepared by the fusion of appropriately mutagenized mouse plasmacytoma cells with splenic B cells of MRL/ℓ mice (2). This strain was used because it spontaneously develops a severe form of SLE and produces high levels of anti-DNA and other lupus autoantibodies (7). Immunization of the animal, as routinely employed in the preparation of conventional hybridomas, was unnecessary because MRL/ℓ mice spontaneously produce autoantibodies. This feature of the system allows us to examine the repertoire of spontaneously produced autoantibodies.

Products of the MRL/ℓ hybridomas were screened by solid-phase radioimmunoassays (RIAs) that detect antibodies to dDNA or nDNA. These assays may be carried out in test tubes or entirely within 96-well microtiter plates, in which case autoradiography of the test plate is used to reveal specific binding of the radiolabeled second-step antibody. The latter should detect both IgG and IgM antibodies, an important consideration when seeking information about the repertoire of autoantibodies.

Hybridomas that produced anti-DNA antibodies were transferred to 2-ml wells for further growth and then cloned by a limiting dilution technique. The immunoglobulin products of these clones produced patterns of monoclonal immunoglobulins when subjected to isoelectric focusing (10). The cloned hybridomas can be injected intraperitoneally and ascites fluid used for subsequent analyses. We prefer, however, to employ tissue culture fluid for analytical purposes because it is uncontaminated by irrelevant immunoglobulins, aggregates, proteolysed fragments, and other interfering substances. Affinity purification of the tissue culture fluids on antiimmunoglobulin or Protein-A columns further refines the reagents and renders their immunochemical properties sharply defined and highly reproducible. We have made over 40 hybridoma clones that produce anti-DNA autoantibodies. Our analysis of these clones is incomplete and the present report of their properties should not be regarded as definitive.

A competitive RIA was used to analyze the binding preferences of the monoclonal anti-DNA autoantibodies. We have used both solid- and liquid-phase techniques for this purpose. The former is relatively sensitive, but for some hybridoma autoantibodies the less sensitive liquid-phase technique may be preferred. The solid-phase RIA employs DNA-coated polystyrene tubes with the antibody and the competitor in solution. Various polynucleotides, oligonucleotides, and mononucleotides have been tested for their ability to inhibit the binding of monoclonal autoantibodies to DNA (3). In this way it was possible to obtain a spectrum of binding preferences for each autoantibody. In some cases the preferred ligand was an oligonucleotide containing the purine base guanine. In other cases, by contrast, the monoclonal autoantibody was capable of binding to several different polynucleotides. Particularly noteworthy was the ability of many of the hybridoma products to bind to polyinosinic acid, a synthetic polynucleotide that can assume varied helical structures or present the purine hypoxanthine in single-stranded regions.

The ability of several monoclonal autoantibodies to react with a variety of different polynucleotides, including both polypurine and polypyrimidine polymers, suggested that the relevant ligand was located in the sugar phosphate backbone of these molecules. The backbones of all polynucleotides contain repeating phosphate groups in diester linkage with adjoining carbon atoms. This structure could have been the epitope to which the monoclonal autoantibodies bound.

This interpretation was tested by an analysis of molecules that are not polynucleotides, but which possess a backbone structure that contains phosphate groups in diester linkage with adjacent carbon atoms. Phospholipids are molecules of this type and, when in micellar form, they display repeating phosphate groups to the aqueous phase. Several monoclonal "anti-DNA" autoantibodies were tested and found to bind avidly to cardiolipin (diphosphatidyl glycerol), phosphatidic acid, and phosphatidyl glycerol (10). Moreover, the fluorescent antinuclear antibody reaction produced by one of the hybridoma autoantibodies could be completely blocked by prior incubation with cardiolipin micelles.

The lupus anticoagulant is a peculiar autoantibody whose main effect is to prolong the partial thromboplastin time (PTT). In this test, a phospholipid extract of rabbit brain is used to mimic the action of platelets in the coagulation of test plasma. We reasoned that an autoantibody with the ability to bind phospholipids could behave like a lupus anticoagulant.

Monoclonal autoantibody H102, an antibody that binds both DNA and cardiolipin, was tested in this system, and it prolonged the PTT in a manner similar to that of a lupus anticoagulant (10).

Our results demonstrate that a single molecular species of lupus autoantibody can have diverse serological activities. For instance, the product of hybridoma H102 binds to single-stranded DNA, polyinosinic acid, and cardiolipin; it produces the fluorescent antinuclear reaction; and it behaves like a lupus anticoagulant. These reactions, we believe, are due to an epitope present in a variety of biological molecules. This epitope seems to be a phosphate group in diester linkage with carbon atoms. When such groups are favorably arranged, perhaps as repeating units, they can bind avidly with the autoantibody.

An important implication of these findings is that the heterogeneity of lupus autoantibodies is less than previously envisioned. We are currently analyzing a large number of monoclonal autoantibodies in order to determine with greater accuracy the extent of the diversity of lupus autoantibodies. The heterogeneity of the population can be analyzed not only by their binding preferences, but also by idiotypic relationships among them (3). Hypotheses about the immunological abnormalities essential to cause SLE may require revision if the diversity of lupus autoantibodies is found to be relatively restricted.

REFERENCES

1. Andrews, B. S., Eisenberg, R. A., Theofilopoulos, A. N., Izui, S., Wilson, C. B., McConahey, J. P., Murphy, E. D., Roths, J. B., and Dixon, F. J. Spontaneous murine lupus-like syndromes. Clinical and immunopathological manifestations in several strains. *J. Exp. Med. 148*, 1198-1215 (1978).

2. Andrzejewski, C., Jr., Stollar, B. D., Lalor, T. M., and Schwartz, R. S. Hybridoma autoantibodies to DNA. *J. Immunol. 124*, 1499-1501 (1980).

3. Andrzejewski, C., Jr., Rauch, J., Lafer, E., Stollar, B. D., and Schwartz, R. S. Antigen-binding diversity and idiotypic cross-reactions among autoantibodies to DNA. *J. Immunol. 126*, 226-231 (1981).

4. Block, S. R., Winfield, J. B., Lockhsin, M. D., D'Angelo, W. A., and Christian, C. L. Studies of twins with systemic lupus erythematosus. *Am. J. Med. 59*, 533-552 (1975).

5. Budman, D. R. and Steinberg, A. D. Hematologic aspects of systemic lupus erythematosus. *Ann. Intern. Med. 86*, 220-228 (1977).

6. Decker, J. L., Steinberg, A. D., Reinertsen, J. L., Plotz, P. H., Balow, J. E., and Klippel, J. H. Systemic lupus erythematosus: evolving concepts. *Ann. Intern. Med. 91*, 587-604 (1979).

7. Friend, P. S., Kim, Y., Michael, A. F., and Donadio, J. V. Pathogenesis of membranous nephropathy in systemic lupus erythematosus: possible role of non-precipitating DNA antibody. *Br. Med. J. 1*, 25 (1977).

8. Johnson, R. I. and Richardson, E. P. The neurological manifestations of systemic lupus erythematosus. *Medicine (Baltimore) 47*, 337-369 (1968).

9. Koffler, D., Agnello, V., Thoburn, R., and Kunkel, H. G. Systemic lupus erythematosus: prototype of immune complex nephritis in man. *J. Exp. Med. 134*, Suppl., 169-179 (1971).

10. Lafer, E., Rauch, J., Andrzejewski, C., Jr., Stollar, B. D., and Schwartz, R. S. Polyspecific lupus autoantibodies that bind to both polynucleotides and phospholipids. *J. Exp. Med. 153*, 897-909 (1981).

Immunopathology: VIIIth International Symposium, 1980

ALTERATIONS OF ESTROGEN METABOLISM IN SYSTEMIC LUPUS ERYTHEMATOSUS

Robert G. Lahita
Henry G. Kunkel

The Rockefeller University
New York, New York

Many diseases with immune characteristics have a sexual preference for the female. This predilection is not associated with human disease alone, but is also seen in several animal models such as the mouse and the dog. Several diseases in which immune aberrations predominate in the human female (Table I) after puberty are systemic lupus erythematosus (SLE) (10:1 females to males) (25), rheumatoid arthritis (3:1), scleroderma (3:1), Sjogren's syndrome (9:1), myasthenia gravis (3:1), chronic active hepatitis (noninfectious origin) (9:1), primary biliary cirrhosis (9:1), and chronic idiopathic thrombocytopenic purpura (4:1) (1-3, 6).

In addition, the age of the patient seems to play a role in the manifestation of the disease. The ratio of 10:1 for females with SLE applies only to females in the childbearing years, whereas the ratio in rheumatoid arthritis applies largely to the postmenopausal female.

ISBN 0-12-218320-7

TABLE I. Some Diseases That Predominate in the Female[a]

Systemic lupus erythematosus (10:1)
Scleroderma (3:1)
Rheumatoid arthritis (3:1)
Myasthenia gravis (3:1)
Sjogren's syndrome (9:1)
Idiopathic thrombocytopenic purpura (chronic) (4:1)
Chronic active hepatitis (9:1)
Primary biliary cirrhosis (9:1)

[a] *Number in parentheses show the female:male ratio.*

In infectious hepatitis, a disease associated with arthralgias and circulating immune complexes where the etiology is clearly viral, the response of the female is different from that of the male. Such a response sometimes appears to dictate whether the host will become a disease-free carrier or go on to develop chronic active liver disease (4).

Our laboratory has studied the disease SLE with regard to sex steroids and pathogenesis. In this decidedly female illness, clinical manifestations usually occur after puberty and before the middle years (9, 12, 13). The cyclicity of the menstrual period, use of synthetic estrogens (5, 8), and pregnancy (16) have all been thought to affect adversely the clinical course of this disease. Additional reports in the human have suggested that ovarian function might play a role in the morbidity of the illness (19, 24). Studies have also shown that patients with Klinefelter's disease and SLE had a pattern of estrogen metabolism toward more feminine metabolites (23).

Work by others in murine systems has implicated female hormones in the morbidity and mortality of the disease (22), autoantibody synthesis (20), immune response to DNA antigen (18), and regulation of lymphocyte populations (21). In addition, some strains of mice are dependent on genetic factors in addition to hormones (15). These effects vary with the strain of mouse. A single strain of mouse, the BXSB, shows an association of disease only with the Y chromosome and seems to depend little if any on sex hormone influences (17).

Work in this laboratory has shown an abnormality of estrogen metabolism in the human with SLE. These studies have shown that estrogen metabolism in the human with SLE is associated with an abnormal pattern of hydroxylation. Starting with the pivotal compound estradiol, we measured the extent of enzymatic hydroxylation at C-16 and C-2 and also looked at the metabolites excreted in the urine as glucuronides. Hydroxylation at C-16 leads to the formation of the very estrogenic metabolites 16 α-hydroxyestrone and estriol. Hydroxylation at C-2 leads to the metabolites 2-hydroxyestrone and 2-methoxyestrone which are the catechol estrogens shown to have significant activity in the brain (Fig. 1). The *in vivo* sites of this metabolism are not known. In past work patients with Klinefelter's disease and SLE were shown to have increased levels of estriol as found by urinary metabolites, suggesting that 16-hydroxylation was increased.

In recent studies normals and SLE patients were examined to see whether 16-hydroxylation was identical for both groups. This was accomplished using two methods of study. Patients were hospitalized for four to six days in the research hospital of the Rockefeller University. In the study of the extent of hydroxylation, patients were hospitalized for six days. Total body water was determined by measuring 24-hr urine creatinines (14) and by administration of deuterated water (D_2O) with subsequent determination of body water by mass spectroscopy at 3 hr. Tritiated estradiol was administered iv and the extent

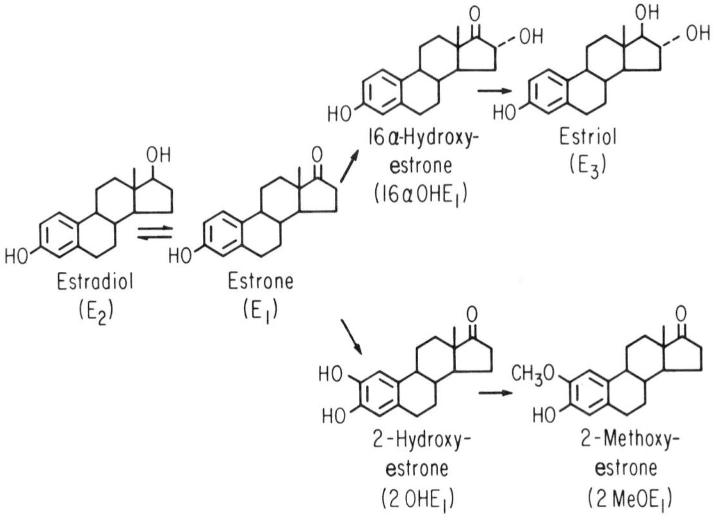

FIGURE 1. Estradiol metabolism in the human.

of hydroxylation determined using the formula:

$$\frac{\text{BW} \times \text{cpm/ml (blood) } 3\text{H}_2\text{O}}{\text{wt of dose} \times \text{cpm/mg dose}} = \%\text{ hydroxylation.}$$

Tritium is located at either C-16, C-2, or C-17. After injection of the isotope, blood samples are taken at timed intervals and lyophilized. The lyophilized, tritiated water then becomes the index of the reaction. A curve is derived and the maximal percentage of hydroxylation is calculated from the curve. Figure 2 indicates that SLE males and females hydroxylate significantly more estradiol at C-16 than do normal controls (male SLE $\overline{x}$ = 13.2% ± 3.0, range 8.8-18.0%) (nℓ male $\overline{x}$ = 8.3% ± 2.1, range 5.3-14.4%) (female SLE $\overline{x}$ = 15.7% ± 5, range 9-30%) (nℓ female $\overline{x}$ = 9.92% ± 2.2, range 5.9-14.1%) (10). The differences between the disease groups and normals are significant to $p < .001$. Minor differences in hydroxylation at C-2 were noted between normal female patients and female SLE patients. No association with 16-hydroxylation and clinical

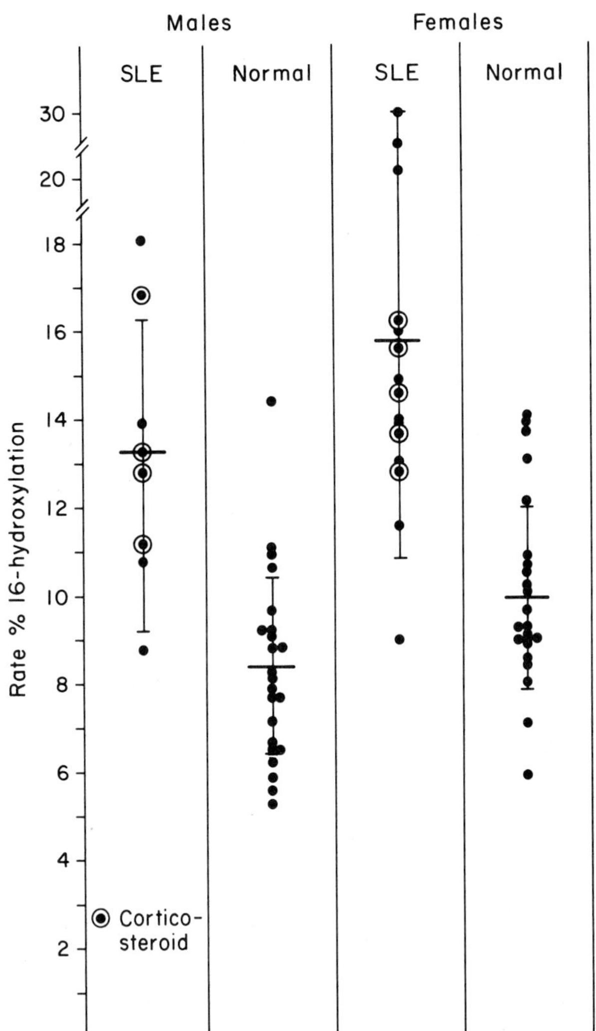

FIGURE 2. Males and females with SLE compared to normals when studied for extent of hydroxylation of estradiol at C-16. Means and standard deviations are given.

activity was evident (Fig. 3) as measured by anti-nDNA and total hemolytic complement values. In addition, the use of corticosteroids did not alter the extent of hydroxylation (Fig. 2). Many other acute and chronic diseases have been studied by this

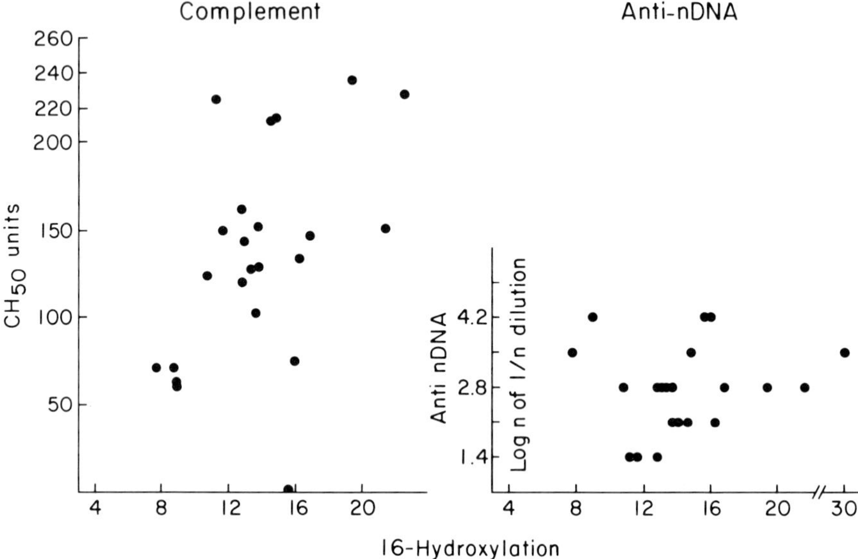

FIGURE 3. Clinical activity correlated with 16-hydroxylation of estradiol measured using total hemolytic complement and anti-nDNA antibodies (CH_{50} $R = .49$, $n = 23$, $p < .01$) (anti-nDNA $R = .02$, $n = 23$, $p < .001$).

method (Table II) and none as a group shows the extent of hydroxylation observed for patients with SLE. These data were supported by intravenous administration of [6,7-^{3}H]estradiol to patients and subsequent measurement of urinary metabolites after hydrolysis of glucuronidase (Fig. 4). Data derived from such studies indicated that 16-hydroxylation was increased. One metabolite (Fig. 1), 16 α-hydroxyestrone, was elevated in both males and females with SLE (Fig. 5) whereas in females estriol was also elevated (Fig. 6) (11). These findings stimulated work in other laboratories on properties of the compound 16 α-hydroxyestrone; it is a potent estrogen, binding tightly to the cytosol receptor and poorly to testosterone-estrogen binding globulin (TEBG) (7).

TABLE II. Disease Controls for 16 α-Hydroxylation of Estradiol

Disease	Number	Extent of 16 α-hydroxylation
SLE (female)	15	15.8(4.9)
SLE (male)	8	13.2(3.1)*
Lead poisoning	5	7.7(4.0)
Cancer (breast)	11	9.4(2.4)
Cancer (endometrial)	7	10.6(2.3)
Obesity	14	9.2(2.6)
Porphyria (acute intermittent porphyria)	5	9.1(5.3)
Porphyria (porphyria cutanea tarda)	3	10.7(4.7)
Chronic liver disease	5	11.5(3.5)**
Rheumatoid arthritis	2	12.3(0.7)
Normal female	21	9.9(2.2)
Normal male	23	8.3(2.1)

*Mean (±SD).

**All on high dose corticosteroids.

The exact significance of these findings with respect to the disease manifestations of SLE remains to be determined. The extent of hydroxylation of estradiol at C-16 is increased toward the more feminizing metabolites, 16 α-hydroxyestrone and estriol, in patients with SLE. In addition, fractionation of urine from patients with SLE reveals elevation of 16 α-hydroxyestrone in males and females and elevation of estriol in females.

Increases in estradiol which can occur via ingestion of oral contraceptives, during pregnancy or prior to menstruation would be expected to result in increased amounts of

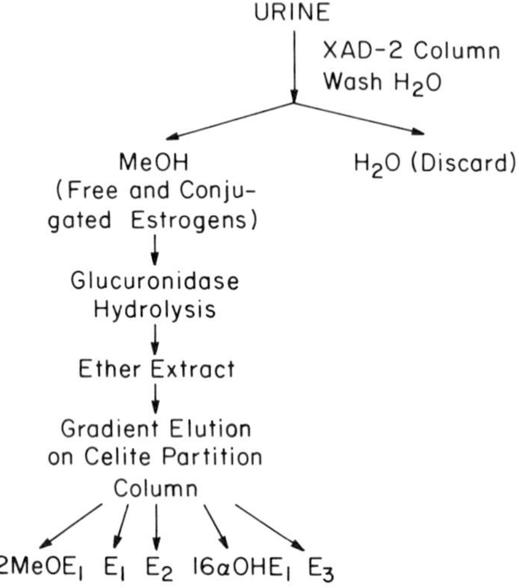

FIGURE 4. Flow diagram for isolation of 16-hydroxylated metabolites from urine after iv injection of [6,7-^{3}H]estradiol.

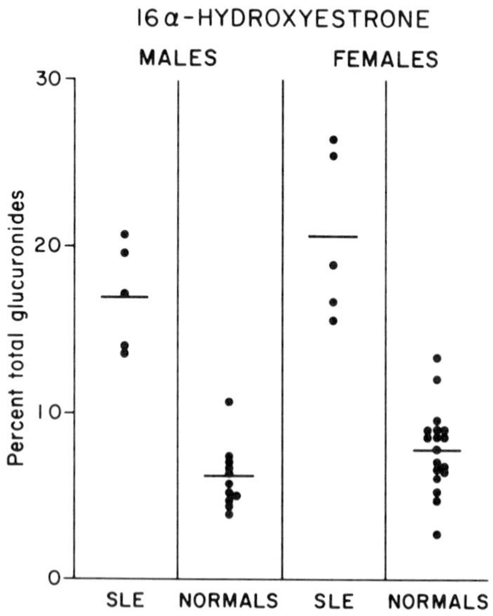

FIGURE 5. Comparison of levels of 16 α-hydroxyestrone in SLE and normals.

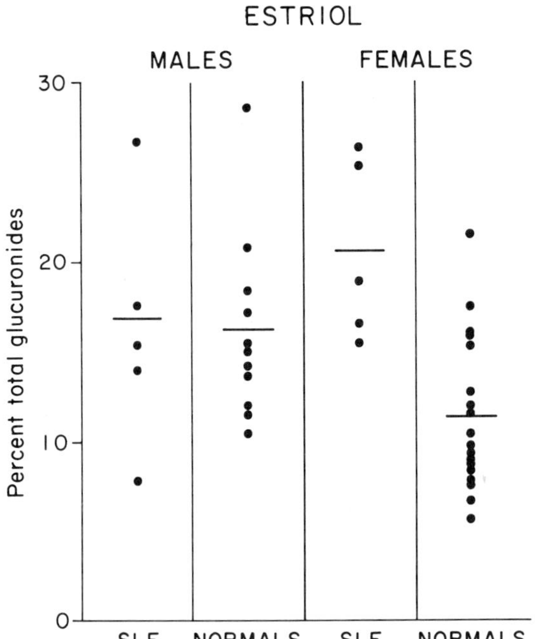

FIGURE 6. Comparison of levels of estriol in SLE and normals.

16-hydroxylated metabolites. These metabolites might contribute to the pathogenesis of the disease. 16 α-Hydroxyestrone has already been shown to have unique estrogenic properties. Additional evidence of the importance of these metabolites to disease processes is the age relationship of these diseases. The fact that certain diseases become apparent during sexual stages such as the childbearing years or senescence gives added importance to the role of these hormones. The effects of the 16-hydroxylated metabolites on the immune system are unknown and experiments are in progress to illuminate the role of these metabolites in the regulation of the immune system. Studies to link these alterations with known histocompatibility associations also need to be done. It is clear that differences between patients with SLE and normals with regard to sex hormone metabolism do exist, and an understanding of their significance might enhance our insight of the etiology of disease and others showing a high female incidence.

REFERENCES

1. Ahrens, E. H., Jr., Payne, M. A., Kunkel, H. G., Eisenmenger, W. J., and Blandheim, S. H. Primary biliary cirrhosis. *Medicine (Baltimore) 29*, 299 (1950).

2. Baldini, M. G. Idiopathic thrombocytopenic purpura and the ITP syndrome. *Med. Clin. North Am. 56*, 47 (1972).

3. Bearn, A. G., Kunkel, H. G., and Slater, R. J. The problem of liver disease in young women. *Am. J. Med. 21*, 3 (1956).

4. Blumberg, B. S. Sex differences in response to hepatitis B virus. I. History. *Arthritis Rheum. 22*, 1261 (1979).

5. Chapel, T. A. and Burns, R. E. Oral contraceptives and exacerbations of lupus erythematosus. *Am. J. Obstet. Gynecol. 110*, 366 (1971).

6. Dubois, E. L. and Tuffanelli, D. L. The clinical picture of systemic lupus erythematosus. *In* "Lupus Erythematosus"(E. L. Dubois, ed.), p. 232. Univ. of Southern California Press, Los Angeles, 1974.

7. Fishman, J. and Martucci, C. Biological properties of 16 α-hydroxyestrone: Implications in estrogen physiology and pathophysiology. *J. Clin. Endocrinol. Metab. 51*, 611 (1980).

8. Garovich, M., Agudelo, C., and Pisko, E. Case report: Oral contraceptives and SLE. *Arthritis Rheum 23*, 1396 (1980).

9. Kornreich, H. Systemic lupus erythematosus in childhood. *Clin. Rheum. Dis. 2*, 429 (1976).

10. Lahita, R. G., Bradlow, H. L., Kunkel, H. G., and Fishman, J. Increased 16 α-hydroxylation of estradiol in SLE. *J. Clin. Endocrinol. Metab. 53*, No. 1, 174-178 (1981).

11. Lahita, R. G., Bradlow, H. L., Kunkel, H. G., and Fishman, J. Alterations of estrogen metabolism in systemic lupus erythematosus. *Arthritis Rheum. 22*, 1195 (1979).

12. Maddock, R. K. Incidence of systemic lupus erythematosus by age and sex. *J. Am. Med. Assoc. 191*, 137 (1965).

13. Masi, A. T. and Kaslow, R. A. Sex effects in systemic lupus erythematosus: A clue to pathogenesis. *Arthritis Rheum. 21*, 480 (1978).

14. Miller, A. T. and Blythe, C. S. Estimation of lean body mass and body fat from basal oxygen consumption and creatinine excretion. *J. Appl. Physiol. 5*, 73 (1951).

15. Moyes, E. and Fuchs, S. Linkage between immune response potential to DNA and X chromosome. *Nature (London) 249*, 167 (1974).

16. Mund, A., Simson, J., and Rothfield, N. Effect of pregnancy on course of systemic lupus erythematosus. *J. Am. Med. Assoc. 183*, 917 (1963).

17. Murphy, E. D. and Roths, J. B. A Y-chromosome associated factor in strain BXSB producing accelerated autoimmunity and lymphoproliferation. *Arthritis Rheum. 22*, 1188 (1979).

18. Raveche, E. S., Tjio, J. H., Boegel, W., and Steinberg, A. D. Studies of the effects of sex hormones on autosomal and X linked genetic control of induced and spontaneous antibody production. *Arthritis Rheum. 22*, 1177 (1979).

19. Rose, E. and Pillsbury, D. M. Lupus erythematosus (erythematodes) and ovarian function: Observations on a possible relationship, with a report of 6 cases. *Ann. Intern. Med. 21*, 1022 (1944).

20. Roubinian, J. R., Talal, N., Greenspan, J. S., Goodman, J. R., and Siiteri, P. K. Effect of castration and hormone treatment on survival, antinucleic acid antibodies and glomerulonephritis in NZB/NZW F_1 mice. *J. Exp. Med. 147*, 1568 (1978).

21. Seaman, W. and Gindhardt, T. Estrogen and its effects on natural killer cells. *Arthritis Rheum. 22*, 1234 (1979).

22. Siiteri, P. K., Jones, L. A., Roubinian, J., and Talal, N. Sex steroids and the immune system. I. Sex difference in autoimmune disease in NZB/NZW hybrid mice. *J. Steroid Biochem. 12*, 425 (1980).

23. Stern, R., Fishman, J., Brusman, H., and Kunkel, H. G. Systemic lupus erythematosus associated with Klinefelter's syndrome. *Arthritis Rheum. 20*, 18 (1977).

24. Yocum, M. W., Grossman, J., Waterhouse, C., Abraham, G. N N., May, A. G., and Condemi, J. J. Monozygotic twins discordant for systemic lupus erythematosus. *Arthritis Rheum. 18*, 193 (1975).

25. Zvaifler, N. Etiology and pathogenesis of systemic lupus erythematosus. *In* "Rheumatology" (W. N. Kelly, ed.), p. 1085. Saunders, Philadelphia, Pennsylvania, 1981.

DISCUSSION

DR. I. S. JOHNSON: Have antiestrogens been used in an effort to control this disease in man?

DR. LAHITA: Not to our knowledge.

DR. NEIL COOPER: Would materials that act at the level of the liver, that is, drugs that stimulate microsomal oxidation, affect hydroxylation?

DR. LAHITA: It is plausible that agents which increase microsomal oxidation might adversely affect the disease if these metabolites are important to fluctuations in disease activity.

DR. SAMUEL STROBER: Are disorders of target organs responsible for these abnormalities?

DR. LAHITA: Patients were selected for study who were free of liver and thyroid disease. Females were also studied in the mid-follicular phase of their cycles. Renal disease did not seem to affect the data. Urine values of $3H_2O$ paralleled those seen for blood when urines were lyophilized.

Immunopathology: VIIIth International Symposium, 1980

ANTIBODY-MEDIATED TUBULOINTERSTITIAL NEPHRITIS[1]

B. Noble
J. R. Brentjens
G. A. Andres

Departments of Microbiology,
Pathology, and Medicine,
State University of New York at Buffalo,
Buffalo, New York

I. INTRODUCTION

Antibodies are known to play an important part in the pathogenesis of most human glomerular diseases. Damage to glomeruli may result either from the deposition of immune complexes along the glomerular basement membrane (GBM) or from the fixation of specific anti-GBM antibodies to the GBM. These two mechanisms are usually readily distinguished by direct immunofluorescence tests which reveal the pattern of distribution of immune reactants within the diseased kidney. Immune complex deposits have a characteristic discrete,

[1]*This work has been supported by Grants AM-26394 and AI-10334 of the National Institutes of Health, U.S. Public Health Service.*

ISBN 0-12-218320-7

granular appearance which can be detected by staining with fluorescein-labeled antibodies to immunoglobulins (Ig), complement (C), or the relevant antigen. In contrast, binding of anti-GBM antibody is recognized by a continuous, finely linear staining pattern. It is now well established that the tubules and interstitium of the kidney are also susceptible to injury initiated by the deposition of immune complexes or antibodies to the tubular basement membrane (TBM) (2, 22, 25). Interstitial inflammation and abnormalities of the tubular epithelium and the TBM may result when Ig, with or without C, is present in granular or linear deposits in renal tubules and interstitium.

A great deal of our present appreciation of the contribution of antibody-mediated injury to tubulointerstitial pathology is based on studies with animal models. The recognition of immunological processes in the pathogenesis of human interstitial nephritis has tended to follow observations made in the laboratory, although human disease can still be only partly explained by the available animal models. This chapter will review salient features of animal models of antibody-mediated experimental tubulointerstitial nephritis. Evidence for similar mechanisms in human interstitial nephritis will be evaluated and compared with the findings in laboratory animals.

II. TUBULOINTERSTITIAL NEPHRITIS ASSOCIATED WITH ANTIBODIES TO TBM

Active immunization of guinea pigs with TBM antigens prepared from rabbit kidneys produces a severe tubulointerstitial nephritis within several weeks (37). The sera of nephritic guinea pigs contain antibodies that stain guinea pig TBM in indirect immunofluorescence tests. Deposition of Ig and C in a linear pattern along the TBM of cortical tubules can be demonstrated in the kidneys of nephritic animals by direct immunofluorescence tests within a few weeks of immunization. The central importance of antibodies to TBM in the induction of this form of interstitial nephritis has been established by successful passive transfer experiments (38). From passive transfer experiments it has also been determined that classical or alternative complement-pathway activation is required for the full development of interstitial and tubular lesions (34, 36). Although antibodies to TBM are essential for development of the disease, they alone appear not to be a sufficient cause. Recipients of TBM antiserum that have been depleted of circulating leukocytes by prior irradiation do not develop characteristic tubulointerstitial nephritis despite substantial deposition of Ig and C along TBM (35). Full expression of the disease appears to require the participation of radiosensitive cells derived from bone marrow as well.

Anti-TBM nephritis in guinea pigs is characterized histologically by a mononuclear cell infiltration of the interstitium in which multinucleated giant cells have come to be recognized as a hallmark (3). Therefore, although a great deal of evidence suggests that antibody to TBM is an essential factor in the pathogenesis of the disease, the histology of the interstitial cellular infiltration is consistent with a cell-mediated immune reaction. In an attempt to evaluate the interplay of humoral and cellular responses in the pathogenesis of this renal disease a study of the morphology of the interstitial lesion at different stages of development of nephritis has been made (3). Deposits of Ig in a thin, interrupted linear pattern are seen along the TBM of some proximal tubules as early as two weeks after immunization. Interstitial lesions detected at that time consist primarily of focal peritubular accumulations of monocytes and macrophages and are limited to

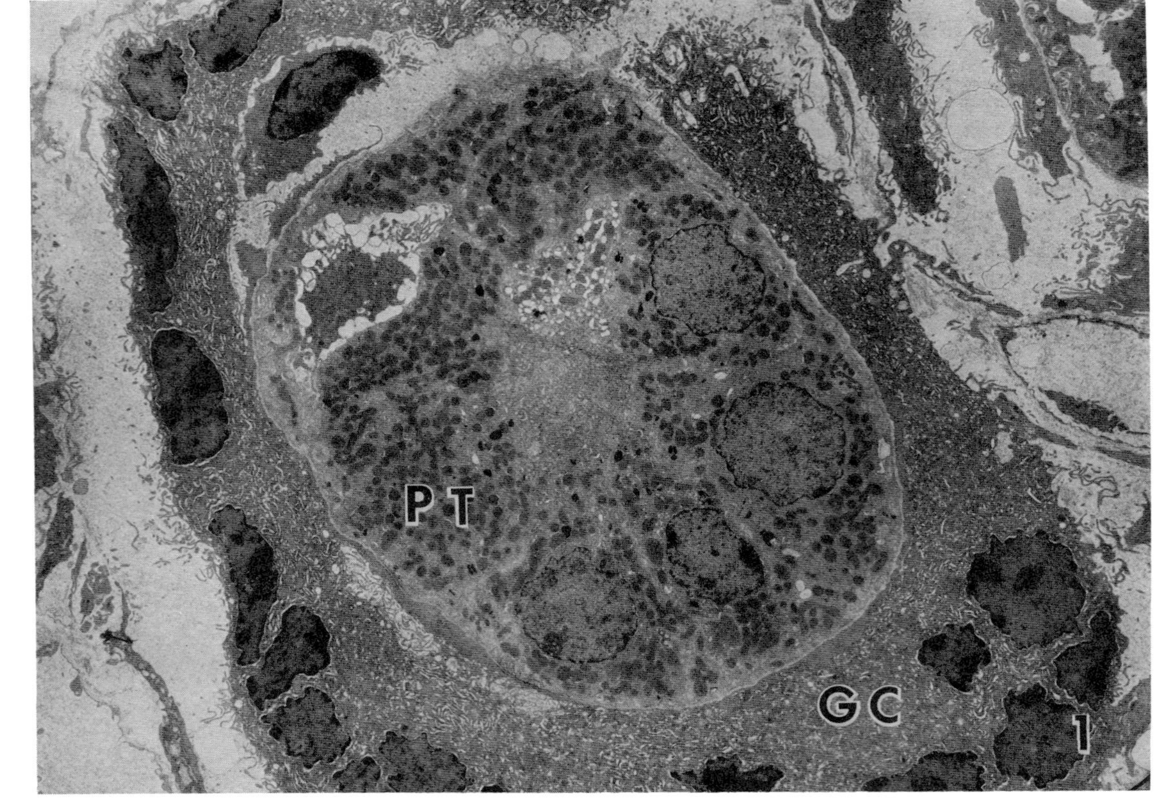

FIGURE 1. Electron micrograph of a proximal tubule (PT) completely surrounded by a multinucleated giant cell (GC) in the kidney of a guinea pig with tubulointerstitial nephritis mediated by antitubular basement membrane (TBM) antibodies (×3000).

the outer cortex. A high frequency of mitotic figures in the proximal tubules attests to an increased rate of epithelial cell proliferation. By electron microscopy, the TBM in this early stage of disease is seen to be normal or only slightly swollen, with minimal irregularities.

After two to three weeks, clinical manifestations of the disease such as renal glucosuria and uremia are exhibited by many animals, and an increasing severity of tubulointerstitial lesions is observed in tissue specimens. The cortex is found to be diffusely infiltrated with mononuclear cells, principally monocytes and macrophages. Epithelioid cells are present in small numbers. By electron microscopy the epithelioid cells are seen to be engaged in active pinocytosis and phagocytosis and are frequently associated and interlocked by pseudopodia.

In the final stage of renal disease, approximately three to five weeks after the initial immunization, TBM is seen to be missing at the base of many tubules. Multinucleated giant cells with central nuclei are distributed throughout the cortex. Giant cell formation seems to result from contact of plasma membranes of adjacent epithelioid cells, leading to the formation of cytoplasmic bridges and, eventually, to fusion. The giant cells are frequently in direct contact with the TBM. The cell cytoplasm near the point of contact is homogeneous, containing only bundles of microfilaments and no cytoplasmic organelles (Fig. 1). Contact of giant cells with the TBM may be followed by lysis, perforation, and phagocytosis of the TBM. Pseudopodia of the giant cells penetrate gaps in the TBM. These observations suggest that direct contact of the giant cells with the TBM, and not secretory activity, is a prerequisite for TBM destruction. The process seems analogous in many histologic features to a number of cytotoxic reactions studied *in vitro*, including antibody-dependent lymphocytotoxicity. Therefore, it has been proposed that an antibody-dependent cell-mediated immune reaction could be the important mode of tissue damage in this model of tubulointerstitial nephritis. The requirement for radiosensitive, bone marrow-derived cells, as well as specific antibody, for complete expression of the disease could be explained by such a mechanism.

The results of several experiments suggest that humoral factors may play an important, if complicated and as yet poorly understood, role in the pathogenesis of anti-TBM nephritis in guinea pigs. Active immunization of guinea pigs with rabbit TBM elicits production of anti-TBM antibodies of both IgG_1 and IgG_2 isotypes. The separate transfer of either isotype induces tubulointerstitial nephritis, but also stimulates the synthesis, by the recipient, of anti-TBM autoantibodies of both immunoglobulin subclasses (14). The mechanism by which transferred antibody might stimulate the synthesis of autoantibody of the same reactivity is not understood. One possibility is that the injected antibodies cause the modification or release of TBM antigens sufficient to provoke an autoimmune response by the recipient. This kind of autoimmune amplification could explain the progressive nature of the disease.

Significant inhibition of tubulointerstitial nephritis can be achieved by the intraperitoneal administration of small amounts of an antiidiotypic antiserum at the time of active immunization with TBM antigens (9). The antiidiotypic antibodies obtained from rabbits are directed against guinea pig antibodies to TBM. Although the mechanism of suppression of interstitial nephritis has not been explained, similar effects in other systems have been ascribed to clonal deletion of B cells or the production of T suppressor cells. The relative amounts of idiotypic and antiidiotypic antibody make it unlikely that a simple molecular reaction of those two antibody populations is sufficient to explain the result.

An interstitial nephritis characterized by production of antibodies to TBM and deposition of Ig along TBM has also been studied in BN and LEW/BN rats (21, 39). Many aspects of the immunopathology of anti-TBM disease in rats are similar to the disease produced in guinea pigs. However, an important difference is the influx of polymorphonuclear leukocytes seen in the early stages of tubulointerstitial nephritis in rats. The peritubular giant cells which appear to be important in the destruction of the TBM in guinea pigs are not a conspicuous feature of the histopathology of the interstitial inflammation seen in rats.

Antibodies to TBM may be found in rare cases of human disease. The observation of antibodies to TBM as an isolated phenomenon, comparable to the animal models, is very unusual. Antibodies to TBM in humans have been described in methicillin-related interstitial nephritis (5, 6), in association with immune complex glomerulonephritis (23, 24, 28, 40), and following renal transplantation (42). Antibodies to TBM are detected most frequently in patients with concomitant anti-GBM glomerulonephritis (1, 22). The reactivity of circulating or eluted anti-TBM antibodies in anti-GBM anti-TBM disease is not always restricted to the basement membrane of proximal tubules (41). In some cases the antibodies only react with the basement membrane of more distal segments of the nephron (Figs. 2A and 2B). This may explain why extensive binding *in vivo* of the anti-TBM antibodies is observed in some patients, whereas in others the binding is confined to just a few tubules.

In order to evaluate the relative importance and specific contribution of anti-TBM responses to human renal disease, the histopathology of the interstitium in tissues obtained from patients with anti-GBM anti-TBM disease has been compared to that of specimens from patients with isolated anti-GBM disease

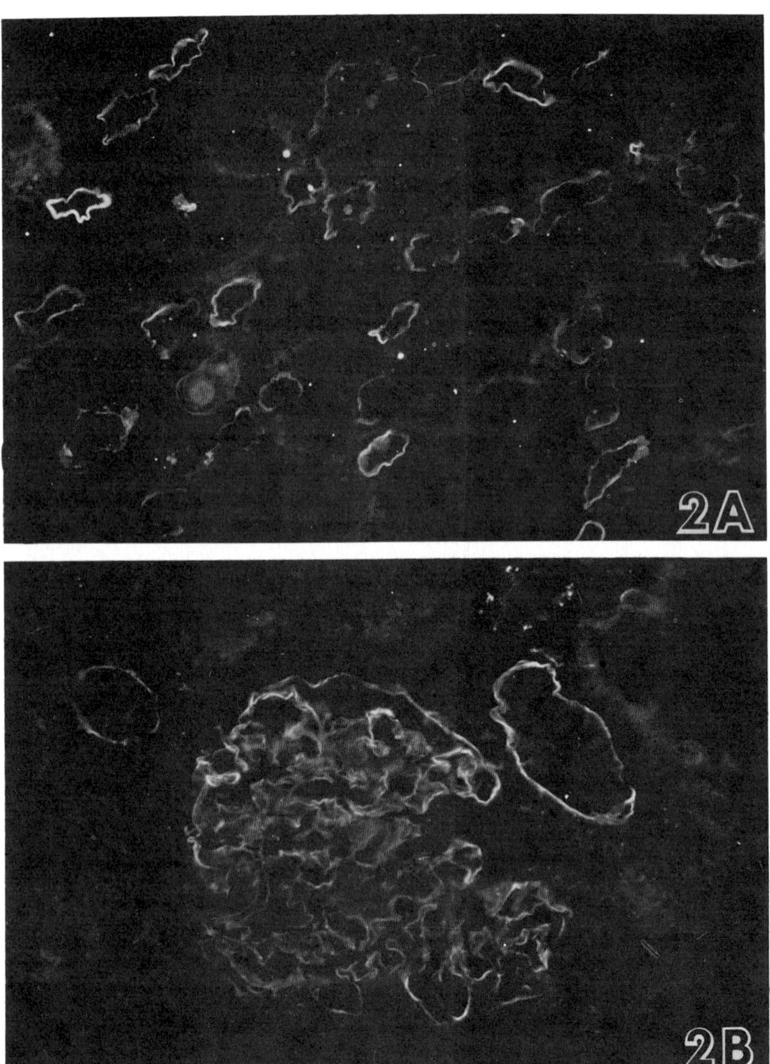

FIGURE 2. (A) Section of medulla of frozen kidney of a patient with anti-GBM anti-TBM nephritis stained by the direct immunofluorescence technique for human IgG. IgG is present in a linear pattern along the basement membrane of Henle's loops. The collecting tubules are free from deposits. In the cortex (not shown) only a few tubules had linear deposition of IgG along the basement membrane (×500). (B) Section of frozen normal human kidney incubated first with serum of the same patient whose kidney is shown in A, followed by staining with a fluoresceinated antiserum to human IgG. There is linear binding of IgG along GBM and along the basement membrane of distal tubules. No binding is seen along the basement membrane of proximal tubules (×500).

and other forms of crescentic nephritis (1). It was found that tubulointerstitial nephritis was most frequent and severe in patients with antibodies to both GBM and TBM. The tubulointerstitial lesions appear typically as peritubular and perivascular infiltrations composed of polymorphonuclear and mononuclear cells. Occasionally, multinucleated giant cells may be present. Cell proliferation and degeneration may be discerned in the epithelium of the tubules. The TBM can be thin and disrupted in some areas; in other places it may be thickened or duplicated. Mononuclear cells may be found between cells of the proximal tubular epithelium. The proliferation of epithelial cells seen in this human disease is not a prominent feature of anti-TBM nephritis in guinea pigs or rats, nor do the giant cells seen in human anti-GBM anti-TBM nephritis appear to function as those described in the guinea pig model.

The differences in histopathology of interstitial lesions seen in association with deposits of Ig along TBM in guinea pigs, rats, and humans may reflect differences in the immunopathogenetic mechanisms responsible for the production of those lesions. On the other hand, it is also possible that with similar underlying mechanisms, species differences produce different patterns of inflammatory cell accumulation within the interstitium.

The detection of anti-TBM antibodies in a few cases of methicillin-associated interstitial nephritis has led to the suggestion that anti-TBM antibodies may play a part in the pathogenesis of drug-related nephritis (5, 6). It was proposed that the dimethylpenicylloyl group, which is secreted by proximal tubules, may, when bound to the TBM as a hapten protein conjugate, stimulate an immune response that results in linear fixation of Ig along the TBM (6). Interstitial damage would be presumed to be the consequence of antibody deposition.

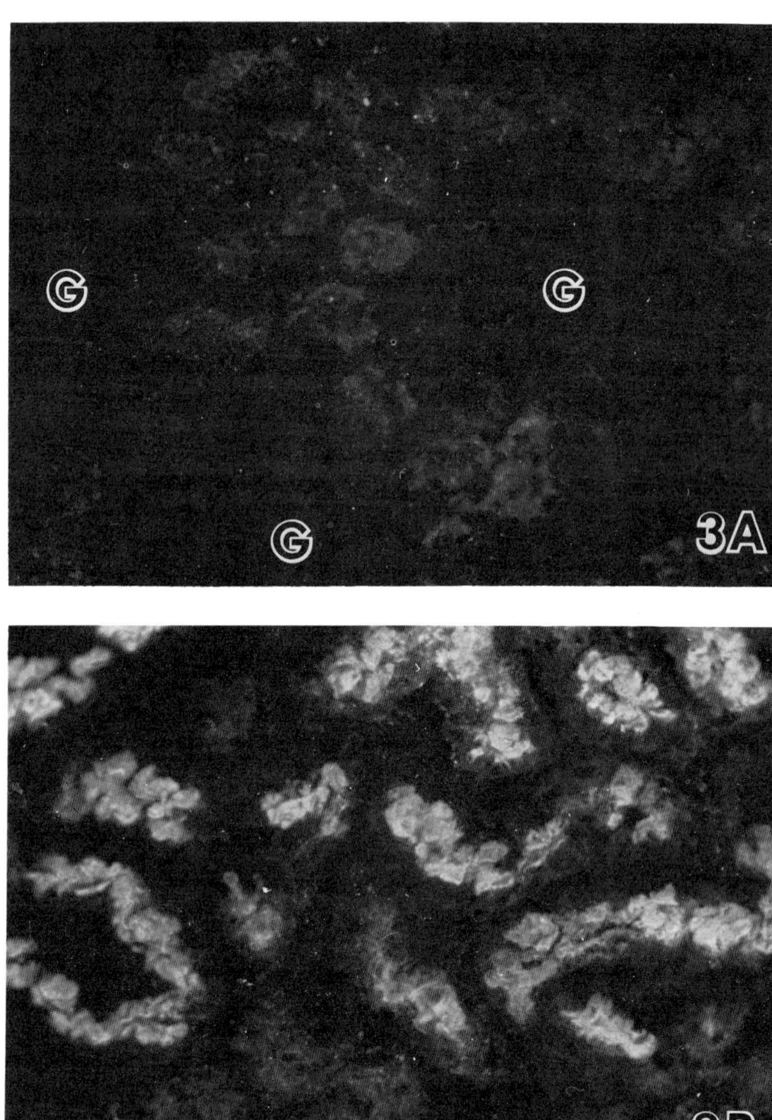

FIGURE 3. Acetone-fixed sections of outer cortex (A) and outer medulla (B) of frozen kidney of a normal rat, incubated first with serum from a rat in Stage 1 of Heymann nephritis (HN), followed by staining with a fluoresceinated antiserum to rat IgG. Binding of IgG is observed along the brush border of proximal tubules (S3 segments) present in the outer medulla only. G: glomerulus (×500).

However, as anti-TBM antibodies are not present in most cases of drug-related nephritis, including many in which penicillin analogs are implicated, anti-TBM antibodies most probably are not directly responsible for the majority of cases of interstitial nephritis associated with drug hypersensitivity (11, 27, 32). Taken together, the clinical manifestations of hypersensitivity, the elevated circulating IgE concentrations and the distinctive eosinophil component of the interstitial cellular infiltration seen in many cases of drug-associated interstitial nephritis provide some evidence that IgE-mediated hypersensitivity may contribute to renal pathology. For this intriguing and perplexing disease an animal model would be invaluable and is lacking.

III. INJURY TO PROXIMAL TUBULES ASSOCIATED WITH ANTIBODIES TO BRUSH BORDER (BB) MEMBRANES

Damage to proximal tubules may result from deposition of specific antibodies along the luminal border of proximal tubule cells (26). Antibodies to BB are elicited in an autoimmune disease of rats called Heymann nephritis (HN) (13) produced by immunization with a glomerulus-free extract of rat kidneys, designated FxlA (12). The disease is characterized by membranous glomerulonephritis with typical granular deposits of Ig and C along the GBM (12). Antibodies present in the undiluted sera of rats with HN stain the BB of all normal proximal tubule cells in indirect immunofluorescence tests. At high dilutions the sera frequently stain BB of the S3 segments of the proximal tubules only (Fig. 3A and 3B). A similar pattern of binding may be observed *in vivo*. This phenomenon may reflect heterogeneity of the antigenic specificity of antibodies to BB or it may be the consequence of differences in distribution of a single antigen which is present in higher concentrations in the microvilli of the S3 segments of proximal tubules, located mainly in the outer medulla.

In an attempt to evaluate the contribution of specific antibody-mediated cytotoxicity to damage of renal tubules in HN, a study has been made of immunopathology in proximal tubules throughout the natural course of the disease (26). From this study a division of the natural history of HN into four discrete stages could be made. In Stage 1, titers of circulating antibodies to BB rise and granular deposits of Ig and C begin to accumulate at the subepithelial side of the GBM. During this period the morphology of renal tubules is normal as judged by examination of kidney tissue fixed by *in situ* perfusion to ensure optimal preservation of the architecture of tubules and interstitium. Occasionally, focal, very fine granular deposits of Ig may be seen along the TBM of proximal tubules in direct immunofluorescence tests, but tubules are otherwise free of Ig deposits. Abnormal urinary protein excretion, the consequence of progressive glomerular pathology, marks the beginning of Stage 2, six to eight weeks after the initial immunization. The onset of proteinuria coincides with the maximum titers of antibody to BB seen during the course of HN. With significant elevation of protein excretion, antibodies pass the glomerular filter, gain access to the proximal tubules and bind *in vivo* to the microvilli of the luminal membrane. Ig deposits may be found in all proximal tubule segments or they may be limited in this early stage to the S3 segments present in the outer medulla. Deposition of Ig along BB is correlated with extensive alteration of the normal morphology of the epithelial lining. Aspects of tissue damage seen in Stage 2 include extensive loss of microvilli, flattening of epithelial cells, increased mitotic activity of epithelial cells, accumulation of cells within the lumen of proximal tubules, and significant reduction in the number of pinocytotic apical vesicles.

Stage 3 of HN, defined as the second six weeks of proteinuria, is characterized by a declining antibody titer. During this period, proximal tubules have been chronically exposed to specific antibodies. Kidneys taken from rats in Stage 3 are seen, by light microscopy, to be essentially devoid of microvilli in proximal tubules. Deposits of Ig along the luminal border of proximal tubules are focal in distribution and weak in intensity, or entirely absent. Indirect immunofluorescence tests confirm the absence of BB antigen(s). In contrast, conspicuous granular deposits of Ig are present along the TBM of many proximal tubules in most animals. These deposits will be described and discussed in Section IV.

In the natural course of HN, antibodies to BB eventually fall to undetectable concentrations in serum. Stage 4 of HN is that period, more than twelve weeks after the onset of proteinuria, when antibodies to BB are present in insignificant titers in circulation. Despite persistent proteinuria, in the absence of antibody-mediated immunologic attack, proximal tubules seem to recover partially from injury. Direct immunofluorescence tests show immune deposits to be limited to the GBM. Both BB and TBM are free of Ig. Light and electron microscopy reveal substantial regeneration of microvilli and restoration of a near normal appearance of epithelial cells.

These observations of the natural history of HN are consistent with the hypothesis that damage to the proximal tubules results from a cytotoxic injury mediated by antibodies to BB. When specific antibodies have access to the tubules, Ig is deposited along the BB. Deposition of Ig is accompanied by drastic alteration of proximal tubule morphology. In the absence of antibodies, substantial regeneration may take place.

Furthermore, the limitation of damage to proximal tubules is identical to the specificity exhibited by the antisera.

Reimmunization with FxlA of rats in the recovery phase (Stage 4) of HN stimulates a secondary immune response which produces high titers of antibody to BB within a few days and has the result of exposing cells of the proximal tubules to specific antibodies once again (29). This exposure causes severe damage to the epithelium, similar in kind but more devastating in extent than that seen in rats in early HN. Most of these rats develop renal glucosuria and a further decrease in glomerular filtration rate.

Study of the association of damage to the proximal tubules with deposition of Ig along BB in rats with active HN provides indirect evidence of the ability of antibodies to BB to produce injury to the tubular epithelium. For direct demonstration of the cytotoxicity of BB antiserum it was necessary to perform passive transfer experiments (30). Rats with chronic serum sickness induced by daily immunization with bovine serum albumin (BSA) (4) served as recipients of high-titered sera obtained from rats with HN. Chronic serum sickness produces proliferative glomerulonephritis with markedly elevated urinary protein excretion in rats. The morphology of proximal tubules in rats with early chronic serum sickness is essentially normal, however (26). The injection over a 24-hr period of 4.5 ml of BB antiserum is associated with extensive deposition of Ig along the luminal border of proximal tubules. Preferential staining of tubules in the inner cortex is observed. Examination of the morphology of the tubular epithelium, following *in situ* perfusion fixation, reveals extensive loss of microvilli from the luminal surface. Dramatic proliferation of epithelial cells is also observed in some kidneys. The accumulation of many cells in the lumen of tubules suggests that at least some of the intraluminal cells seen in active HN are of epithelial origin. It had not been previously possible on morphologic grounds to identify, as blood borne or epithelial, any of the cells that accumulate in the lumen of tubules of rats actively immunized with FxlA.

A role of antibodies to BB in human interstitial nephritis has not yet been demonstrated. However, from the natural history of HN in rats it is now apparent that immune deposits in the tubules may be transitory. Furthermore, tubule cell damage may be difficult to evaluate in all but optimally fixed tissue specimens. For these reasons, it is possible that similar immune mechanisms operating in human disease have been overlooked or improperly interpreted in the past.

IV. INTERSTITIAL NEPHRITIS ASSOCIATED WITH DEPOSITION OF IMMUNE COMPLEXES

Deposition of immune complexes in the renal interstitium may also be associated with interstitial inflammation and pathology. That phenomenon has been described in a number of animal models and is also a feature of many cases of nephritis in systemic lupus erythematosus (SLE).

A. *Immune Complexes Containing Nonrenal Antigens*

Rabbits, rats, and mice immunized daily with high doses of BSA develop glomerulonephritis with deposits of immune complexes containing BSA, Ig, and C along the GBM (4, 10, 31). In addition, granular immune deposits containing all three reactants may be found in many organs and tissues, as well as in extraglomerular sites within the kidney (4, 7, 31). The extraglomerular renal deposits are distributed in the walls of peritubular capillaries, in the interstitium, along Bowman's capsule and along the TBM. The TBM deposits are not restricted to cortical tubules but are found along all tubule segments, in the medulla as well as the cortex. Cells of the tubular epithelium are frequently damaged and may become atrophic. The TBM is often thickened and split. Accumulation of immune deposits within the renal interstitium can be associated with mononuclear cell infiltration and with interstitial fibrosis. It is generally believed that the immune complex deposits seen in animal models of chronic serum sickness form in circulation and deposit nonspecifically in many highly vascularized tissues, including the renal interstitium.

A similar phenomenon is observed in a high percentage of patients with SLE nephritis (8). Granular to ribbon-like immune deposits of Ig and C may be found in extraglomerular sites, including the TBM of all tubule segments, the walls of peritubular capillaries and larger vessels, and the interstitium. These deposits have, in some cases, been shown to contain denatured DNA and probably arise as DNA/anti-DNA immune complexes, deposited in tissues after formation in circulation. The histologic abnormalities seen in the renal interstitium of patients with SLE are similar to those observed in animals with systemic immune complex disease produced by chronic immunization with BSA. That pathology includes inflammatory cell infiltration of the interstitium, degeneration of tubule cells, and thickening and splitting of the TBM. Granular extraglomerular renal immune deposits have occasionally been observed in association with other renal diseases, but are so characteristic of SLE nephritis that their demonstration is of diagnostic significance.

B. *Immune Complexes Containing Renal Antigens*

Rabbits immunized with nonglomerular components of rabbit kidney develop an interstitial nephritis that is characterized by focal lymphocytic infiltration, tubule degeneration, and extensive fibrosis of the interstitium (18). The immunization elicits production of autoantibodies that stain the cytoplasm of normal proximal tubule cells in indirect immunofluorescence tests. In the kidneys of affected rabbits, Ig and C are found to be deposited in a granular pattern along the TBM of proximal tubules. Passive transfer of serum from rabbits with interstitial nephritis to normal rabbits results in focal deposition of Ig along TBM in a pattern identical to that seen in the donors. Eluates of the kidneys of immunized rabbits stain antigens located primarily in the BB of proximal tubules of normal kidneys (20). In addition, the eluates contain antibodies that stain antigens present in the granular TBM deposits. These observations are consistent with a hypothesis that immune complexes along the TBM may form by the local or *in situ* reaction of circulating antibodies with antigen(s) of the proximal tubule "leaking" from the base of the epithelial cell.

Granular immune deposits along the TBM of proximal tubules are also a feature of HN (19, 26). Although they may be detected in an early stage of disease, before the onset of proteinuria, they are particularly prominent in kidney tissue obtained from rats in Stage 3 of HN. At that time extensive damage to epithelial cells of the proximal tubules has been sustained. By electron microscopy, dense deposits, corresponding to the granules seen by fluorescence microscopy, are found exclusively in a subepithelial location along TBM and proximal tubules (Fig. 4A). The TBM is wrinkled and thickened; basal infoldings of the epithelial cell are absent. In Stage 4

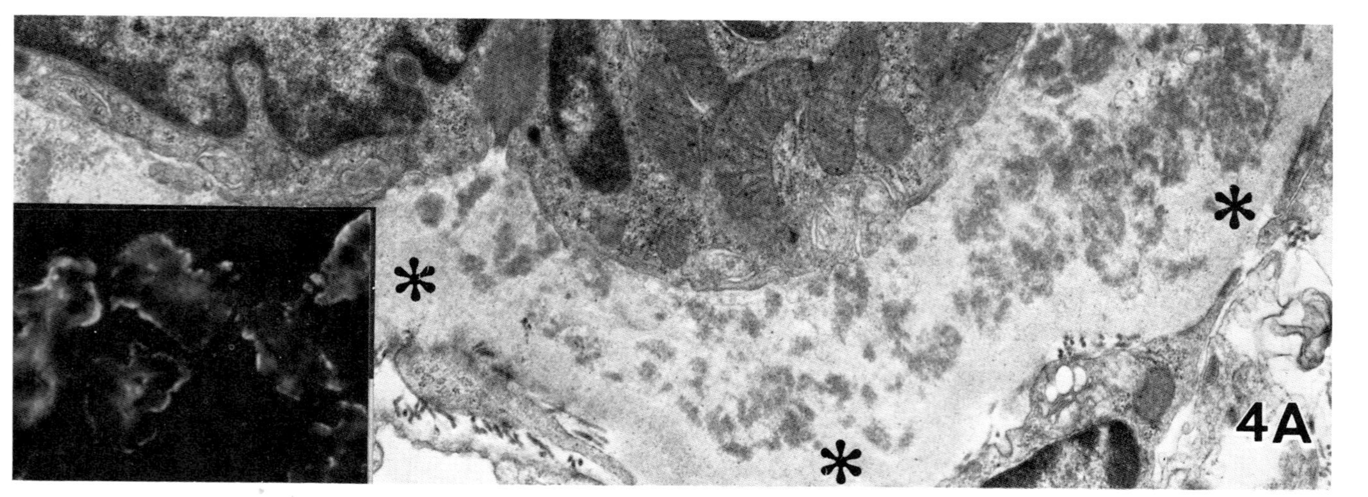

FIGURE 4A. Electron micrograph of the base of a proximal tubule of a rat in Stage 3 of HN. Large dense deposits are seen exclusively on the epithelial side of the TBM (asterisks). The space between the TBM and the epithelium is greatly widened (×6000). Inset: A section of frozen kidney from the same rat stained with a fluoresceinated antiserum to rat IgG. There is granular deposition of IgG along TBM (×500).

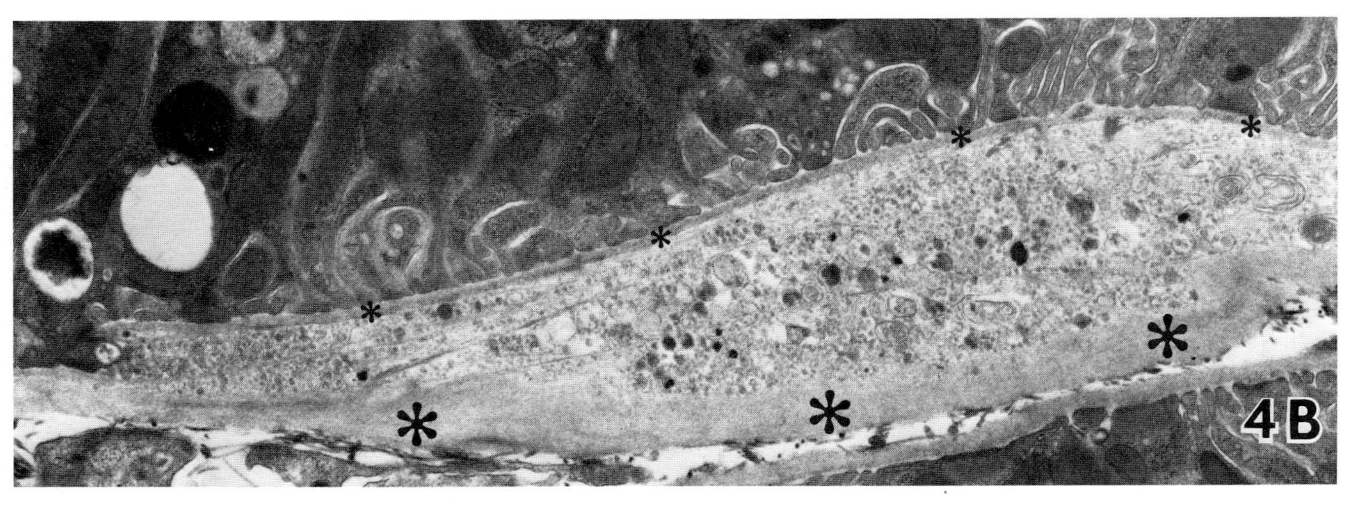

FIGURE 4B. Electron micrograph of the base of a proximal tubule of a rat in Stage 4 of HN. The original TBM (large asterisks) is separated from the epithelium by debris. What appears to be newly formed TBM (small asterisks) is visible directly underneath the epithelium. Electron dense deposits are no longer present. The basal infoldings of the epithelial cells have reappeared (×6000).

of HN, when antibodies to BB are no longer present in serum, TBM deposits of Ig are also no longer detectable by direct immunofluorescence. Studies by electron microscopy of kidneys from rats in Stage 4 show that substantial recovery of the normal morphology of the basal portion of tubular epithelium may occur. A newly formed TBM lies just below the basal membrane of the epithelial cells, to which characteristic infoldings are restored. A layer of cellular debris lies between the new TBM and the thickened, wrinkled original TBM (Fig. 4B).

Following reimmunization of animals in Stage 4 of HN with FxlA, electron dense deposits accumulate again in a subepithelial site between the newly formed TBM and the base of epithelial cells, resulting in a multilayered TBM and producing a very thickened aspect at the basal side of the epithelium. The subepithelial location of TBM immune deposits in HN and the strict limitation of those deposits to the TBM of proximal tubules suggests that a local antibody reaction specific for antigen(s) of the proximal tubule is responsible for their formation. Because the deposits are not present elsewhere in the interstitium or the tubules, it seems unlikely that they originate as immune complexes preformed in circulation like those in chronic serum sickness. It is rather more probable that they arise by reaction of antibodies present in HN serum with fixed antigens of the proximal tubules or with antigens "leaking" from the cell as a consequence either of normal metabolic processes or of the extensive cytotoxic damage suffered by the interaction of the epithelial cell with antibodies to BB.

Immune deposits along the basement membrane of cells in the thick ascending limb of Henle's loop have been described to be associated with selective leukocytic infiltration around that distal nephron segment (17). The immune deposits, which contain Ig, C, and Tamm-Horsfall (T-H) protein, appear following immunization of rats with T-H protein, an antigen limited in distribution to the thick ascending limb of the loop of Henle. In this animal model of tubulointerstitial nephritis it has also been proposed that immune complex formation is a consequence of the *in situ* reaction of antibodies in circulation with molecules of T-H protein associated with the tubule cell membrane.

There is an indication that T-H protein may be involved in the pathogenesis of some human renal diseases. Deposits of T-H protein, sometimes associated with inflammatory cell infiltration, have been seen in a number of tubulointerstitial diseases (33, 43). Autoantibodies to T-H protein have been described in patients with pyelonephritis (15) and in reflux nephropathy (16). However, until now, there is no evidence that immune deposits containing Ig as well as T-H protein occur in any form of human renal disease.

V. SUMMARY

The pathogenic significance of the deposition of antibody or immune complexes in tubular and interstitial nephritis is incompletely understood. The application of immunofluorescence techniques to the study of renal biopsy specimens has increased the ability to recognize tubulointerstitial pathology associated with antibody deposition. Animal models of tubulointerstitial renal disease have demonstrated some of the possible relationships of immunologic injury to tissue damage and renal dysfunction. Furthermore, elucidation of the natural history of tubulointerstitial disease mediated by specific antibodies or immune complexes in animals has aided the recognition of similar nephropathies in man. Until now, however, immunopathogenic mechanisms associated with specific antibodies or immune complexes have been implicated in only a small fraction of human interstitial nephritides. Although antibody-mediated interstitial nephritis in man appears rare, it seems likely that an immune pathogenesis has not yet been identified in some instances in which it is important. The contribution of humoral immune factors to tissue damage, which has been greatly clarified by study of animal models, may have been overlooked in tissue specimens obtained at late stages of disease. The mechanisms by which tubule injury could lead to anti-TBM autoimmunization have not been identified, nor has a counterpart of anti-BB damage to tubules been recognized in man. In addition, animal models of tubulointerstitial disease mediated by antibodies of the IgE class are not available.

REFERENCES

1. Andres, G., Brentjens, J. R., Kohli, R., Anthone, R., Anthone, S., Baliah, T., Montes, M., Mookerjee, B., Prezyna, A., Sepulveda, M., Venuto, R., and Elwood, C. Histology of human tubulo-interstitial nephritis associated with antibodies to renal basement membranes. *Kidney Int. 13*, 480-491 (1978).

2. Andres, G. A. and McCluskey, R. T. Tubular and interstitial renal disease due to immunologic mechanisms. *Kidney Int. 7*, 271-289 (1975).

3. Andres, G. A., Szymanski, C., Albini, B., Brentjens, J. R., Milgrom, M., Noble, B., Ossi, E., and Steblay, R. Structural observations on epithelioid and giant cells in experimental autoimmune tubulointerstitial nephritis in guinea pigs. *Am. J. Pathol. 96*, 21-29 (1979).

4. Arisz, L., Noble, B., Milgrom, M., Brentjens, J. R., and Andres, G. Experimental chronic serum sickness in rats. A model of immune complex glomerulonephritis and systemic immune complex deposition. *Int. Arch. Allergy Appl. Immunol. 60*, 80-88 (1979).

5. Baldwin, D. S., Levine, B. B., and McCluskey, R. T. Renal failure and interstitial nephritis due to penicillin and methicillin. *N. Engl. J. Med. 279*, 1245-1252 (1968).

6. Border, W., Lehman, D., Egan, J., Sass, H., Glode, J., and Wilson, C. Antitubular basement membrane antibodies in methicillin-associated interstitial nephritis. *N. Engl. J. Med. 291*, 381-384 (1974).

7. Brentjens, J. R., O'Connell, D. W., Pawlowski, I. B., and Andres, G. A. Extraglomerular lesions associated with deposition of circulating antigen-antibody complexes in kidneys of rabbits with chronic serum sickness. *Clin. Immunol. Immunopathol. 3*, 112-126 (1974).

8. Brentjens, J., Sepulveda, M., Baliah, T., Bentzel, C., Erlanger, B., Elwood, C., Montes, M., Hsu, K., and Andres, G. Interstitial immune complex nephritis in patients with systemic lupus erythematosus. *Kidney Int. 7*, 342-350 (1975).

9. Brown, C. A., Carey, K., and Colvin, R. B. Inhibition of autoimmune tubulointerstitial nephritis in guinea pigs by heterologous antisera containing anti-idiotype antibodies. *J. Immunol. 123*, 2102-2107 (1979).

10. Dixon, F. J., Feldman, J., and Vazquez, J. Experimental glomerulonephritis: the pathogenesis of a laboratory model resembling the spectrum of human glomerulonephritis. *J. Exp. Med. 113*, 899-919 (1961).

11. Galpen, J., Shinaberger, J., Stanley, T., Blumenkrantz, M., Bayer, A., Friedman, G., Montgomerie, J., Guze, L., Coburn, J., and Glassock, R. Acute interstitial nephritis due to methicillin. *Am. J. Med. 65*, 756-765 (1978).

12. Glassock, R. J., Edgington, T. S., Watson, J., and Dixon, F. J. Autologous immune complex nephritis induced with renal tubular antigen. II. The pathogenetic mechanism. *J. Exp. Med. 127*, 573-587 (1968).

13. Grupe, W. E. and Kaplan, M. Demonstration of an antibody to proximal tubular antigen in the pathogenesis of experimental autoimmune nephrosis in rats. *J. Lab. Clin. Med. 74*, 400-409 (1969).

14. Hall, C. H., Colvin, R. B., Carey, K., and McCluskey, R. Passive transfer of autoimmune disease with isologous IgG_1 and IgG_2 antibodies to the tubular basement membrane in Strain XIII guinea pigs. *J. Exp. Med. 146*, 1246-1260 (1977).

15. Hanson, L. A., Fasth, A., and Jodal, U. Autoantibodies to Tamm-Horsfall protein, a tool for diagnosing the level of urinary-tract infection. *Lancet 1*, 226 (1976).

16. Hodson, J., Maling, T. M. J., McManamon, P. J., and Lewis, M. G. Reflux nephropathy. *Kidney Int. 8*, S50 (1975).

17. Hoyer, J. Tubulointerstitial immune complex nephritis in rats immunized with Tamm-Horsfall protein. *Kidney Int. 17*, 284-292 (1980).

18. Klassen, J., McCluskey, R. T., and Milgrom, F. Non-glomerular renal disease produced in rabbits by immunization with homologous kidney. *Am. J. Pathol. 63*, 333-350 (1971).

19. Klassen, J., Sugisaki, T., Milgrom, F., and McCluskey, R. T. Studies on multiple renal lesions in Heymann nephritis. *Lab. Invest. 25*, 577-585 (1971).

20. Klassen, J., Milgrom, F., and McCluskey, R. T. Studies of the antigens involved in an immunologic renal tubular lesion in rabbits. *Am. J. Pathol. 88*, 135-141 (1977).

21. Lehman, D. H., Wilson, C. B., and Dixon, F. J. Interstitial nephritis in rats immunized with heterologous tubular basement membrane. *Kidney Int. 5*, 187-195 (1974).

22. Lehman, D. H., Wilson, C. B., and Dixon, F. J. Extraglomerular immunoglobulin deposits in human nephritis. *Am. J. Med. 58*, 765-786 (1975).

23. Levy, M., Gagnadoux, M. F., Beziau, A., and Habib, R. Membranous glomerulonephritis associated with antitubular and anti-alveolar basement membrane antibodies. *Clin. Nephrol. 10*, 158-165 (1978).

24. Makker, S. Tubular basement membrane antibody-induced interstitial nephritis in systemic lupus erythematosus. *Am. J. Med. 69*, 949-952 (1980).

25. McCluskey, R. T. and Klassen, J. Immunologically mediated glomerular, tubular and interstitial renal disease. *N. Engl. J. Med. 288*, 564-569 (1973).

26. Mendrick, D., Noble, B., Brentjens, J. R., and Andres, G. Antibody-mediated injury to proximal tubules in Heymann nephritis. *Kidney Int. 18*, 328-343 (1980).

27. Mery, J.-P. and Morel-Maroger, L. Acute interstitial nephritis. *Proc. Int. Congr. Nephrol., 6th, Florence,* p. 524-529 (1976).

28. Morel-Maroger, L., Kourilsky, O., Mignon, F., and Richet, G. Antitubular basement membrane antibodies in rapidly progressive poststreptococcal glomerulonephritis. *Clin. Immunol. Immunopathol. 2*, 185-194 (1974).

29. Noble, B., Brentjens, J. R., Andres, G., and VanLiew, J. B. Damage to renal proximal tubules in rats with Heymann nephritis following reimmunization with FxlA. *Kidney Int. 18*, 188 (1981).

30. Noble, B., Mendrick, D., Brentjens, J. R., and Andres, G. Damage of proximal tubules in the rat kidney by passive transfer of homologous anti-brush border serum. *Clin. Immunol. Immunopathol. 19*, 289-301 (1981).

31. Noble, B., Olson, K. A., Milgrom, M., and Albini, B. Tissue deposition of immune complexes in mice receiving daily injections of bovine serum albumin. *Clin. Exp. Immunol. 42*, 255-263 (1980).

32. Ooi, B., Ooi, Y., Mohini, R., and Pollak, V. Humoral mechanisms in drug-induced acute interstitial nephritis. *Clin. Immunol. Immunopathol. 10*, 330-334 (1978).

33. Resnick, J., Sisson, S., and Vernier, R. L. Tamm-Horsfall protein: Abnormal localization in renal disease. *Lab. Invest. 38*, 550-555 (1980).

34. Rudofsky, U. H., McMaster, P. R., Ma, W.-S., Steblay, R. W., and Pollara, B. Experimental autoimmune renal cortical tubulointerstitial disease in guinea pigs lacking the fourth component of complement (C4). *J. Immunol. 112*, 1387-1393 (1974).

35. Rudofsky, U. H. and Pollara, B. Studies on the pathogenesis of experimental autoimmune renal tubulointerstitial disease in guinea pigs. I. Inhibition of tissue injury in leukocyte-depleted passive transfer recipients. *Clin. Immunol. Immunopathol. 4*, 425-439 (1975).

36. Rudofsky, U. H., Steblay, R. W., and Pollara, B. Inhibition of experimental autoimmune renal tubulointerstitial disease in guinea pigs by depletion of complement with cobra venom factor. *Clin. Immunol. Immunopathol. 3*, 396-407 (1975).

37. Steblay, R. and Rudofsky, U. H. Renal tubular disease and autoantibodies against tubular basement membrane induced in guinea pigs. *J. Immunol. 107*, 589-594 (1971).

38. Steblay, R. and Rudofsky, U. H. Transfer of experimental autoimmune renal cortical tubular and interstitial disease in guinea pigs by serum. *Science 180*, 966-968 (1973).

39. Sugisaki, T., Klassen, J., Milgrom, F., Andres, G. A., and McCluskey, R. T. Immunopathologic study of an autoimmune tubular and interstitial renal disease in Brown Norway rats. *Lab. Invest. 28*, 658-671 (1973).

40. Tung, K. and Black, W. Association of renal glomerular and tubular immune complex disease and antitubular basement membrane antibody. *Lab. Invest. 32*, 696-700 (1975).

41. Wilson, C. B. and Dixon, F. J. Renal injury from immune reactions involving antigens in or of the kidney. *In* "Immunologic Mechanisms of Renal Disease" (C. B. Wilson, B. M. Brenner, and J. H. Stein, eds.), pp. 35-66. Churchill Livingstone, New York, 1979.

42. Wilson, C. B., Lehman, D., McCoy, R., Gunnells, J., and Stukel, D. Antitubular basement membrane antibodies after renal transplantation. *Transplantation 18*, 447-452 (1974).

43. Zager, R., Cotran, R., and Hoyer, J. Pathologic localization of Tamm-Horsfall protein in interstitial deposits in renal disease. *Lab. Invest. 38*, 52-57 (1978).

Immunopathology: VIIIth International Symposium, 1980

HUMAN LYMPHOPLASMACYTIC PROLIFERATIONS WITH PRODUCTION OF STRUCTURALLY ABNORMAL IMMUNOGLOBULINS

Jean-Louis Preud'homme
Maxime Seligmann

Laboratoire d'Immunochimie
et d'Immunopathologie (INSERM U 108),
Institut de Recherches sur les Maladies
du Sang de I'Université Paris VII,
Laboratoire d'Oncologie et d'Immuno-Hématologie
du C.N.R.S., Hôpital Saint-Louis,
75475 Paris Cedex 10, France

I. INTRODUCTION

Myeloma globulins were long believed to be aberrant proteins and the term "paraprotein" coined by Apitz was for a time very popular. Fifteen to twenty years ago, several laboratories including our own showed that these components were in fact homogeneous populations of normal immunoglobulin (Ig) molecules, reflecting the expansion of a single clone of plasma cells. The biochemical and immunological study of such myeloma globulins has provided very valuable data on the structure, antigenic markers, and functions of human and

ISBN 0-12-218320-7

murine normal immunoglobulins. However, structurally altered Ig molecules have now been characterized in the serum of patients and mice with various B-cell neoplasias. They are occasionally found in common cases of myeloma or macroglobulinemia where they are considered rare mutants. They are invariably present in some other conditions such as heavy-chain diseases. Recent studies of Ig biosynthesis performed in our laboratory have demonstrated its production by the proliferating plasma cells of structurally abnormal Ig chains, which are rapidly degraded and therefore not detectable in the serum or urines, in Bence-Jones and nonsecretory myeloma, and in a new condition featured by visceral Ig deposits. The purpose of this chapter is to summarize roughly these findings and underline their biological and clinical implications.

II. HEAVY-CHAIN DISEASES

Heavy-chain disease(s) (HCD) [reviewed in Seligmann *et al.* (17)] are defined by the production of Ig molecules devoid of light chains and made of incomplete heavy chains. The structural defect of most HCD proteins is an internal deletion of the heavy chain [reviewed in Franklin and Frangione (6) and Seligmann *et al.* (17)]. As illustrated in Fig. 1, the site of resumption of the normal sequence of the heavy chain of the same class is not random. In most γ-chain disease proteins, the gap following an aminoterminal segment varying in length from 2 to about 100 residues ends at position 216, at the very beginning of the hinge. In both α-chain disease proteins studied in our laboratory normal sequence resumes at a similar position. As shown in Fig. 1, the resumption of normal sequence occurs at other sites in a few other HCD proteins. For each of the three μ-chain disease proteins for which structural data are available, the resumption of normal sequence

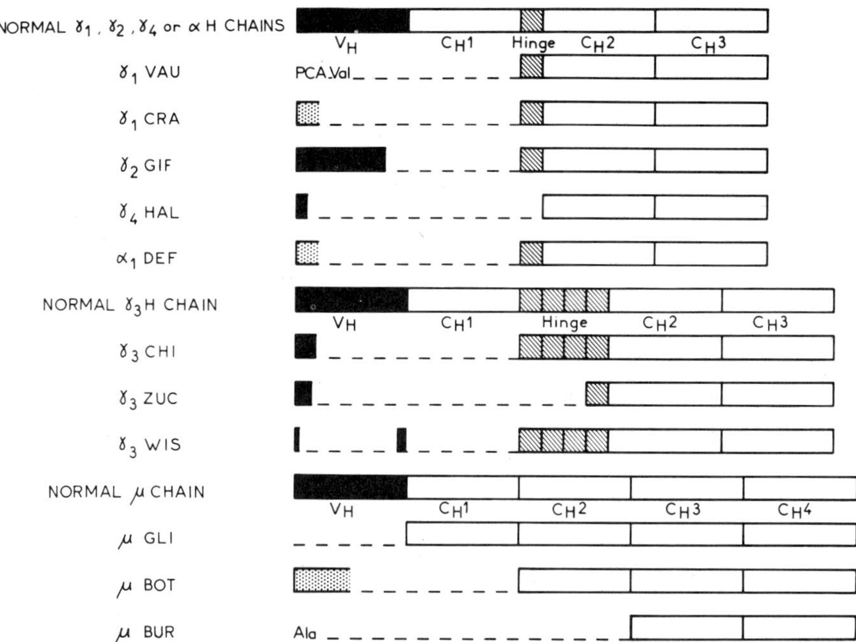

FIGURE 1. Schematic diagram of the structure of selected heavy chain disease proteins compared to normal heavy chain of the same class or subclass. The black bars represent sequences of unknown origin. The broken lines represent the gaps. [From Seligmann *et al.* (17, p. 152), with permission of the publisher.]

occurs at the beginning of the constant domain, CH1, CH2, or CH3. These findings fit well the notion of genetic discontinuity.

The deletions in HCD proteins usually affect two or even three heavy-chain domains and the reason they skip one or two potential joining regions is not yet understood. The study of DNA and RNA of proliferating cells producing these HCD proteins should help us understand the nature of the recognition signals needed for splicing and elucidate the nature of the genetic defect responsible for the synthesis of these abnormal chains. It has recently been shown that a murine variant IF2, with a deletion of only the CH1 domain, has a corresponding deletion of the DNA (5). This simple explanation may be true, but only for some human heavy-chain diseases, which represent a heterogeneous group. For instance, as shown in Fig. 1, the amino terminus can often be identified as VH, whereas in some other proteins the amino terminal stretch preceeding the deletion represents sequences of unknown origin, possibly due to abnormal splicing. It is of interest in this regard that the internally deleted κ variant of MPC11 that lacks the V region results from aberrant DNA- and RNA-splicing events due to a structural gene abnormality with absence of the J segment and of the site for V - C_{κ} splicing (4, 15).

The other main feature of HCD proteins is the lack of light chains. The failure of light-chain synthesis is demonstrated in some (3) but not all (10) cases of heavy-chain diseases. It is probably due to some regulatory rather than structural defect. The absence of the light-chain gene with a double defect at the DNA level is difficult to visualize since the genes coding for heavy and light chains are not linked. The DNA defect responsible for the heavy-chain deletion could possibly result in an error in light-chain RNA splicing and processing.

Another intriguing structural feature of HCD proteins is their high carbohydrate content and particularly the presence of unusual carbohydrate moieties (such as galactosamine in γ or μ chains) located at the amino terminal end of these proteins. It is worth noting that abnormal glycosylation was found in a mouse myeloma mutant with short heavy chains (18).

The production of human HCD proteins is not necessarily linked to overt malignant lymphoid proliferation. In some patients with γ or μ HCD it has been impossible to detect an underlying truly neoplastic B-cell proliferation, and the presence of the HCD proteins may even be transient.

Alpha-chain disease proceeds in two stages. The second stage is characterized by an immunoblastic lymphoma and the sarcomatous cells were shown to be derived from the HCD protein producing clone. The first stage is characterized by a diffuse plasma cell infiltration of the gut and mesenteric nodes, which is possibly preneoplastic and not truly malignant since it can revert completely after administration of antibiotics.

III. MYELOMA

Several serum myeloma globulins with various deletions (e.g., a deletion of the hinge) have been described [reviewed in Franklin and Frangione (6)]. Human and murine myeloma IgA or IgG half-molecules usually appear to be associated with a heavy-chain deletion [reviewed in Seligmann *et al.* (16)]. We would like to focus here on cases where the study of immunoglobulin biosynthesis by the malignant plasma cells allows one to demonstrate the production of unreleased or degraded structurally abnormal Ig chains.

Bence-Jones myeloma is defined by the presence in serum and urine of monotypic free light chains without detectable whole monoclonal Ig molecules. We have shown several years ago that the immunofluorescence study of the plasma cells of such patients revealed the presence of apparently unreleased intracytoplasmic heavy chains in 10 of 36 cases studied (9). We have discussed the possibility of a structural abnormality of the heavy chain leading to a block in secretion and/or to proteolysis. Biosynthesis experiments were recently performed in one such patient with intracellular IgG (11). They showed that γ chains were produced with a heavy-to-light chain ratio of about 0.7, that these heavy chains were abnormally short (45,000 daltons), and that their assembly with light chains was blocked. Whereas the light chains were rapidly secreted as free light chains and light-chain dimers, heavy-chain containing molecules were secreted more slowly and were degraded after secretion, a finding consistent with the lack of detectable monoclonal IgG in this patient's serum. The degradation is probably related to the structural abnormality since a rapid intra- or extracellular proteolysis featured several murine myeloma producing deleted heavy chains (2, 7, 11, 19).

Analogous findings have been made in some cases of so-called nonsecretory myeloma. In a series of 30 patients with overt myeloma and the absence of any monoclonal Ig in serum and urine (9, Preud'homme *et al.*, unpublished observations) we have found by direct immunofluorescence monoclonal immunoglobulin chains (IgG, IgA or light chains) in the cytoplasm of the plasma cells of all patients studied. The occurrence of true nonproducers, which is well documented in murine myeloma variants (1), is therefore very low in human myeloma. Biosynthesis studies were performed in some of these patients. Synthesis of normal-sized Ig chains followed by very slow or absent secretion appears to be very rare (one single case in our series). In another patient we demonstrated the production of an abnormally short heavy chain with a normal-sized light chain, a block in assembly, intracellular degradation, and the absence of detectable secretion even in the early samples. The most common situation in our experience is the synthesis of abnormally short or large heavy or light chains followed by postsecretory proteolysis. It should be noted that structural alterations in the Ig chains have also been found in nonsecreting variant clones of murine myeloma (8, 20).

IV. IMMUNOGLOBULIN DEPOSITION DISEASE

In our laboratory we have recently studied 12 patients affected with a syndrome closely resembling that described in 1976 by Randall *et al.* (14) under the designation of light-chain deposition disease. These patients had systemic tissue deposition of an amorphous material which was clearly different from amyloidosis and which was stained by anti-Ig serum in immnofluorescence studies. In several of these patients we showed the synthesis of structurally abnormal Ig not detectable in serum and urine (or in trace amounts) and which may result in severe systemic disease (12, 13).

Most of these patients presented with proteinuria and renal failure. Biopsy of the kidney lead in most instances to diagnosis showing both glomerular and tubular lesions. The most constant feature was a marked thickening of the tubular basement membranes by a nonfibrillar material strongly positive for PAS staining. A similar material was found in the mesangial matrix. A thickening of the glomerular basement membrane was present in some but not all patients and a nodular glomerulosclerosis was observed in about 50% of cases. The deposits lacked the histochemical properties of the amyloid substance, showed no fibrillar structure in electron microscopy, and were stained with anti-Ig conjugates. Hepatomegaly was noted in several patients and liver biopsy showed deposits of anti-Ig reactive material along the sinusoids. One patient presented with major portal hypertension and peliosis hepatis at histopathologic examination. Cardiac failure and polyneuropathy, presumably due to tissue Ig deposits, were also observed in some patients.

Table I summarizes several important features in these patients. The tissue deposits may contain both heavy- and light-chain determinants. The term "light-chain deposition"

TABLE I. Monoclonal Immunoglobulin Deposition Disease: Hematological and Immunological Data

Patient	Hematological diagnosis	Monoclonal Ig in serum and/or urine	CIg positive marrow plasma cells (%)	Tissue I fluorescence
Mo	Myeloma (preceding Ig deposition disease)	IgA (sharp decrease when Ig deposition)	40-95 $\alpha\kappa$	$\alpha\kappa$
Sa	Myeloma	κ BJ	22-99 κ	κ
Lev	Myeloma	Small IgG λ + λ BJ	50-70 $\gamma\lambda$	λ
Mi	Myeloma	Transient small IgG λ	10-15 $\gamma\lambda$	$\gamma\lambda$
Be	Myeloma (diagnosis after follow up)	IgG κ	6-12 $\gamma\kappa$	κ
Lau	Myeloma (diagnosis after follow up)	None (transient traces of free κ chains)	1-58 κ	κ
Po	Plasmocytoma of both kidneys	IgA κ	1 $\alpha\kappa$	$\alpha\kappa$
Ro	Pleomorphic lympho-plasmacytic proliferation	None	5 κ	κ
Cai	Questionable myeloma (stable for 3 yr without treatment)	None	2-10 κ	κ
Laa	No overt lymphoplasmacytic malignancy	Traces of free κ chains	5 κ	κ
Cap	No overt lymphoplasmacytic malignancy	None	2- 4 κ	κ
Uz	No overt lymphoplasmacytic malignancy	None	3- 5 κ	κ

is therefore inappropriate and we preferred to call this condition "monoclonal immunoglobulin deposition disease." Some of the patients were affected with overt myeloma. It is worth noting that in one of these patients, who was treated for IgAκ myeloma, bone marrow relapse and a sharp drop in the serum IgA level paralleled tissue deposition (13). In some other patients myeloma, which was not detectable when progressive renal failure with nephrotic syndrome led to the diagnosis of Ig deposition disease, was diagnosed some time later. One patient was affected with a diffuse malignant plasmacytoma of both kidneys without evidence of other plasma cell proliferation. The patient presenting with hepatic peliosis had a pleiomorphic lymphoplasmacytic malignance analogous to Waldenström's macroglobulinemia (12). Some of the patients showed no evidence of overt malignant lymphoplasmacytic proliferation after thorough investigation and, in some cases, reasonable follow-up. However, a monoclonal population of bone marrow plasma cells was easily detectable in every case by immunofluorescence. In many patients the serum or urine did not contain a monoclonal Ig in appreciable amounts, and several of these cases might be classified as nonsecretory myeloma. Ig chains formed in the plasma cells were the same as those revealed by the immunofluorescence study of tissue biopsies except in two patients whose plasma cells contained IgG, whereas only light chains were detectable in the kidney deposits.

The major finding in our study is that of the synthesis of structurally abnormal Ig chains in 5 of 7 patients studied (Table II). Biosynthesis experiments were critical in these patients since the abnormal chains were not detectable in reasonable amounts in their serum or urine. We found abnormally short light chains in two cases and abnormally large light chains in three cases. Additionally, patient Mos heavy chains were short, lacking about one domain. In this patient the

TABLE II. Monoclonal Immunoglobulin Deposition Disease: Biosynthesis Experiments*

	Immunofluorescence		Biosynthesis experiments			
			Molecular weight of Ig chains			
			L			
Patient	Tissues	Plasma cells	cyto.	sec	H	L-Chain polymerization
Lau	κ	κ	*28,000*	31,000	None	Trimers
Cai	κ	κ	*30,000*	31,000	None	160,000
Ro	κ	κ	*12,000*	20,000	None	150,000
Mo	ακ	ακ	*20,000* 23,000	23,000 25,000	*43,000*	?**
Be	κ	γκ	*29,000*	32,000	57,000	?**
Sa	κ	κ	23,000	23,000	None	Dimers
Lev	λ	γλ	29,000***	29,000	55,000	Dimers

**Immunoglobulin chains with abnormal size are shown in italics.*

***Not appreciable because of the presence of assembled molecules with H and L chains.*

****Estimation of the molecular weight of λ chains by SDS-gel electrophoresis is not reliable.*

tissue deposition probably corresponded to the emergence of a variant clone producing the abnormal Ig chains and was possibly due to the mutagenic action of Melphalan. The abnormal light chains were secreted as polymers in three of our patients. Striking differences in apparent molecular weights between cytoplasmic and secreted light chains were observed in all five patients; this feature might be related to abnormal glycosylation. Lack of material precluded biosynthesis experiments with radiolabeled carbohydrates.*

Our results suggest that the structural abnormality of the Ig chains may play a direct role in tissue deposition. Indeed, the deposits contained the very same chains as the abnormal chains found in biosynthesis experiments. Strikingly, in patient Be, whose cells produced normal heavy chains and abnormal light chains, only the latter were detectable by kidney immunofluorescence. The mechanism of tissue precipitation is unknown. The tendency to light-chain polymerization may play a role. It is likely that the secretion of abnormal immunoglobulin chains is not the unique mechanism responsible for Ig deposition disease since, in two patients, the results of biosynthesis experiments were similar to those obtained in common cases of BJ myeloma without deposition, with no abnormal light-chain polymers. The possibility that in these two patients a minor subclone, undetected in the biosynthesis experiments, might produce abnormal chains cannot be excluded but appears rather unlikely.

V. CONCLUSION

It appears that in heavy-chain diseases as well as in immunoglobulin depostion disease, a clone producing the structurally abnormal immunoglobulin chains is not always malignant.

**Recent studies in 2 patients showed that abnormal light chains contained a high percentage of carbohydrates.*

Thus, the structural abnormality is probably not directly linked to malignant transformation. On the other hand, there is much evidence that most malignant B-cell proliferations in leukemias, lymphomas, and myelomas originate in B cells that produce normal immunoglobulin molecules. In order to explain the relative frequency of monoclonal lymphoplasmacytic proliferations with production of structurally abnormal immunoglobulin, we are left with two main possibilities: (a) some normal B cells do produce aberrant immunoglobulin chains; they are only recognized when they undergo monoclonal proliferation and these variants may be more susceptible to ultimate malignant transformation than cells producing normal immunoglobulin molecules and (b) proliferating B cells display genetic instability and therefore have an increased chance to produce aberrant immunoglobulin molecules.

REFERENCES

1. Baumal, R., Birshtein, B. K., Coffino, P., and Scharff, M. D. Mutations in immunoglobulin-producing mouse myeloma cells. *Science 182*, 164-166 (1973).

2. Birshtein, B. K., Preud'homme, J. L., and Scharff, M. D. Variants of mouse myeloma cells that produce short immunoglobulin heavy chains. *Proc. Natl. Acad. Sci. U.S.A. 71*, 3478-3482 (1974).

3. Buxbaum, J. N. and Preud'homme, J. L. Alpha and gamma heavy chain diseases in man: intracellular origin of the aberrant polypeptides. *J. Immunol. 109*, 1131-1137 (1972).

4. Choi, E., Kuehl, M., and Wall, R. RNA splicing generates a variant light chain from an aberrantly rearranged κ gene. *Nature (London) 286*, 776-779 (1980).

5. Dunnick, W., Rabbitts, T. H., and Milstein, C. An immunoglobulin deletion mutant with implications for the heavy-chain switch and RNA splicing. *Nature (London) 286*, 669-675 (1980).

6. Franklin, E. C. and Frangione, B. Structural variants of human immunoglobulins. *Contemp. Top. Mol. Immunol. 4*, 89-125 (1975).

7. Morrison, S. L., Baumal, R., Birshtein, B. K., Kuehl, W. M., Preud'homme, J. L., Frank, L., Jasek, T., and Scharff, M. D. The identification of mouse myeloma cells which have undergone mutations in immunoglobulin production. *In* "Cellular Selection and Regulation in the Immune Response" (G. M. Edelman, ed.), pp. 233-244. Raven, New York, 1974.

8. Mosmann, T. R. and Williamson, A. R. Structural mutations in a mouse immunoglobulin light chain resulting in failure to be secreted. *Cell 20*, 283-292 (1980).

9. Preud'homme, J. L., Hurez, D., Danon, F., Brouet, J. C., and Seligmann, M. Intracytoplasmic and surface bound immunoglobulins in "nonsecretory" and Bence-Jones myeloma. *Clin. Exp. Immunol. 25*, 428-436 (1976).

10. Preud'homme, J. L., Brouet, J. C., and Seligmann, M. Cellular immunoglobulins in human γ and α-chain diseases. *Clin. Exp. Immunol. 37*, 283-291 (1979).

11. Preud'homme, J. L., Labaume, S., and Praloran, V. Synthesis of abnormal heavy chains in Bence-Jones plasma cell leukemia with intracellular IgG. *Blood 56*, 1136-1140 (1980).

12. Preud'homme, J. L., Morel-Maroger, L., Brouet, J. C., Cerf, M., Mignon, F., Guglielmi, P., and Seligmann, M. Synthesis of abnormal immunoglobulins in lymphoplasmacytic disorders with visceral light chain deposition. *Am. J. Med. 69*, 703-710 (1980).

13. Preud'homme, J. L., Morel-Maroger, L., Brouet, J. C., Mihaesco, E., Mery, J. P., and Seligmann, M. Synthesis of abnormal heavy and light chains in multiple myeloma with visceral deposition of monoclonal immunoglobulin. *Clin. Exp. Immunol. 42*, 545-553 (1980).

14. Randall, R. E., Williamson, W. C., Mullinax, F., Tung, M. Y., and Still, W. J. S. Manifestations of light chain deposition. *Am. J. Med. 60*, 293-299 (1976).

15. Seidman, J. G. and Leder, P. A mutant immunoglobulin light chain is formed by aberrant DNA- and RNA-splicing events. *Nature (London) 286*, 779-783 (1980).

16. Seligmann, M., Mihaesco, E., Chevalier, A., and Miglierina, R. Immunochemical study of a human myeloma IgG1 half molecule. *Ann. Immunol. (Paris) 129C*, 855-870 (1978).

17. Seligmann, M., Mihaesco, E., Preud'homme, J. L., Danon, F., and Brouet, J. C. Heavy chain diseases: current findings and concepts. *Immunol. Rev. 48*, 145-167 (1979).

18. Weitzman, S., Nathenson, S. G., and Scharff, M. D. Abnormalities in the glycosylation of immunoglobulin heavy chains and an H-2 transplantation antigen in a mouse myeloma mutant. *Cell 10*, 679-687 (1977).

19. Weitzman, S., Palmer, L., and Grennon, M. Serum decay and placental transport of a mutant mouse myeloma immunoglobulin with defective polypeptide and oligosaccharide structure. *J. Immunol. 122*, 12-18 (1979).

20. Winberry, L., Marks, A., and Baumal, R. Immunoglobulin production and secretion by variant clones of the MOPC 315 mouse myeloma cell line. *J. Immunol. 124*, 1174-1182 (1980).

Immunopathology: VIIIth International Symposium, 1980

TREATMENT OF AUTOIMMUNE DISEASES WITH TOTAL LYMPHOID IRRADIATION (TLI)

Samuel Strober
Brian L. Kotzin
David J. Schurman

Departments of Medicine and Surgery,
Stanford University School of Medicine,
Stanford, California

I. INTRODUCTION

Total lymphoid irradiation (TLI) is a routine and safe treatment for Hodgkin's disease (10). The critical features of TLI that differ from single-dose whole body irradiation are (a) the use of lead shielding to protect vital radiosensitive tissues such as the central nervous system, lungs, kidneys, and bone marrow and (b) the use of fractionated irradiation such that large cumulative doses (4400 rads) are achieved by administering multiple small doses (150-250 rads each). Figure 1 shows the radiation ports used to administer TLI to patients with Hodgkin's disease (10). The "mantle" field includes the cervical, axillary, and mediastinal lymph nodes as well as the thymus. The "inverted Y" field includes the paraaortic iliac and inguinal lymph nodes. The spleen is also

ISBN 0-12-218320-7

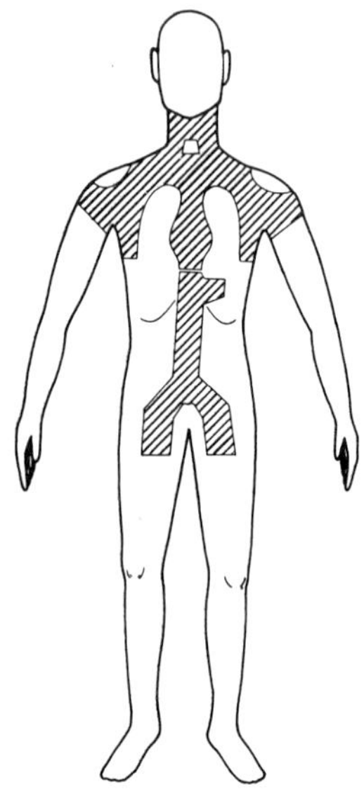

FIGURE 1. Total lymphoid irradiation in man. Shaded areas show ports for X irradiation in patients with Hodgkin's disease.

included in the fields if it has not been removed during the staging laparotomy. Irradiation is given to the mantle field in doses of 150-250 rads per fraction until a total dose of 4400 rads is achieved over a period of four to six weeks (10). A similar course of fractionated radiotherapy (4400 rads) is administered to the abdominal fields to complete the regimen.

II. IMMUNE DEFICITS IN PATIENTS WITH HODGKIN'S DISEASE AFTER TLI

In the course of investigating the cellular basis of the immunodeficiency of patients with Hodgkin's disease, we examined the number and function of T lymphocytes in the peripheral blood before and after treatment with TLI (6). Before radiotherapy, the total lymphocyte count and percentage of T and B cells in patients with Hodgkin's disease were not significantly different from those observed in normal controls (6). However, at the completion of TLI (4400 rads above and below the diaphragm), the mean total peripheral blood lymphocyte (PBL) count of $503/mm^3$ was 4 standard deviations below the mean of normal. Recovery of the lymphocyte count began shortly after completion of radiotherapy and reached pretreatment levels about 2 years later (6). After full recovery of the total count, the percentage of T cells as measured by an *in vitro* cytotoxicity assay with anti-T cell antiserum was approximately half the pretreatment value and remained at that level for at least 10 years (6). The T lymphocytopenia was associated with a B lymphocytosis, and marked reduction of the normal T:B ratio.

The peripheral blood lymphocytes of untreated patients with Hodgkin's disease showed a decreased response to PHA *in vitro*, measured by $[^3H]$thymidine or $[^3H]$leucine incorporation, as compared to normal controls. After radiotherapy, the PHA response of patients with Hodgkin's disease fell significantly below that of the pretreatment level (6). The further reduction in the response persisted for at least 10 years after radiotherapy without disease recurrence.

The mixed leukocyte response (MLR) of untreated patients with Hodgkin's disease was similar to that of normals as measured by incorporation of $[^3H]$thymidine. However, after radiotherapy the MLR was virtually eliminated, and fell to background levels for about 20 months (6). Thereafter, a slow recovery was observed such that normal responses were uniformly observed five or more years after treatment. The minority (27%) of untreated patients with Hodgkin's disease showed a delayed hypersensitivity skin reaction to dinitrochlorobenzene (DNCB). Of the responding group, almost all lost their skin reactivity immediately after the completion of TLI (6). More than half of these treated patients showed a delayed hypersensitivity response to DNCB by one year after treatment. However, 29% of these patients remained anergic for at least eight years after radiotherapy.

III. SIDE EFFECTS OF TLI

Despite the potent immunosuppression induced by TLI, it is an outpatient procedure that is tolerated extremely well. Less than 1% of Hodgkin's disease patients given TLI to a total dose of 4400 rads required hospitalization for irradiation complications (10). Mild self-limited constitutional symptoms were frequent and included fatigue, anorexia, and nausea. Severe thrombocytopenia or leukopenia (less than 50% of baseline) which persisted beyond 2 months after treatment was observed in less than 1% of patients with Hodgkin's disease (10). The incidence of severe bacterial infection requiring hospitalization was less than 1% and was not significantly increased above that associated with the splenectomy performed at the time of staging of disease (10). There have been no cases of acute leukemia or non-Hodgkin's lymphoma in several hundred patients treated with TLI alone at the Stanford Medical Center during the past 10 years (2, 13). Approximately 20% of patients treated with TLI developed Herpes zoster within 2 years after the completion of therapy. Less than 1% of this group progressed to disseminated zoster requiring hospitalization (10). Further possible complications of subdiaphragmatic irradiation include gastric ulcer, bleeding, chronic radiation enteritis, and azospermia. Each was seen in less than 1% of patients treated with TLI for Hodgkin's disease (10).

IV. IMMUNE DEFICITS IN MICE AND RATS AFTER TLI

In view of the potent immunosuppression in humans without severe side effects, we investigated the effects of TLI in mice and rats. Accordingly, adult (six-month-old) BALB/c mice were given high dose, fractionated lymphoid irradiation. The lymph nodes, as well as the spleen and thymus were exposed to radiation. The skull, long bones, tail and lungs were shielded with lead. Each animal was given 17 fractions of 200 rads each to achieve a total dose of 3400 rads within a period of approximately three weeks. Mice were anesthetized with pentobarbital during each treatment. The survival of skin grafts from C57BL/Ka (H-2^b) donors on BALB/c (H-2^d) recipients treated with TLI (17 fractions of 200 rads each) was prolonged about five times as compared to that of untreated recipients (mean of 49.1 versus 10.5 days) (20). The prolongation was related to the total dose of irradiation, and graft survival fell to a mean of 18.4 days after 1400 rads (7 fractions) was administered to the recipients. Thymic irradiation alone (17 fractions of 200 rads each) produced a negligible increase in the mean survival time (21).

The effect of TLI on the humoral antibody response of BALB/c mice to sheep red blood cells (SRBC) injected at different time intervals after radiotherapy was also studied (26). Antibody responses were eliminated for about one month after TLI and recovered during the second month. However, only IgM antibody was produced for at least four months after radiotherapy. IgG antibody was first detected at about seven months, but the response remained six $\log_2$ units below that of normal controls for at least nine months after treatment (26).

Irradiation of the thymus alone or just the subdiaphragmatic tissues had little effect on the anti-SRBC response as compared to normals (26).

V. INDUCTION OF TISSUE TRANSPLANTATION TOLERANCE IN MICE AFTER TLI

In several experiments, BALB/c mice were given TLI, and an intravenous injection of bone marrow cells from C57BL/Ka donors one day later (20, 21). Of 27 recipients given BM cells 24 were chimeras as judged by the presence of donor-type lymphocytes in the peripheral blood more than 100 days after BM transplantation. The majority of lymphocytes in the lymph nodes, spleen, and bone marrow (exposed to irradiation) were of donor type, and chimerism was also found in the erythrocytes. Although allogeneic BM engraftment was achieved in this strain combination, no clinical eveidence of graft-versus-host disease (GVHD) was observed in the recipients (21).

VI. HUMORAL ANTIBODY TOLERANCE AFTER TLI

The induction of humoral tolerance was also studied in mice treated with TLI (27). At various time intervals after TLI, mice were given two intraperitoneal injections of non-deaggregated bovine serum albumin (BSA) (40 mg in 0.5 ml saline) 2 days apart. Approximately one month later, animals were challenged with DNP-BSA in complete Freund's adjuvant (CFA), and the anti-DNP antibodies in the serum were measured by a modified Farr assay for three weeks thereafter (27). Untreated mice or mice given TLI alone made a similar anti-DNP response to DNP-BSA in CFA. Mice given TLI and BSA in saline made a minimal anti-DNP response after challenge with DNP-BSA. The unresponsiveness of the latter mice was due to specific tolerance to BSA, since a similarly treated group of animals made a normal response to DNP-bovine gamma globulin (DNP-BGG) in CFA (27). Mice given TLI and BGG in saline responded poorly to DNP-BGG, but made abnormal response to DNP-BSA (27). Tolerance could be induced to BSA in saline for at least 100 days after the completion of TLI, and appeared to be mediated by antigen-specific suppressor T cells (27).

VII. TREATMENT OF THE LUPUS-LIKE DISEASE OF NZB/NZW MICE WITH TLI

NZB/NZW F_1 mice spontaneously develop an autoimmune disease characterized by antinuclear antibodies and a fatal immune complex glomerulonephritis (9). These features are similar to those seen in human SLE. These F_1 mice offer an excellent model in which to study therapeutic regimens possibly applicable to human disease. Many studies have demonstrated the efficacy of immunosuppressive drug therapy before clinical NZB/NZW disease appears, but few have been effective in mice with established or advanced disease (7, 8, 14, 15, 18, 22). We recently determined whether TLI could produce a remission in mice with moderate or advanced disease.

One large group of forty-eight 4-7-month-old (mean age 6.0 months) NZB/NZW female mice with documented proteinuria were randomly allocated to a treatment (TLI) or control group (11). The mice tolerated the irradiation (3400 rads in 17 fractions of 200 rads each) extremely well and there were no deaths during irradiation in the treated group. At age 8 months (2 months after irradiation), the difference in survival of the two groups became statistically significant, and the difference continued to widen so that by 12 months of age, 2 of the 24 treated animals and 18 of the 24 control animals had died ($p < .0001$). Neither death in the treated group was secondary to NZB/NZW renal disease. In contrast, 16 of the 18 control group deaths were secondary to the lupus-like kidney disease. There was a significant reduction in the progression to high grade proteinuria in the treated group, and by 12 months of age 75% of the controls had progressed to high grade proteinuria compared to less than 19% in the irradiated group (11). Suppression of anti-DNA antibodies was also observed in the treated group (11). The levels of antibody in the treated and control groups were significantly different at 8, 9, 10, and 11 months of age. By the completion of the study (16 months of age), there was no difference in the incidence of tumors between the irradiated and control groups.

A follow-up study was performed which compared the effects of TLI (3400 rads in 17 fractions), whole body irradiation (WBI) (500 rads in one fraction), and no treatment. Twelve 6-month-old NZB/NZW female animals with proteinuria were randomly

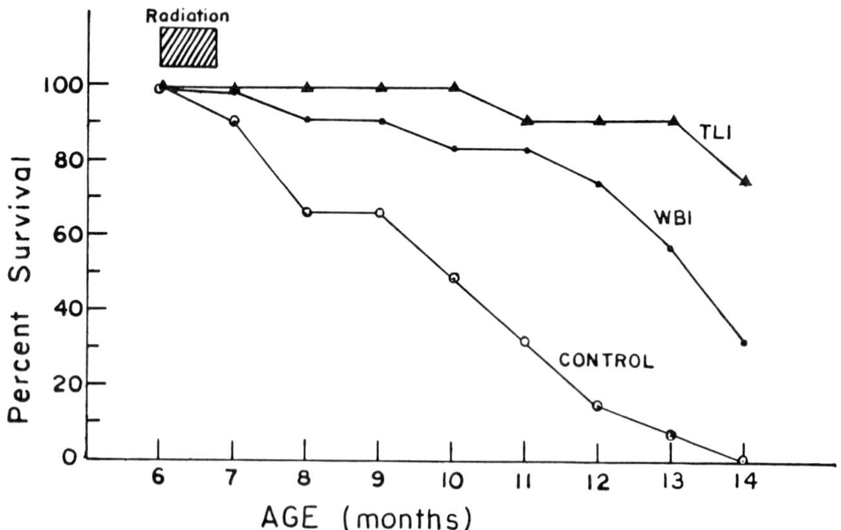

FIGURE 2. Effect of treatment on the survival of NZB/NZW mice up to 14 months of age. (▲) TLI group, (●) WBI group, (○) control group.

allocated to each group. Figure 2 shows the improved survival rate of irradiated animals, both TLI and WBI, compared to no treatment. At 12 months of age (6 months after irradiation), more than 80% of the control animals had died compared to 25% of the WBI and less than 10% of TLI animals. At 14 months of age, 100% of the control animals were dead compared to 67% of the WBI and 25% of the TLI animals. The more profound and longer lasting suppression of NZB/NZW renal disease by TLI compared to WBI is better illustrated in Fig. 3 which shows the progression to high grade proteinuria. Although 58% of WBI mice had progressed by 12 months, more than 90% had progressed by the conclusion of the study at 14 months of age. In contrast, only 8% and 33% of the TLI animals had progressed by 12 and 14 months, respectively. Suppression of antinative DNA antibodies was also greatest in the TLI group, but significant suppression was seen in the WBI group as well.

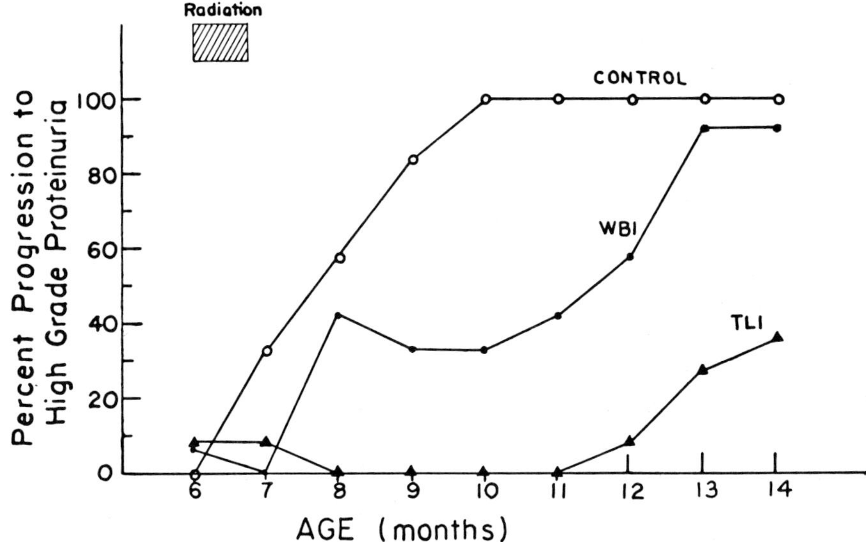

FIGURE 3. Effect of treatment on the cumulative progression to high grade proteinuria (>2^+, >100 mg%) up to 14 months of age. (▲) TLI group, (●) WBI group, (O) control group.

In another study designed to demonstrate the potency of TLI, seven-month-old female NZB/NZW mice were selected for advanced proteinuria and placed in treatment or control groups (11). Prolongation of survival and reversal of proteinuria was observed in the TLI group. Even clinically ill mice (ascitic or wasted) actually showed clinical improvement during the irradiation period, but all control mice died within six weeks.

In summary, we demonstrated that TLI reversed well-expressed disease in NZB/NZW mice with a prolongation in survival, decrease in proteinuria, and decrease in anti-DNA antibodies as compared to control animals. Few side effects were observed in the treated groups. WBI was also capable of disease suppression, but suppression was greater and longer lasting after TLI. It is unclear at this time whether the mechanism of suppression by TLI and WBI is similar, and studies are underway to investigate this question. TLI also prolonged survival in animals with very advanced renal disease. Few studies have shown a similar suppression of disease after the development of proteinuria (7, 8, 14, 15, 18, 22).

VIII. TREATMENT OF THE AUTOIMMUNE DISEASE OF MRL/ℓ MICE WITH TLI

MRL/ℓ mice spontaneously develop massive nonmalignant T-cell proliferation and autoimmune disease that kills 50% of animals by 5-6 months of age (1). Of such mice, 100% given total lymphoid irradiation (TLI 3400 rads) at 3 months of age (time of clinical onset of disease) and 82% given whole body irradiation (WBI 300 rads) remained alive at 9 months of age when the experiment was terminated (24). At that age 92% of unirradiated controls were dead with massive lymph node hyperplasia, splenomegaly, and severe glomerulonephritis. In contrast, none of the TLI or WBI animals had enlarged lymph nodes or splenomegaly and only 11 to 15% of them developed glomerulonephritis (24). Irradiated mice had less serum IgG and total immune complexes than controls, and no gp70-anti-gp70 complexes. However, levels of serum IgM and anti-double-stranded DNA antibodies were minimally reduced in irradiated animals as compared to controls. Anti-single-stranded DNA antibodies were the same in all groups. Because of the lack of T-cell proliferation, TLI and WBI mice had 10-fold fewer lymphocytes in their lymph nodes and 4- to 7-fold fewer mononuclear cells in their spleens than unmanipulated age-matched diseased mice. TLI and WBI mice had 14- and 33-fold, respectively, fewer spontaneous splenic Ig-secreting cells than controls (24). At 6 months after irradiation, treated animals had normal suppressor T-cell function (Con A-induced), but the helper T-cell activity found on a cell-to-cell basis was much below that of the controls. Further studies are underway to determine whether remissions induced by TLI will be longer lasting than those induced with WBI.

IX. TREATMENT OF ADJUVANT ARTHRITIS IN RATS WITH TLI

We investigated the effect of TLI with or without local joint irradiation on adjuvant arthritis in rats induced by a subcutaneous injection of mineral oil with M.butyricum (19). Four groups of rats with adjuvant arthritis were formed: (a) an untreated group, (b) a group treated only with TLI, (c) a group given only paw irradiation, and (d) a group given both TLI and paw irradiation.

The interval arthritis scores for the four groups of Lewis rats are summarized in Fig. 4. There were no statistical differences between any of the groups at the time the groups

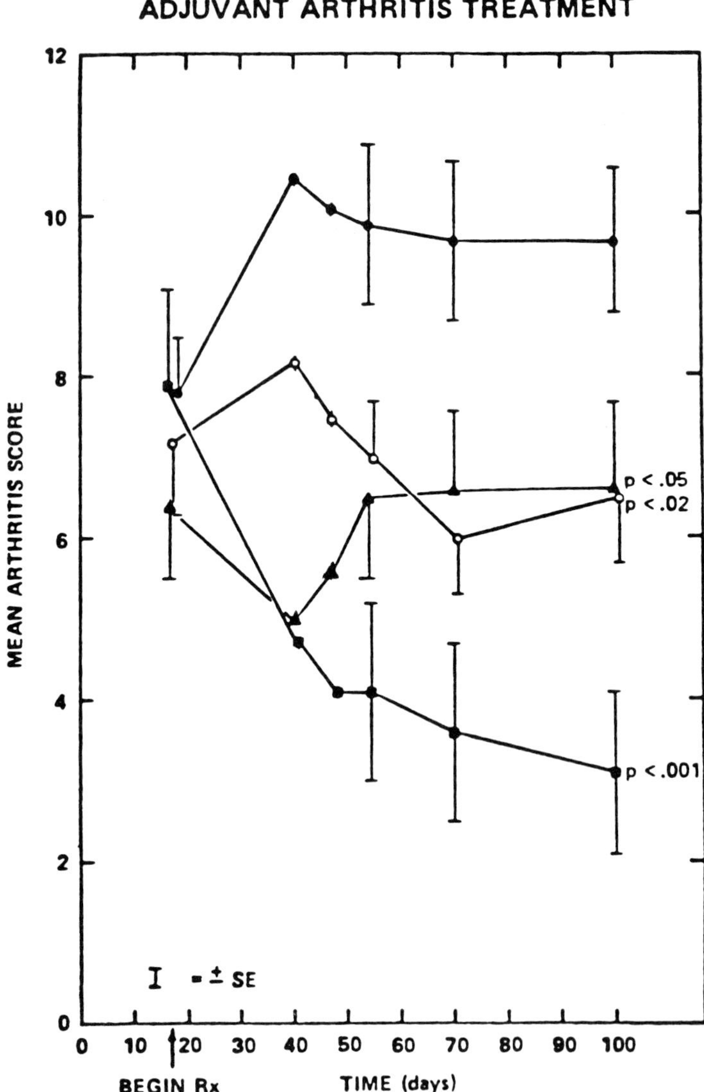

FIGURE 4. Effect of irradiation on arthritis scores in adjuvant arthritis. *p* values (2-sample *t*-test with 2-tail criterion) indicate the significance of the difference between the indicated group and the control group. (♦) untreated group, (○) paw irradiation group, (▲) TLI group, (■) TLI plus paw irradiation group.

were formed and treatment initiated (i.e., 17 days after adjuvant injection). The untreated animals' clinical course of inflammation and deformity steadily worsened from the time of the first appearance of clinical arthritis 11 to 15 days after adjuvant inoculation until day 40 when the maximum mean score was recorded. At this time there was little or no inflammation, but ankylosis was now well established. For all four experimental groups, the individual arthritis ratings remained unchanged after day 100. Most of the animals were followed for at least several months after day 100 and some of them were followed for one year.

At the conclusion of irradiation the group receiving TLI had significantly less inflammation than the control group ($p < .001$). However, very soon after treatment ended, the arthritis scores of the TLI group rose to their pretreatment levels. The scores then stabilized at this grade. There was a persistent benefit from TLI as compared to controls, although 60 days after TLI ended, the difference between the group receiving TLI and controls was modest ($p < .05$) (Fig. 4).

The time course of inflammation and deformity in the rats treated with only local irradiation paralleled that of the control rats, but the severity was reduced. The final effect of this treatment was modest, although significant ($p < .02$) and similar in magnitude to the effect of TLI.

The arthritis scores of animals treated with both TLI and local paw irradiation fell dramatically when treatment was begun (Fig. 4). The response was most pronounced during treatment, but appeared to continue during the first several months after treatment. Control animals improved somewhat in the period from 40 to 100 days. The improvement in the arthritis score was mirrored in the clinical observation of increased use of extremities and improved paw function.

Roentgenographic findings correlated very closely with the arthritis rating score (19). One animal was selected from each of the four groups whose arthritis scores were close to the group average of each of the time intervals. The roentgenographic findings of each paw in all groups at day 17 were similar, showing soft tissue swelling, but either minimal or no abnormalities of the bones or joints. The rats which received no irradiation treatments had rapid destructive changes during the period between 17 and 40 days. Soft tissue swelling persisted and bony erosions, demineralization, and joint space widening and narrowing occurred to a marked degree during this period. By day 100, cartilage space narrowing and ankylosis of the involved joinings were typical, with remineralization of the bones and subperiosteal new bone formation. Soft tissue swelling had largely subsided. Roentgenographs taken up to one year showed little or no further change. In rats treated with either TLI or local paw irradiation only, joint abnormalities on X rays were similar to controls except that changes were less marked and areas of involvement were fewer. When erosions, demineralization, joint narrowing or widening, remineralization, periosteal new bone formation, or ankylosis occurred, these events took place in the same time sequence as for control animals. Rats treated with a combination of TLI and local paw irradiation had very few significant radiologic abnormalities, but those that did occur were similar to controls except diminished in degree. The severity of changes on X ray were always parallel to the arthritis score (19).

X. TREATMENT OF INTRACTABLE RHEUMATOID ARTHRITIS WITH SUBDIAPHRAGMATIC LYMPHOID IRRADIATION

Recently, we investigated the use of total lymphoid irradiation in selected patients with rheumatoid arthritis. Cytotoxic drugs such as azathioprine and cyclophosphamide have been used in the past few years to treat rheumatoid arthritis refractory to conventional therapy. Although these drugs are efficacious in controlling even severe disease, the frequency of dangerous side effects is so great as to restrict their widespread use (3-5, 16, 17, 25). During clinical trials using cyclophosphamide in rheumatoid arthritis, several investigators reported a high incidence of short-term complications including leukopenia, infection, hemmorhagic cystitis, alopecia, amenorrhea, and azospermia (3). Long-term complications include the development of leukemia and other neoplasms (3-5, 16, 17, 25). In a literature comparison, complications associated with the use of total lymphoid irradiation (TLI) in the treatment of Hodgkin's disease are substantially less than that associated with the chronic use of cytotoxic drugs such as azathioprine and cyclophosphamide in rheumatoid arthritis (2-5, 10, 13, 16, 17, 25).

Six patients with intractable rheumatoid arthritis were treated with fractionated irradiation of the subdiaphragmatic lymphoid tissues including the para-aortic, iliac, and inguinal lymph nodes in a feasibility phase 1 study. All had long-standing erosive disease and were severely disabled by unremitting active synovitis. All patients were treatment failures with gold compounds and penicillamine and were considered candidates for the use of cytotoxic drugs before entering the study.

Four of the six patients showed an objective decrease in joint disease activity which persisted for at least six months after radiotherapy (23). Three of the four patients also showed a marked decrease in morning stiffness and considerable functional improvement (23). Except for mild fatigue and nausea, radiotherapy was well tolerated. No severe or chronic complications of irradiation have been identified during a two- to three-year follow-up (23). As expected, all patients developed marked lymphocytopenia during or shortly after irradiation (23). The absolute lymphocyte counts remained markedly decreased during the six-month follow-up period after treatment. Patients with a normal pretreatment response to PHA showed a marked persistent decrease after high dose irradiation (23).

In view of the improvement in disease activity in the majority of patients and lack of severe side effects with subdiaphragmatic irradiation, we recently initiated another feasibility study investigating the use of total lymphoid irradiation (cumulative dose 2000 rads) instead of subdiaphragmatic irradiation in a patient population similar to that used in the initial study. These results suggest that TLI is considerably more effective than subdiaphragmatic irradiation in reducing disease activity (12).

REFERENCES

1. Andrews, B. S., Eisenberg, R. A., Theofilopoulos, A. N., Izui, S., Wilson, C. B., McConahey, P. J., Murphy, E. D., Roths, J. B., and Dixon, F. J. Spontaneous murine lupus-like syndromes. Clinical and immunopathological manifestations in several strains. *J. Exp. Med.* *148*, 1198 (1978).

2. Coleman, C. N., Williams, C. J., Flint, A., Glatstein, E., Rosenberg, S., and Kaplan, H. S. Hematologic neoplasia in patients treated for Hodgkin's disease. *N. Engl. J. Med. 297*, 1249 (1977).

3. Davis, J. D., Muss, H. B., and Turner, R. A. Cytotoxic agents in the treatment of rheumatoid arthritis: *South. Med. J. 71*, 58 (1978).

4. Fosdick, W. M., Parsons, J. L., and Hill, D. F. Long-term cyclophosphamide therapy in rheumatoid arthritis. *Arthritis Rheum. 11*, 151 (1968).

5. Fosdick, W. M., Parsons, J. L., and Hill, D. F. Long-term cyclophosphamide therapy in rheumatoid arthritis, a progress report, six years' experience. *Arthritis Rheum. 12*, 663 (1969).

6. Fuks, Z., Strober, S., Bobrove, A. M., Sasazuki, T., McMichael, A., and Kaplan, H. S. Long-term effects of radiation on T and B lymphocytes in peripheral blood of patients with Hodgkin's disease. *J. Clin. Invest. 48*, 803 (1976).

7. Gelfand, M. C., Steinberg, A. D., Nagle, R., and Knepshield, J. Therapeutic studies in NZB/NZW mice. I. Synergy of azathioprine, cyclophosphamide, and methylprednisolone in combination. *Arthritis Rheum. 15*, 239 (1972).

8. Gelfand, M. C. and Steinberg, A. D. Therapeutic studies in NZB/NZW mice. II. Relative efficacy of azathioprine, cyclophosphamide, and methylprednisolone. *Arthritis Rheum. 15*, 247 (1972).

9. Howie, J. B. and Helyer, B. J. The immunology and pathology of NZB mice. *Adv. Immunol. 9*, 215 (1968).

10. Kaplan, H. S. "Hodgkin's Disease." Harvard Univ. Press, Cambridge, Massachusetts, 1972.

11. Kotzin, B. L. and Strober, S. Reversal of NZB/NZW disease with total lymphoid irradiation. *J. Exp. Med. 150*, 371 (1979).

12. Kotzin, B. L., Strober, S., Hoppe, R., Calin, A., and Kaplan, H. S. Treatment of intractable rheumatoid arthritis with total lymphoid irradiation. *N. Engl. J. Med. 305*, 969 (1981).

13. Krikorian, H. G., Burke, J. S., Rosenberg, S. A., and Kaplan, H. S. Occurrence of non-Hodgkin's lymphoma after therapy for Hodgkin's disease. *N. Engl. J. Med. 300*, 452 (1979).

14. Lehman, D. H., Wilson, C. B., and Dixon, F. J. Increased survival times of New Zealand hybrid mice immunosuppressed by graft versus host reactions. *Clin. Exp. Immunol. 25*, 297 (1976).

15. Morris, A. D., May, C., and Esterly, J. Mechanisms and quantitation of reduction in NZB/NZW nephritis by cyclophosphamide. *Arthritis Rheum. 15*, 119 (1972).

16. Parsons, J. L., Strong, J. S., and Fosdick, W. M. The causes of death in patients with rheumatoid arthritis treated with cytotoxic agents. *J. Rheumatol., Suppl.* No. 1, 76 (1974).

17. Pollock, B. H., Blair, J. H., Stolzer, B. L., Eisenbeis, C. H., Agawall, A., and Margolis, H. M. Neoplasia and cyclophosphamide. *Arthritis Rheum. 16*, 524 (1973).

18. Russel, P. J. and Hicks, J. D. Cyclophosphamide treatment of renal disease in NZB/NZW F_1 hybrid mice. *Lancet 1*, 440 (1968).

19. Schurman, D. J., Hirshman, P., and Strober, S. Total lymphoid irradiation and local joint irradiation in the treatment of adjuvant arthritis. *Arthritis Rheum. 24*, 38 (1981).

20. Slavin, S., Strober, S., Fuks, Z., and Kaplan, H. S. Induction of specific tissue transplantation tolerance using fractionated total lymphoid irradiation in adult mice: Long-term survival of allogeneic bone marrow and skin grafts. *J. Exp. Med. 146*, 34 (1977).

21. Slavin, S., Fuks, Z., Kaplan, H. S., and Strober, S. Transplantation of allogeneic bone marrow without graft-versus-host disease using total lymphoid irradiation. *J. Exp. Med. 147*, 963 (1978).

22. Steinberg, A. D., Gelfand, M. C., Hardin, J. A., and Lowenthal, D. T. Therapeutic studies in NZB/NZW mice. III. Relationship between renal status and efficacy of immunosuppressive drug therapy. *Arthritis Rheum. 18*, 9 (1975).

23. Strober, S., Kotzin, B. L., Hoppe, R. T., Slavin, S., Gottlieb, M., Calin, A., Fuks, Z., and Kaplan, H. S. The treatment of intractable rheumatoid arthritis with lymphoid irradiation. *Int. J. Radiat. Oncol. Biol. Phys. 7*, 1 (1981).

24. Theofilopoulos, A. N., Balderas, R., Shawler, D. L., Izui, S., Kotzin, B. L., Strober, S., and Dixon, F. J. Inhibition of T cell proliferation and SLE-like syndrome of MRL/ℓ mice by whole body or total lymphoid irradiation. *J. Immunol. 125*, 2137 (1980).

25. Townes, A. S., Sowa, J. M., and Shulman, L. E. Controlled trial of cyclophosphamide in rheumatoid arthritis. *Arthritis Rheum. 19*, 563 (1976).

26. Zan-Bar, I., Slavin, S., and Strober, S. Effect of total lymphoid irradiation (TLI) on the primary and secondary antibody response to sheep red blood cells. *Cell. Immunol. 45*, 167 (1979).

27. Zan-Bar, I., Slavin, S., and Strober, S. Induction and mechanism of tolerance to bovine serum albumin in mice given total lymphoid irradiation (TLI). *J. Immunol. 121*, 1400 (1978).

DISCUSSION

The potential long-term complications of radiotherapy were discussed, including the development of neoplasms, in patients with intractable rheumatoid arthritis. Although several groups of patients treated with only TLI for Hodgkin's disease have shown no increased risk of additional neoplasia during a 10-year follow-up, it is possible that a more prolonged follow-up (20-30 years) would reveal an increased risk. In addition, the risk in the treated rheumatoid arthritis population might be different from that of the Hodgkin's disease population. It was noted that protocalized studies for the treatment of arthritis patients excludes all individuals under 40 years of age in order to minimize these potential risks. Dr. Miescher suggested that some younger patients with intractable disease may benefit from the use of the antihelminthic drug, Levamisole.

Immunopathology: VIIIth International Symposium, 1980

COMPLEMENT DEFECTS, IMMUNOLOGICAL HEALTH, AND IMMUNOLOGICAL DISEASE

Peter Lachmann

MRC Unit on Mechanisms in Tumour Immunity,
MRC Centre,
Cambridge CB2 2QH, England

I. INTRODUCTION

The complement system has a respectable evolutionary history, being present in all vertebrate groups since and including the elasmobranch fishes (2). It can therefore scarcely be doubted that the system is maintained by selective advantage. It thus came as a surprise when it was found that genetic deficiencies of isolated complement components and sometimes acquired abnormalities that lead to widespread decompensation of complement, are not necessarily associated with obvious clinical problems. However, as more such patients have been studied it has become clear that whereas indeed there is no necessary association with disease, complement-deficient subjects are at substantially higher risk of developing certain diseases. These diseases are in the main either infections of some kind, which came as no surprise

ISBN 0-12-218320-7

since all the most obvious functions of the complement system are in relation to resistance to infection; or immune complex diseases which was indeed surprising since complement plays a large part in the mediation of immune complex damage.

The topic of this chapter is to discuss clinical associations of genetic variants of the complement system and of the defects of complement, both genetic and acquired. In particular the question to be addressed is whether the disease associations found with complement defects are due to consequences of complement deficiency *per se* or whether they are due to the genetic linkage of true disease susceptibility genes to the genes coding for complement components.

A. *Complement Genetics*

I have argued elsewhere (17, 18) that the complement system has evolved by a process of gene duplication from simpler precursors. This is particularly clearly seen in the reactions leading up to the formation of the two C3 converting enzymes of the classical and alternative pathways, respectively. This is shown schematically in Fig. 1. C4 and C2 of the classical pathway are the homologs of Factor B and C3 of the alternative pathway, and there is now growing biochemical evidence to show the close similarity of C2 to Factor B (16) and of C4 to C3. The latter family contains a further component C5, the first acting component of the terminal pathway or membrane attack complex.

The membrane attack pathway has properties quite distinct from the phlogistic enhancement produced by the complement enzyme cascade. The membrane attack complex is a self-associating, multiprotein complex which, in its finally assembled form, is capable of insertion into membranes which it causes

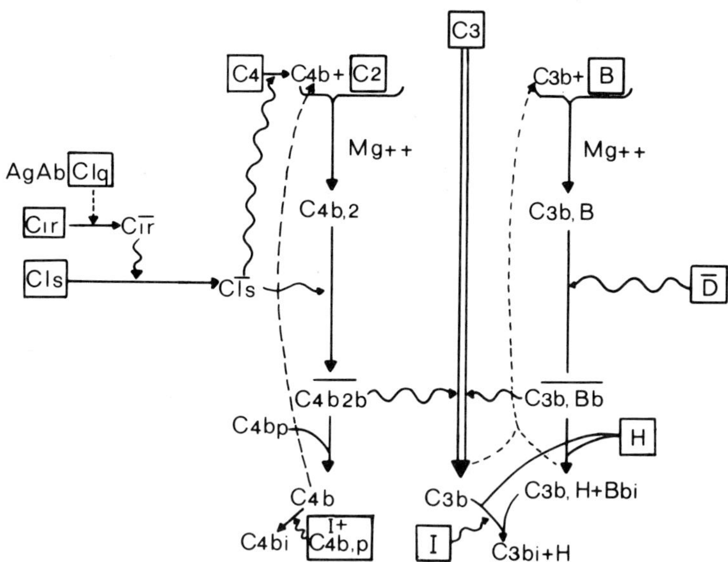

FIGURE 1. The complement pathways shown as homologs.

to leak (9). There is no obvious homolog of this activity in other plasma systems, although there are striking analogies between this type of membrane damage and the cytotoxic activity of lymphocytes. Except for C5, which is clearly closely similar to C3 and C4, the remaining components of the membrane attack complex are not clearly related to other complement components. The two components reacting after C5 i.e., C6 and C7, are extremely similar to one another and are clearly tandem gene duplicates. There is some degree of similarity between C6 and C7 on the one hand, and Factor B and C2, or even Factor H, on the other hand, but there is insufficient evidence to suggest that they are homologs. The final two components, C8 and C9, do not obviously resemble any other complement components.

B. *The Gene Loci Coding for Complement Components*

There are three loci known where there is extensive mapping data.

1. A locus close to the B locus of HLA and probably on the side toward the D locus. Here are coded C4, C2, and Factor B.

2. The C3 locus. In man this is not within mapping distance of HLA and the only genes for which positive linkage has been claimed are the Lewis blood groups and genes controlling cholesterol metabolism.* However, in the mouse the structural locus for C3 is on the 17th chromosome and about 11 centimorgans from H2 (25, 28). There is furthermore a recent report [cited in Kaidoh *et al.* (15)] that the C4 binding protein in mice is also coded at 16 centimorgans from H2, although curiously enough a linkage to C3 was not ascertained.

3. A locus coding for C6 and C7. These two loci are very closely linked but are not within mapping distance of any other genetic locus that has been investigated (12, 13).

TABLE I. Complement Loci

Components	Linkage data
C4, C2, Factor B	Very close to B locus of HLA
C6, C7	Unassigned
C3	Loose linkage to Lewis Blood groups (NB in mice loose linkage to *H-2*)
C1	Unassigned and show no linkage to any of the three loci above. (Insufficient data to exclude linkage within this group of components)
C5	
C8	
Factor D	
$C\overline{1}$ inhibitor	
C3b inactivator	

**Note added in proof.* *It has recently been demonstrated that the human C3 gene is on chromosome 19 (31).*

There is more limited genetic information on a number of other components as shown in Table I. With these loci it is generally clear that they are not within close mapping distance of the three loci discussed above. There are insufficient data to know whether any of these other loci are linked with each other.

II. COMPLEMENT POLYMORPHISMS AND DISEASE

Genetic polymorphism was defined by Ford (10) as the occurrence together in the same habitat of two or more forms of a species in such proportions that the rarest of them cannot be maintained by recurrent mutation. If the second-most-frequent allele has a frequency of 1% or more this is generally taken as evidence that such an allele is not maintained by recurrent mutation. It has frequently been held that polymorphisms so defined are maintained by selective pressures generally because the disadvantages of homozygosity for the rare allele is balanced by some advantage of the heterozygote over the homozygote for the common allele. This interpretation, however, is not established beyond doubt in all such cases and will be discussed again in relation to the polymorphisms of C6 and C7. There are a surprisingly large number of complement components that do show polymorphisms and four of them show polymorphisms where the second-most-frequent allele has a frequency in excess of 10%. These include two components linked to the HLA locus (Factor B and C4) and two that are not so linked (C3 and C6). In view of the postulated selective pressure maintaining such polymorphisms, it is pertinent to enquire whether there are functional differences between the alleles (which are normally recognized only by differences in electrophoretic charge) which could form the basis of some form of selective pressure. It is also of interest to inquire whether there are disease associations with any particular allele, possibly reflecting the selective disadvantage. It has, of course, become apparent from the extensive work on disease associations with HLA alleles that a disease association with a particular allele at one locus may reflect some physiological consequence of that allele; but on the other hand it may also reflect linkage disequilibrium with an allele at a closely linked locus. In the former case the gene under study is itself the disease-susceptibility gene, whereas in the latter, it is a genetic marker for a linked disease-susceptibility gene.

It is by no means always easy to distinguish between these situations. However, one good piece of evidence that the effect is physiological occurs when the same disease susceptibility is found in association with alleles at separate and unlinked loci whose products are physiologically related. A very good example of this situation exists in the association of duodenal ulcers with blood groups. There is an association both with Group O and with nonsecretor status. Now the ABH locus and the secretor locus are not genetically linked and it therefore seems inescapable that the association is with the

TABLE II. Allelic Frequencies of C3 and C6

	Population group	Allele frequencies		
		Commonest	Second	Others
C3	Caucasoids	0.77 (C3S)	0.22 (C3F)	Rare
	Mongoloids	0.99 (C3S)	<0.01 (C3F)	Rare
	Negroids	0.93 (C3S)	0.06 (C3F)	Rare
C6	All groups	0.6 (C6A)	0.35 (C6B)	0.05

secretion of blood group substances within the gut rather than by genetic linkage to other disease-susceptibility genes. In the complement system a similar argument would apply if disease susceptibilities were found to be associated with particular alleles of C3 and C6 and one of the HLA-linked complement components, since these are known not to be linked to each other. It is particularly, of course, in the HLA-linked loci that the problem arises of distinguishing disease susceptibility due to the complement allotypes themselves from those due to linked alleles at the other loci of the HLA supergene.

A. The C6 Locus

It is perhaps convenient to consider first the case of C6, since the two major C6 variants are of equal hemolytic activity and since no functions for C6 other than its involvement in the membrane attack complex of complement are known. The frequency of C6 alleles are shown in Table II where it can be seen that there is remarkably close agreement for all racial groups studied. This state of affairs is unusual for complement allotypes and in fact of the major, frequent polymorphisms, C6 is the only one to show the same gene frequency in all major racial groups. One explanation for this would be that the selective pressure of C6 variation works equally in all groups, and that this maintains a balanced polymorphism of this kind, by heterozygote advantage. The difficulty with this explanation is that there are no known functional differences between the two alleles nor has any disease association for either allele so far been described. It is also possible that the explanation given for these high-frequency polymorphisms as due to heterozygote advantage may not always be correct and that some polymorphisms are selectively neutral.

TABLE III. C6 and C7 Polymorphism in Various Mammalian Species (Numbers of Species)*

C7 Polymorphism	C6 Polymorphism		
	+	-	Assay failed
+	4	5	0
-	8	8	1
Assay failed	4	3	

*From Eldridge and Hobart (8).

Some evidence in favor of this view of the C6 polymorphism can be obtained from looking at the polymorphism of C6 and the closely linked complement component C7 in a variety of different species. Such data are shown in Table III which is taken from Eldridge and Hobart (8). Here it can be seen that looking at a substantial number of mammalian species, polymorphism may be found in C6 or C7, or both, or neither, in an apparently random fashion. It must be pointed out that the number of members of these species studied is usually small, and the statement that there is no polymorphism can only be taken to mean that it does not occur at a high frequency. It is a little difficult to imagine what selective pressure could be maintaining a balanced polymorphism of either or both of these components in quite such a random way among a group of species and, although it is difficult to draw certain conclusions from this sort of study, this evidence probably does point toward a neutral explanation for C6 polymorphism.

Whereas the electrophoretic variants of C6 appear to be functionally equivalent there are disease associations reported with heterozygous C6 deficiency even though this has only a minor effect on the hemolytic titer of serum. This will be discussed again below.

B. The C3 Locus

The situation with regard to C3 polymorphism is rather different. The two major alleles of C3, C3S and C3F, are not uniformly distributed throughout all races (see Table II) and C3F is a predominantly Caucasian gene. Furthermore, there are functional differences between the two alleles. Although it has been reported that their hemolytic activity is equal, it has more recently been shown that C3F has a higher hemolytic efficiency (21). Furthermore, it has been claimed that C3F gives better rosetting with macrophages than does C3S (1). Since C3 has multiple functions and its adherence reactions are perhaps as important *in vivo* as its hemolytic activity these differences give a basis on which a balanced polymorphism could exist. There is also a hypomorphic allele of C3 which behaves to some extent like a null allele, i.e., heterozygotes for this hypomorphic variant behave rather as if they

TABLE IV. Disease Association of C3 Alleles*

1. The hypomorphic C3 Fast Variant (C3f) and familial hypocomplementaemia
    a. Arthritis and focal glomerulonephritis in proband; haematuria in sibling
    b. Partial lipodystrophy in proband, C3f in family members
    c. Cutaneous vasculitis, SLE-like syndrome and proteinuria in proband; C3f in cousin
2. Increased frequency of C3F allele
    a. Membranoproliferative glomerulonephritis
    b. Partial lipodystrophy
    c. Juvenile systemic lupus erythematosus

*From McLean et al. (20, 21, 23).

TABLE V. Diseases Associated with C6 Deficiency*

Diseases in the families	Number of families	Number of heterozygotes with disease/total heterozygotes	Number of homozygotes with disease/total homozygotes
Healthy	(4)	(0/27)	(0/1)
Neisserial infection	8	0/18	8/9
Infection other than Neisseria	1	0/10	2/4
MCGN	3	2/12	1/1
Totals with diseases	16	2/67	11/15

*From *Coleman* et al. *(4)*.

had heterozygous C3 deficiency. The disease associations of the different C3 alleles have been studied by McLean and are listed in Table IV.

It is interesting that the associations of the hypomorphic variant C3f and the second-most-common allele C3F overlap. Both are associated with the curious conditions of partial lipodystrophy where partial loss of body fat may follow a virus infection and which is most characteristically associated with the presence of the so-called C3 nephritic factor or NeF. NeF is an autoantibody to the alternative pathway C3 convertase ($\overline{\text{C3b,Bb}}$) which it stabilizes against dissociation by Factor H. Membranoproliferative glomerulonephritis is the other major clinical correlate of NeF. This again is found more frequently in subjects carrying the C3F allele. To a lesser extent both are also associated with systemic lupus erythematosus. Mesangiocapillary glomerulonephritis (MCGN) has been known for some time to be a predominantly Caucasian disease, and since C3F is also a predominantly Caucasian gene, this association makes sense. It is still possible to ask whether the association of MCGN with C3F is due to linkage to a true disease susceptibility gene or whether it is due to some effect of complement action itself or possibly to the fact that the $\overline{\text{C3b,Bb}}$ complex made with C3F is more antigenic and more likely to give rise to nephritic factor. Evidence against the idea that it is due to a linked disease-susceptibility gene unrelated to complement comes from the observation of Coleman *et al.* (4) that there is also an association of MCGN with heterozygous C6 deficiency (see Table V). This somewhat surprising observation would make one believe that the pathogenesis of MCGN must involve complement function even after the C3 stage.

From clinical observations of patients with partial lipodystrophy (PLD), some of whom go on after a period of years to develop MCGN, (29) it would seem that the presence of NeF predates, often considerably, the development of the renal disease since most children with PLD have NeF when they are first seen. It therefore seems likely that the hypocomplementemia due to NeF or perhaps on a genetic basis, predisposes to the changes that bring about MCGN. It is not known whether the partial lipodystrophy itself is a consequence of having NeF and therefore perhaps of hypocomplementemia or whether the relationship is the other way around. The genetic association of partial lipodystrophy with the hypomorphic C3 allele as well as with C3F would again suggest that perhaps the hypocomplementemia predisposes also to PLD and perhaps causes children to react to virus infections like measles in this rather strange way. However, no details of the pathological processes that bring about partial lipodystrophy are known.

C. *The HLA Associated Complement Locus*

There are many diseases that show associations with alleles of the various loci at HLA and, especially for those that show the best association with HLA DR alleles, it is widely believed that immune response genes may be the true disease-susceptibility genes. This topic has a vast literature [see, e.g. (5)]. It is therefore probable that most of the disease associations seen with alleles of the complement components within the MHC will be due to their linkage disequilibrium with alleles at closely linked loci. It is nevertheless interesting that in certain diseases, notably insulin-dependent diabetes mellitus, the average relative risk is higher for certain rare complement alleles, for example Bf F1 (26), than for alleles at the other loci. It remains likely that these associations are due not to the physiological effects of the rare complement allotypes but rather to other disease-susceptibility genes occurring in these haplotypes carrying the rare complement allotypes; and that the complement allotype is the best marker for the haplotype that carries the susceptibility to the disease (27).

What these findings would therefore suggest is that the true disease-susceptibility genes for insulin-dependent diabetes are none of these that at present can be serologically or electrophoretically typed within the HLA region and that all the associations so far discovered, including those of the complement components, are due to allelic associations with other hitherto undescribed gene loci. There is another interesting example of this nature. Increased susceptibility to multiple sclerosis is associated with the HLA-DR allele, DRW2. The DRW2-containing haplotype that is most common in patients with MS in northern Europe is A3, B7, Bfs, DRW2 and these patients do not show abnormalities of the complement system. However, increased incidence of MS has also been shown in association with the HLA haplotype A10, B18, Bfs, DRW2, especially in France (30). There is an association between this haplotype and heterozygous C2 deficiency, i.e., haplotypes of this kind are not infrequently A10, B18, $C2^0$, Bfs DRW2 and such patients will be hypocomplementemic. Here again, it is likely that the true disease-susceptibility gene for multiple sclerosis is not DRW2 itself but an allele in linkage disequilibrium with DRW2 at a closely linked locus within HLA.

III. COMPLEMENT DEFICIENCY AND DISEASE

Isolated complement component deficiencies have now been described for almost all the complement components. Homozygous deficiencies of Factors B, D, and Properdin have not yet been described; this almost certainly is because deficiency of these components would not be picked up by the measurement of total hemolytic complement, and for this reason far smaller numbers of patients have been screened for such deficiencies. However, the heterozygous Factor B-deficient state is known by the presence of a silent allele (11), and there is therefore no reason to believe that homozygotes will not in due course be found. Table VI shows in outline form the deficiencies that have been described and the diseases associated with them. These diseases fall into two major categories. First there are infections. These may be either a generalized increased susceptibility to bacterial, and often pyococcal, infections, or more commonly a rather specific immune defect with regard to Neisserial infections, either recurrent meningococcal meningitis or disseminated gonococcal infections.

The second group is a number of immune complex diseases of which systemic lupus erythematosus or diseases closely resembling it are most common but which include glomerulonephritis, polymyositis, polyarthritis nodosa, Henoch Shonlein purpura, and others. No complement deficiency (with the exception of $C\bar{1}$ inhibitor deficiency which is really a rather

TABLE VI. Clinical Associations of Complement Deficiency

Bacterial infection	
General (especially pyococcal)	C1 (2:3); C3 (4:5); I (1:4)
Neisserial	I (2:4); C5 (2:4); C6 (4:5); C7 (4:9); C8 (2:9)
Immune complex disease	C1r (3:3); C1s (1:1); C C4 (2:2); C2 (c. 50%); C5 (1:4); C8 (3:9); C1-inhibitor (raised incidence, c. 18 described cases)

separate condition) is invariably associated with a disease. What the complement deficiency does is to raise susceptibility to the diseases with which they are associated, i.e., complement deficiency is a "diathesis." There are good reasons to believe that the associations are physiological and not due to linked susceptibility genes. This is true both for the infections found both with genetic deficiencies of C3 and with genetic deficiencies such as those of the C3b inactivator which gives rise to a secondary deficiency of C3. In fact, a similar predisposition to generalized infection is found in patients with C3 nephritic factor (NeF) who have an acquired C3 deficiency. There is therefore every reason to believe that it is the C3 deficiency itself and not any linked gene that gives rise to the susceptibility to infection.

The susceptibility to neisserial infection is again seen with deficiencies of a variety of complement components that are not linked to each other. Neisserial infections have been described in most of the terminal complement component deficiencies as well as in C3b-inactivator deficiency. Since it is believed that complement is concerned largely with resistance to infection it is not surprising that complement deficiency should lead to an increased susceptibility to infection. It is, however, more surprising that there should be this increased susceptibility to immune complex disease, and it is the nature of this association that has given rise to most speculation. The arguments have been previously rehearsed (18). The earlier suggestions that the association is due to an ascertainment artifact appear now fairly clearly to be untenable; and one can calculate, albeit from rather unreliable incomplete data, that the average relative risk for lupus in C2-deficient subjects is in the region of 50.

Since easily the most common isolated complement component deficiency in man is C2 the largest number of disease associations are also known for this component. Since C2 is coded within HLA, the possibility that this is linked to another disease susceptibility gene is a real one. It nevertheless seems unlikely that this explains the association with the immune complex disease. For one thing the C2-deficient gene seems to be in strong linkage disequilibrium with a particular haplotype A10, B18, C4 A4B2, $C2^0$, BfS, DRW2 which haplotype is not associated with C4 deficiency. However, C4 deficiency is associated with the same diseases. So is Cl deficiency and occasionally C5 and C8 deficiency, which are not linked to HLA. Finally and most importantly, there is also an excess incidence of immune complex diseases in association with Cl esterase inhibitor deficiency (hereditary angioedema or HAE) where the deficiency of C4 and C2 are secondary to their increased catabolism. Donaldson *et al.* (7) described patients with systemic LE and herediatary angioedema and the author is aware of two siblings with HAE and nephritis and several further cases of SLE and HAE.

A. *Critical Stage Complement Deficiency*

The discussion so far has been of genetic complement deficiencies that are essentially permanent. It is, however, possible that complement deficiency or depletion at critical times in relation to experience of infective organisms may be able to give rise to important consequences which become manifest only much later. Two possible examples may be given. In neither case is the relationship of the pathogenesis to complement depletion established but the hypotheses have a certain plausibility.

B. *EB Virus and Burkitt's Lymphoma*

It is known that in areas where there is holoendemic malaria a small percentage of children, all of whom can be considered as having encountered the EB virus, develop Burkitt's lymphoma. It is recognized from a large prospective study that the children who subsequently develop Burkitt's lymphoma have unusually high antibody levels to EB virus antigens long before the tumour develops (6), and one can be fairly confident that there is an abnormality occurring at the time of their original encounter with the virus. It has been suggested (19) that this abnormality may reside in the children's having severely depleted complement systems due to malaria at the time they first encounter the virus. It is known (18) that EB virus-transformed cells activate the alternative pathway of complement in the absence of antibody and can be destroyed in this way. It is conceivable that if at the time the initial cell transformation is taking place there is insufficient complement to produce this activation, a small number of cells may be able to establish themselves at extravascular sites where they are protected from complement activation and where they can provide a persistent nidus of infection making it possibile both for excessive immunization and for development of tumors.

C. *The Measles Virus and SSPE*

A somewhat analogous situation exists in relation to the measles virus and subacute sclerosing panencephalitis. This chronic neurological infection with the measles virus occurs in a very small minority of children (about one in a million) most commonly in those who have measles before the age of two. Although its exact pathogenesis remains unknown the best available explanation has been offered by Joseph and Oldstone (14) who pointed out that if measles virus-infected cells are grown in the presence of antibody and in the absence of complement, measles virus antigens normally present on the cell surface of the infected cell become modulated and are shed from the cell; and no further synthesis of these surface antigens takes place. In this way the infection can be sequestered within the cell in a form where it is no longer susceptible to immune attack, again providing the opportunity for prolonged hyperimmunization and persistent shedding of virus. If this is indeed the cause of SSPE then one must envisage that in the children who will develop the disease there is antibody formation but no efficient complement system at the time of the initial infection. It is known that measles virus infection itself can severely deplete complement in some children (3). It is therefore possible that in rare children there may be sufficient complement depletion such that even at the time when antibody appears there is insufficient complement to lyse the infected cell.

REFERENCES

1. Arvilommi, H. Capacity of complement C3 phenotypes to bind onto mononuclear cells in man. *Nature (London) 251*, 740 (1974).

2. Ballow, M. Phylogenetics and ontogenetics of the complement system. *Compr. Immunol. 2*, 183 (1977).

3. Charlesworth, J. A., Pussell, B. A., Roy, L. P., Robertson, M. R., and Beveridge, J. Measles infection: involvement of the complement system. *Clin. Exp. Immunol. 24*, 401 (1976).

4. Coleman, T. H., Forristal, J., and West, C. D. Hereditary C6 deficiency in membranoproliferative glomerulonephritis Type 1. Submitted for publication (1981).

5. Dausset, J. and Svejgard, A. (eds.). "HLA and Disease." Munksgaard, Copenhagen, 1977.

6. de The, G., Geser, A., Day, N. E., Tukei, P. M., Williams, E. H., Beri, D. P., Smith, P. G., Dean, A. G., Bornkamm, G. W., Feorino, P., and Henle, W. Epidemiological evidence for causal relationship between Epstein-Barr virus and Burkitt's lymphoma from Ugandan prospective study. *Nature (London) 274*, 756 (1978).

7. Donaldson, V. H., Hess, E. V., and McAdams, A. J. Lupus-erythematosus-like disease in three unrelated women with hereditary angioneurotic edema. *Ann. Intern. Med. 86*, 312 (1977).

8. Eldridge, P. and Hobart, M. J. Cited in Lachmann, P. J., and Hobart, M. J. The genetics of the complement system. *Ciba Found. Symp. 66*, 231 (1979).

9. Esser, A. F. Interactions between complement proteins and biological and model membranes. *In* "Biological Membranes" (D. Chapman, ed.), Vol. 4, Academic Press, New York, 1981.

10. Ford, E. B. "Genetics for Medical Students." Methuen, London, 1942.

11. Hauptmann, G., Tongio, M. M., Klein, J., Cinqualbre, J., Jeanblanc, B., Kieny, R., Mauff, G., and Federman, G. Le Facterur B de la Properdine: polymorphisme, lieu de synthese et premier cas de deficit genetique. *Nouv. Presse Med. 9*, 45 (1980).

12. Hobart, M. J., Cook, P. J. L., and Lachmann, P. J. Linkage studies with C6. *J. Immunogenet. 4*, 423 (1977).

13. Hobart, M. J., Joysey, V., and Lachmann, P. J. Inherited structural variation and linkage relationships of C7. *J. Immunogenet. 5*, 157 (1978).

14. Joseph, B. S. and Oldstone, M. B. A. Antibody-induced redistribution of measles virus antigens on the cell surface. *J. Immunol. 113*, 1205 (1974).

15. Kaidoh, T., Natsuume-Sakai, S., and Takahashi, M. Murine C4-binding protein. A rapid purification method by affinity chromatography. *J. Immunol. 126*, 463 (1981).

16. Kerr, M. A. Limited proteolysis of complement components C2 and Factor B. Structural analogy and limited sequence homology. *Biochem. J. 183*, 615 (1979).

17. Lachmann, P. J. An evolutionary view of the complement system. *Behring Inst. Mitt.* No. 63, 23 (1979).

18. Lachmann, P. J. Complement. *In* "The Antigens" (M. Sela, ed.), pp. 283-353. Academic Press, New York, 1979.

19. McConnell, I., Klein, G., Lint, T. F., and Lachmann, P. J. Activation of the alternative complement pathway by human B cell lymphoma lines is associated with Epstein-Barr virus transformation of the cells. *Eur. J. Immunol. 8*, 453 (1978).

20. McLean, R. H., Abeles, M., Weinstein, A., Kennedy, T. L., and Rothfield, N. Increased frequency of the third component of complement (C3) in juvenile systemic lupus erythematosus (SLE). *Annu. Rheum. Assoc. Annu. Sci. Meet., Atlanta, Ga.,* (1980).

21. McLean, R. H. and Hoefnagel, D. Partial lipodystrophy and familial C3 deficiency. *Hum. Hered. 30*, 149 (1980).

22. McLean, R. H., Kennedy, T. L., Ballow, M., and Siegel, N. J. Increased frequency of the BfF gene in the idiopathic nephrotic syndrome (INS). Studies of the alternative pathway in INS. *Int. Pediatr. Nephrol. Symp., 5th, Philadelphia, Pa.,* (1980).

23. McLean, R. H., Weinstein, A., Chapitis, M., and Rothfield, N. Familial partial deficiency of the third component of complement (C3) and the hypocomplementaemic cutaneous vasculitis syndrome. *Am. J. Med. 68*, 549 (1980).

24. McLean, R. H., Weinstein, A., Danjanov, I., and Rothfield, N. Hypomorphic variant of C3 arthritis and chronic glomerulonephritis. *J. Pediatr. 93*, 937 (1978).

25. Natsuume-Sakai, S., Hauakawa, J.-I., Amano, S., and Takahashi, M. Genetic mapping of the locus controlling structural variations of murine C3 in the chromosome 17. *J. Immunol. 123*, 947 (1979).

26. Raum, D., Alper, C. A., Stein, R., and Gabbay, K. H. Genetic marker for insulin-dependent diabetes mellitus. *Lancet ii*, 98, 376 (1979).

27. Rittner, C. and Bertrams, J. On the significance of C2, C4 and Factor B polymorphisms in disease. *Hum. Genet.* (1981).

28. Rubinstein, P., Vienne, K., and Hoecker, G. F. The location of the C3 and GLO (glyoxalase 1) loci of the IXth linkage group in mice. *J. Immunol. 122*, 2584 (1979).

29. Sissons, J. G. P., West, R. J., Fallows, J., Williams, D. G., Boucher, B. J., Amos, N., and Peters, D. K. The complement abnormalities of lipodystrophy. *New Engl. J. Med. 294*, 461 (1976).

30. Trouillas, P., Berthouz, F., Betuel, H., Bosson, D., Aimard, G., and Devic, M. Hypocomplementaemic multiple sclerosis: heterozygous C2 deficiency linked to HLa A10, B18. *Lancet ii*, 1023 (1976).

31. Whitehead, A. S., Solomon, E., Chambers, S. P., Povey, S., and Bodmer, W. F. Assignment of the gene for the third component of hyman complement (C3) to Chromosome 19 using human mouse somatic cell hybrids. *Molec. Immunol.* In press (1982).

Immunopathology: VIIIth International Symposium, 1980

IN VIVO STUDIES OF Fc RECEPTOR DEPENDENT CLEARANCE: DEFECTS IN AUTOIMMUNE DISEASE AND ASSOCIATED WITH THE HLA B8 DRw3 HAPLOTYPE

Michael M. Frank

Laboratory of Clinical Investigation,
National Institute of Allergy and Infectious Diseases,
National Institutes of Health,
Bethesda, Maryland

Detailed studies of the factors that influence the survival of antibody and complement-coated erythrocytes in the circulation of man and animals are now available (5). These show that clearance of sensitized erythrocytes from the circulation is, in general, dependent upon the interaction of antibody and/or complement fragments on the erythrocyte surface with specific receptors for these fragments on the fixed phagocytic cells of the reticuloendothelial system. Early studies focused on the *in vivo* quantitative evaluation of receptor function in normal human volunteers. It was possible to evaluate separately in quantitative terms the functional status of receptors for complement components as distinct from receptors for immunoglobulin. In addition, it was possible to show that

ISBN 0-12-218320-7

these two sets of receptors differ from those responsible for removing aggregated particulate material (albumin, etc.) from the circulation. The details of these studies have been reviewed elsewhere (1, 4, 10).

It was shown that there are some diseases (e.g., primary biliary cirrhosis) where C3b receptors do not appear to function normally (10). It was also shown that certain diseases, particularly those associated with deposition of immune complexes in various organs, are associated with defects in Fc receptor function (4, 8, 9).

In this chapter I would like to review some of these studies, beginning with older observations and concluding with some important new ones. The methods used are not complex. Human anti-Rh_0(D) IgG antibody prepared in an Rh-negative individual to be used as a source of the commercial product Rhogram was separated from the serum and purified free of other classes of immunoglobulins by gel filtration and sucrose density gradient ultracentrifugation. This IgG fraction was utilized to sensitize chromated cells from either normal volunteers or patients who were Rh_0(D) positive. The cells were radio-labeled with about 2 μCi of chromium-51, thus providing little if any risk of radiation toxicity. Following sensitization with about 2500 molecules of IgG per red cell, the cells were transfused into the erythrocyte donor and their survival followed. Figure 1 shows a typical survival curve obtained. When plotted as a semilogarithmic function, a straight line is obtained with relatively little person-to-person variation. Nuclide counting with probes over the liver and spleen demonstrates that the clearance of these IgG-sensitized cells is via splenic sequestration. The cleared cells are destroyed and never return to the circulation. It has been shown by others that cells sensitized with $F(ab)'_2$ antibodies are not

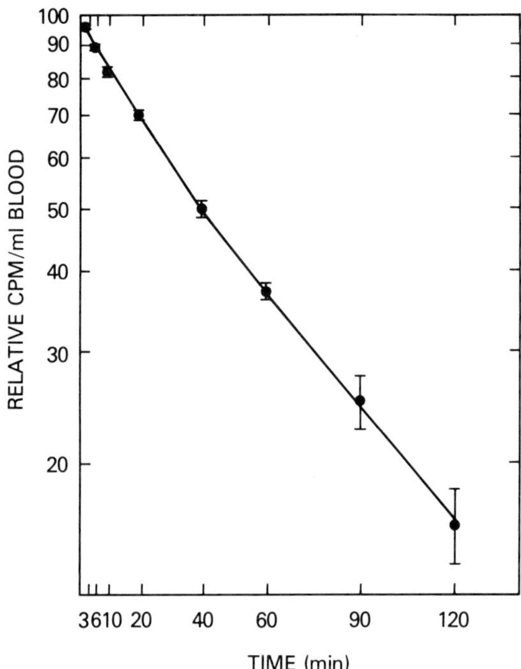

FIGURE 1. Clearance of IgG anti-Rh_0(D)-coated erythrocytes from the circulation of healthy normal human volunteers. Clearance of the red cells follows first-order kinetics. (Reprinted from Jaffe *et al. Journal of Clinical Investigation.*)

cleared at all under these circumstances emphasizing the important role of the Fc fragment of the antibody in mediating clearance (2).

When studies of rates of clearance were performed in normals and compared to rates obtained in patients with systemic lupus erythematosus (SLE), a major defect was noted in Fc receptor-mediated clearance in almost all of the patients with active disease studied (Fig. 2) (4). This defect was quite specific in that the clearance of aggregated albumin in these patients was always normal and, moreover, the Fc receptor defect was not always associated with a defect in C3b receptor-mediated clearance. Some patients with SLE had a defect in

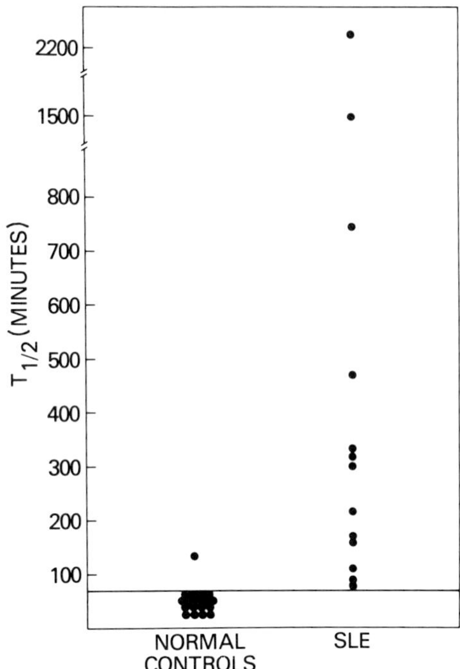

FIGURE 2. Time when half the cells are cleared from the circulation in a group of normal individuals as well as a group of patients with active systemic lupus erythematosus (SLE) with no hematologic manifestations of their disease. The patients with SLE have a profound defect.

C3b receptor-mediated clearance and others did not. Serum Clq binding activity was also studied in these patients as a measure of the presence of circulating immune complexes. High levels of immune complexes as detected by this assay were found in patients with active disease, and the levels tended to correlate in general with disease activity. Patients with more severe disease had higher levels of immune complexes than those with less severe disease. Similarly, the patients with more severe disease had a significantly greater defect in clearance than patients with less severe disease. It was possible to show a statistically significant correlation between the levels of immune complexes in the circulation and the magnitude of the clearance defect, suggesting that circulating immune complexes found in these patients interacted with Fc receptors on the fixed macrophages of the reticuloendothelial system, thereby preventing the clearance of the antibody-sensitized red cells.

In experimental animals immune complexes are rapidly removed from the circulation via the phagocytic cells of the reticulendothelial system (13). For years it has been suspected that patients with SLE might have a defect in the function of the reticuloendothelial system, thereby allowing complexes to continue to circulate and increasing the possibility of their being deposited in tissues. The results of our studies suggested that this hypothesis, that circulating complexes might block Fc receptor function, thereby preventing normal clearance of the IgG sensitized indicator erythrocytes, may be accurate. When patients with circulating immune complexes and Fc receptor-function defects were treated with systemic glucocorticoids it was found that as the patients improved clinically their immune complexes tended to clear from the circulation and, moreover, their clearance defect tended to improve. However, it was noted that very few patients had clearance times return to normal during the course of the study, even though they were completely free of symptoms.

Further studies in our laboratory demonstrated that the relationship between circulating immune complexes and the rate of clearance of IgG-sensitized erythrocytes was considerably more complex. This was shown in a number of diseases. I have chosen our studies of mixed connective tissue disease performed in collaboration with Hamburger and Sharp to make the point (7). If one studies a group of patients with mixed connective tissue disease one finds that an appreciable number have high levels of circulating immune complexes as measured by both Clq binding and Raji cell assays. However, if one studies Fc receptor function in this patient population one finds that the vast majority of patients have perfectly normal Fc receptor function even in the presence of circulating complexes. In fact, of the group of patients studied, only 4 of 18 had a clearance defect, and these 4 appeared to be very different from the 14 patients who did not have a clearance defect. These 4 patients tended to have low complement, glomerulonephritis, anti-Sm antibodies, higher levels of complexes, and high levels of circulating anti-DNA. These patients were much more like patients with SLE than the usual patients with mixed connective tissue disease. Thus, although these patients carried the diagnosis of mixed connective tissue disease, the clearance test separated patients with more typical mixed connective tissue disease from those who were more lupus-like in their manifestations. The patients who were more lupus-like in the manifestations of disease were likely to have the same clearance defect as patients with typical SLE. Those who were less SLE-like in the serologic manifestations of disease did not have a clearance defect. These and other studies demonstrated that circulating immune complexes did not necessarily lead to a clearance defect. It was possible to show that high levels of circulating complexes were completely compatible with normal erythrocyte clearance of Rh-coated cells. Thus, at this point, we had to postulate that the nature or type of complex may differ in various diseases and that this may influence their ability to interact with Fc receptors and their ability to block red cell clearance.

I would like now to turn to some more recent studies which have raised further interesting and important questions. The Dermatology Group of the National Cancer Institute follows a large population of patients with dermatitis herpetiformis. This disease is a chronic papulovesicular eruption thought to be immunologically mediated. Almost all patients have cutaneous IgA deposits in dermal papillae and an asymptomatic gluten sensitive enteropathy. Prior study by Hall *et al.* had shown that this disease is associated in a few cases with circulating immune complexes (6). Rarely, patients had IgG-containing immune complexes by either the Raji or the Clq binding assay. In a modification of the Raji cell assay to allow demonstration of IgA immune complexes, these investigators were able to show that some of the patients also have low levels of IgA-containing complexes as well. It was of interest to determine whether the dermatitis herpetiformis patient population had normal or abnormal clearance.

The studies were performed in a group of 16 patients with typical dermatitis herpetiformis. Most of the patients were well controlled at the time of these studies because of dapsone or sulfapyridine therapy; one patient was free of disease activity on a gluten-free diet. Fifty percent of the patient group were found to have a clearance defect for IgG-sensitized cells, and at times this defect was quite profound (Fig. 2) (12). There was no correlation between the magnitude of the clearance defect and any other parameter that we could measure. Specifically, there was no correlation with disease activity, no correlation with the presence or levels of circulating complexes, and no correlation with complement levels. In this patient group the levels of immune complexes were low. We considered the possibility that the therapy these patients were receiving, particularly the dapsone, might cause a delay in clearance via disturbance of Fc receptor function. Thus, a group of patients were taken off therapy and their studies repeated 48 hr following the cessation of therapy at which time they had undergone relapse of their disease. The study showed no change in clearance in 3 out of 4 patients and a minor change in clearance time in the fourth.

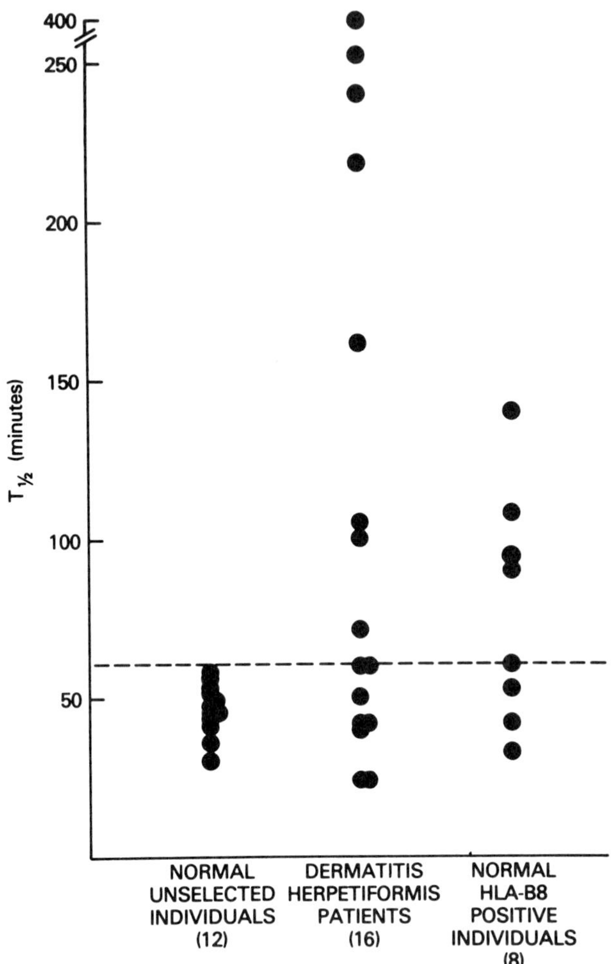

FIGURE 3. Time when half the cells are cleared in a group of normals, a group of patients with dermatitis herpetiformis who uniformly have the HLA type B8/DRw3, and a group of normal individuals with the HLA B8 haplotype. (Reprinted from Lawley *et al. New England Journal of Medicine*.)

These studies demonstrated the fact that measured clearance times were highly reproducible even when studied over a period of several months. They did not answer the question as to the cause of the clearance defect; however, they demonstrated that the clearance defect was not due to the dapsone treatment. Thus, at this point a new problem was apparent. In all diseases we had studied previously, patients with clearance defects had circulating complexes. We know that it was possible to have circulating complexes without a clearance defect, but this was the first instance of a clearance defect in the absence of circulating complexes. We considered certain other aspects of the disease in an attempt to understand the basis for these findings.

We considered the possibility that the patients had hyposplenism (splenic atrophy or failure of splenic perfusion). A technetium sulfur colloid scan demonstrated normal or minimally enlarged spleens in all patients studied. Thus, hyposplenism was not the explanation for the failure to clear the IgG-sensitized erythrocytes. A second possibility was considered. The development of dermatitis herpetiformis is tightly linked to certain HLA determinants. Over 90% of patients with typical dermatitis herpetiformis are HLA B8/DRw3 positive (11). Our studies had compared patients with disease to normals and it seemed important to repeat these studies comparing the patients with dermatitis herpetiformis to normal individuals who were also HLA B8/DRw3 positive. Forty-six normal individuals were screened for HLA type. Of this group 10 were found to have the HLA B8 haplotype. Of these 10 patients 8 were Rh positive and, therefore, suitable candidates for clearance studies. Of this group of 8 individuals considered perfectly normal, 4 had a clearance defect (Fig. 3). Thus, 50% of this normal group of HLA B8 individuals had abnormal functioning of their Fc receptors at a time when they appeared to be free of any disease activity. More careful analysis of this patient group demonstrated that one patient had a history of mild arthralgias, a borderline elevated erythrocyte sedimentation rate, and a low positive ANA titer. Otherwise, none of the patients had any laboratory or clinical features that would lead one to suspect that they were not perfectly normal.

Hematologic parameters of these patients were further analyzed following this important observation. It was shown that both dermatitis herpetiformis patients and normal HLA B8/DRw3 individuals have a slightly lower lymphocyte count than do normal individuals who are not HLA B8. Moreover, studies in Dr. Fauci's laboratory demonstrated that HLA B8 individuals, as well as dermatitis herpetiformis patients, had a number of *in vitro* immunologic abnormalities. These patients and the normals both had significantly depressed levels of T lymphocytes with IgG Fc receptors (T_γ cells) which are thought to function as suppressors in the immune response. Moreover, both the patients and the normal HLA B8 individuals tended to have higher levels of spontaneous immunoglobulin-secreting cells than did normal individuals. The presence of spontaneous immunoglobulin-secreting cells in the circulation is taken as a sign of generalized B-cell activation and is found in a variety of patients with autoimmune as well as certain other illnesses (3).

The HLA B8/DRw3 haplotype is known to be associated with a wide variety of immunologic diseases. Patients with this histocompatibility type are noted to have a high incidence of dermatitis herpetiformis and gluten-sensitive enteropathy. Moreover, patients with systemic lupus erythematosus, Sjögrens syndrome, chronic active hepatitis, and juvenile diabetes all have a higher incidence of HLA B8/DRw3 than do normals. These findings raise the intriguing possibility that the HLA B8/DRw3 haplotype or a closely associated factor is responsible for a defect in Fc receptor function in this patient group and normal HLA B8 individuals and that this defect may predispose to the abnormal clearance of complexes from the circulation as well as abnormal immunoregulation. This defect may provide a proper background for the development of autoimmune disease. When these individuals are exposed to the proper stress, perhaps the presence of a chronic viral infection, they may tend to develop atuoimmunity. Thus, these factors may provide a partial explanation for the defect in these individuals that predisposes them to autoimmune disease under certain circumstances. The nature of the defect leading to abnormal clearance is still unknown. It may be due to a deficiency in Fc receptor number or affinity, or it may be due to an Fc receptor-modulating factor or serum factor in this patient group that affects Fc receptor expression. Further studies will elucidate the basis of this important defect.

REFERENCES

1. Atkinson, J. P. and Frank, M. M. Studies of the *in vivo* effects of antibody, interaction of IgM antibody and complement in the immune clearance and destruction of erythrocytes in man. *J. Clin. Invest. 54*, 339-348 (1974).

2. Engelfriet, C. P., von dem Borne, A. E. G. K., Fleer, A., van der Meulen, F. W., and Roos, D. *In vivo* destruction of erythrocytes by complement-binding and non-complement-binding antibodies. *In* "Immunobiology of the Erythrocyte" (S. G. Sandler, J. Nusbacher, and M. S. Schanfield, eds.), pp. 213-226. Alan R. Liss, New York, 1980.

3, Fauci, A. S. Immunoregulation in autoimmunity. *J. Allergy Clin. Immunol. 66*, 5-17 (1980).

4. Frank, M. M., Hamburger, M. I., Lawley, T. J., Kimberly, R. P., and Plotz, P. H. Defective reticuloendothelial system Fc' receptor function in systemic lupus erythematosus. *N. Engl. J. Med. 300*, 518-523 (1979).

5. Frank, M. M., Schreiber, A. D., Atkinson, J. P., and Jaffe, C. J. Pathophysiology of immune hemolytic anemia. *Ann. Intern. Med. 87*, 210-221 (1977).

6. Hall, R. P., Lawley, T. J., Heck, J. A., and Katz, S. I. IgA containing immune complexes in dermatitis herpetiformis, Henoch-Schonlein purpura, systemic lupus erythematosus and other diseases. *Clin. Exp. Immunol. 40*, 431-437 (1980).

7. Hamburger, M. I., Lawley, T. J., Hall, R. P., Moutsopoulos, H. M., Sharp, G. C., and Frank, M. M. Reticuloendothelial system function in mixed connective tissue disease. Submitted for publication (1981).

8. Hamburger, M. I., Moutsopoulos, H. M., Lawley, T. J., and Frank, M. M. Sjögrens syndrome: A defect in reticuloendothelial system Fc receptor specific clearance. *Ann. Intern. Med. 91*, 534-538 (1979).

9. Hamburger, M. I., Gorevic, P. D., Lawley, T. J., Franklin, E. C., and Frank, M. M. Mixed cryoglobulinemia: Association of glomerulonephritis with defective reticuloendothelial system Fc receptor function. *Trans. Assoc. Am. Physicians 92*, 104-112 (1979).

10. Jaffe, C. J., Vierling, J. M., Jones, E. A., Lawley, T. J., and Frank, M. M. Receptor specific clearance by the reticuloendothelial system in chronic liver diseases: Demonstration of defective C3b specific clearance in primary biliary cirrhosis. *J. Clin. Invest. 62*, 1069-1077 (1978).

11. Katz, S. I. and Lawley, T. J. Dermatitis herpetiformis. *In* "Recent Advances in Immunopathology of the Skin" (E. Beutner, ed.), 2nd ed., pp. 303-313. Wiley, New York, 1979.

12. Lawley, T. J., Hall, R. P., Fauci, A. S., Katz, S. I., Hamburger, M. I., and Frank, M. M. Defective Fc receptor functions associated with the HLA-B8/DRw3 haplotype: Studies in patients with dermatitis herpetiformis and normal subjects. *N. Engl. J. Med. 304*, 185-192 (1981).

13. Mannik, M., Haakenstad, A. O., and Arend, W. P. The fate and detection of circulating immune complexes. *Prog. Immunol. Proc. Int. Congr. Immunol., 2nd, Brighton, Engl. 5*, 91-104 (1974).

Immunopathology: VIIIth International Symposium, 1980

THE UNUSUAL FUNCTIONAL AND STRUCTURAL VERSATILITY OF C3 AND THE INITIATION OF THE ALTERNATIVE COMPLEMENT PATHWAY[1,2]

Hans J. Müller-Eberhard
Robert D. Schreiber
Michael K. Pangburn

Department of Molecular Immunology,
Research Institute of Scripps Clinic,
La Jolla, California

I. INTRODUCTION

The third component of complement C3 was recognized and described in 1960 (1, 2). It is related through evolution to two other components, C4 and C5, because the three proteins share homology in primary structure (3). Along with C3, C4

[1]*This is publication No. 2565 from the Research Institute of Scripps Clinic. This work was supported by United States Public Health Service Grants AI-17354, CA 27489 and HL 16411.*

[2]*Dr. Müller-Eberhard is the Cecil H. and Ida M. Green Investigator in Medical Research, Research Institute of Scripps Clinic. Dr. Schreiber is a recipient of the American Heart Association Established Investigatorship No. 77-202. Dr. Pangburn is a recipient of the American Heart Association Established Investigatorship No. 81-225.*

ISBN 0-12-218320-7

and C5 evolved specific cell surface receptors allowing reaction products of these proteins to communicate with cells involved in host defense and inflammation. C3 may be phylogenetically the older of the three proteins because it is the least specialized, the most versatile, and multifunctional. That complement is essential in host defense against infections has become clear through the occurrence of life-threatening or lethal infections in individuals with homozygous complement deficiencies (4). That complement may participate in disease mechanisms has also become clear, largely through the work done at the Research Institute of Scripps Clinic (5-7). A complement-dependent pathogenesis has been demonstrated for certain experimental disease models such as nephritis, immune vasculitis, immune arthritis, LCM disease, and myasthenia gravis. By analogy and on the basis of clinical investigations, it is probable that the corresponding diseases in man also involve complement in a similar manner.

Complement generates a plethora of biological activities, namely the ability to lyse viral membranes (8), kill gram-negative bacteria (9), kill nucleated cells (10), attract chemotactically inflammatory cells (11), cause the release of their hydrolytic enzymes (12), cause release of SRS-A (13), release histamine from mast cells (14), and opsonize foreign particles so that they may be ingested by phagocytic cells (15, 16). Generation of these activities is accomplished by highly specific protein-protein, protein-carbohydrate, and protein-phospholipid interactions, involving, in part, limited proteolysis and conformational changes.

The system is organized in three pathways: the classical (17), the alternative (18), and that of membrane attack (19). The initial enzyme of the classical pathway C1 is activated by antigen-antibody complexes. The initial enzyme of the alternative pathway is activated by the reaction of native C3 with

H_2O. In the course of complement activation, a unique molecular strategy becomes operative that allows transfer of the system from solution to the solid surface of a target particle (20). The classical pathway establishes firm physical contact with a target particle through C4b; the alternative pathway does so through C3b. The target-bound classical C3 convertase is formed when C2, a proenzyme, binds to C4b and is activated by Cls. The target-bound alternative C3 convertase is formed when Factor B, also a proenzyme, binds to C3b and is activated by Factor D. The action of either enzyme on C3 results in the binding to the target of multiple C3b molecules. C3b is required for the modulation of C5 such that it can be cleaved by the classical or alternative pathway enzyme. Cleavage of C5 initiates the self-assembly of the membrane attack complex. The three activation peptides C3a, C4a, and C5a are released as the phlogogenic anaphylatoxins in the process. It is clear from this description that C3 plays a dominant role.

Early observations indicated that the half-life of C3 hemolytic activity on exposure of the protein to aqueous solvents at 37°C was 111 hours (2). Later, it was observed that chaotropic agents which facilitate access of water to the interior of proteins greatly enhanced the spontaneous decay of C3 (21). In 1961, it was found that treatment of isolated C3 with low concentrations of amines such as hydrazine abolished both its hemolytic activity and its binding ability (22). When, in 1963, hydrazine was shown to abolish the binding capacity of C4, the possibility that the hydrazine effect might be due to nucleophilic attack on an internal ester was considered (23).

II. THE THIOESTER OF C3

Present evidence indicates that C3 contains an internal thioester and that the reactions of this thioester are crucial for two basic events: (a) initiation of the alternative pathway and (b) binding of activated C3 to biological particles. The thioester hypothesis was independently advanced by three laboratories (24-26). Treatment of C3 with radiolabeled methylamine resulted in inactivation of its hemolytic activity and in incorporation of one mole of methylamine into the protein. Concomitant with methylamine incorporation, one mole of sulfhydryl was liberated. Both the liberated sulfhydryl and the methylamine binding site were found in the 35,000-dalton d domain of the α chain of C3, suggesting a close topological relationship between the two sites. Swenson and Howard (27) had reported that serum α_2 macroglobulin is sensitive to treatment with methylamine and that methylamine was bound to the γ-carboxyl group of a glutamyl residue which was contained in the sequence -Gly-Cys-Gly-Glu-Glu-Asn-. Tack *et al.* (24) showed that C3 contained an identical sequence, that the methylamine binding site of C3 was the penultimate glutamic acid residue in the above sequence, and that the sulfhydryl group that was liberated on methylamine binding belonged to the cysteine residue. The occurrence of this sequence in the α chain of C3 was confirmed by Campbell *et al.* (28). The finding that the methylamine reactive glutamyl residue and the iodoacetamide reactive cysteinyl residue were separated only by two amino acid residues, gave much weight to the concept of the existence of an internal thioester. The above hexapeptide was synthesized and the crucial thioester linkage formed by activation of the penultimate glutamyl residue with 1-hydroxybenzotriazol and reaction of the resulting active ester with the cysteinyl thiol group (29). The cyclized hexapeptide resembled native C3 in that it exhibited spontaneous hydrolysis and bound one mole of methylamine with the concomitant liberation of one mole of sulfhydryl. Thus, the 15-membered thiolactone ring may consititute a structural feature of native C3.

III. THE GENERAL STRUCTURE OF C3

Figure 1 (A and B) shows schematic representations of the C3 molecule and its physiological derivatives. C3 has a molecular weight of 185,000 and is composed of two nonidentical polypeptide chains. The molecular weight of the α chain is 110,000 and that of the β chain 75,000. The internal thioester, which constitutes the precursor of the metastable binding site, is located in the α chain and separated from the N-terminus by a mass of approximately 46,000 daltons (30, 31). C3 is activated by cleavage of peptide bond 77 (-Arg-Ser-) of the α chain. Removal of the 9000-dalton activation peptide C3a leads to activation of the metastable binding site in the C3b fragment. C3b consists of the α′ chain and the intact β chain. In its bound or unbound form, C3b is susceptible to attack by Factor I (C3b inactivator) and its cofactor, Factor H (β1H). The product C3bi consists of two α′-chain fragments (67,000 and 40,000 daltons) linked by disulfide bonds to the intact β chain (32, 33). The molecular weight of C3bi is identical to that of C3b, but C3bi has none of the functional properties that characterize C3b. Tryptic plasma enzymes cleave the 67,000-dalton α′ fragment and eventually produce C3c and C3d. C3c has a molecular weight of 150,000 and consists of two α′ fragments (35,000 and 40,000 daltons) and the β chain. The 35,000-dalton C3d fragment contains the liberated sulfhydryl group that in native C3 is part of the thiolactone ring. C3d that is derived from bound C3b remains bound to the

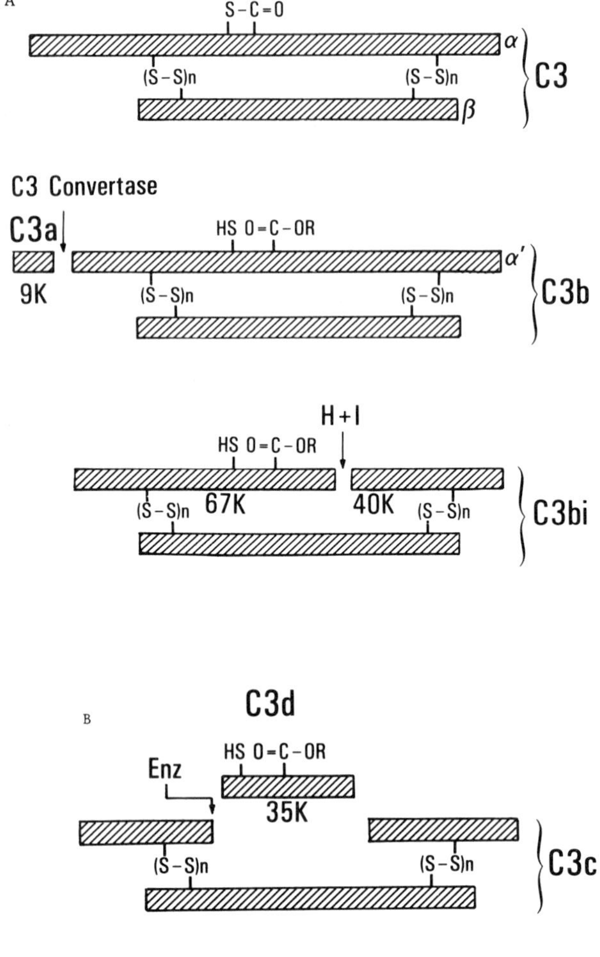

FIGURE 1. (A and B). Chain structure of C3, including approximate topology of the thioester and of the physiological reaction products.

target particle. The 10,000-dalton acidic C3e fragment is derived from C3c, possibly by tryptic attack on the 35,000-dalton α′ fragment (34).

The biological functions of the C3 fragments are indicated in Fig. 2. C3a is one of the three anaphylatoxins. C3b has multiple functions, including the recognition function of the alternative pathway; it constitutes a subunit of the classical C5 convertase and of the alternative C3/C5 convertase and is the ligand for C3b-specific cell surface receptors. C3bi lacks the foregoing activities, but is a ligand for C3bi receptors. C3d also reacts with specific C3d cell surface receptors that occur on K lymphocytes. The interactions of the C3 fragments

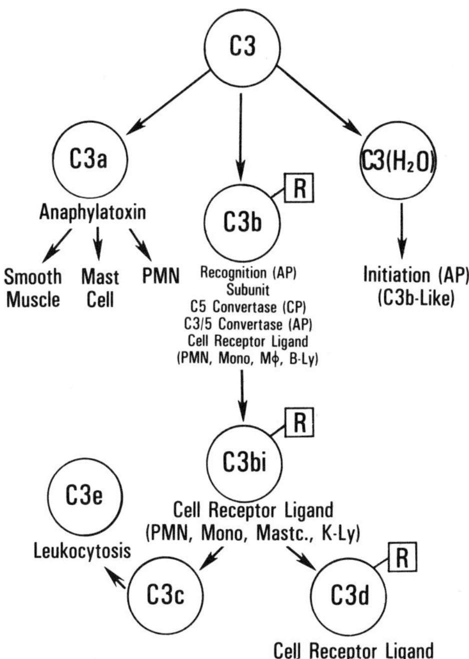

FIGURE 2. Biological activities expressed by the physiological fragments of C3. R indicates cell surface group with which metastable C3b can establish covalent linkage.

with cellular receptors enhance phagocytosis, extracellular killing, and the K-cell dependent ADCC. Finally, C3e is a leukocytosis-producing peptide.

IV. METASTABLE C3b AND ITS THIOESTER SITE

The concept of the metastable binding site of activated C3 was advanced in 1966 (35). It had been known that complement cannot accomplish its opsonic and cytolytic functions unless C3 becomes physically bound to the target particle. Native C3 was unable to bind to targets of complement such as cells. In the classical pathway, C2 and C4 were required for the mediation of C3 binding. One C4,2 complex on the surface of a target cell was capable of mediating the binding of a multiplicity of C3 molecules and many more C3 molecules accumulated in physically and chemically altered form in the fluid phase. These observations not only established the enzymatic nature of the C4,2 complex, but they also led to the realization that the altered C3 molecules in the fluid phase were unable to bind to the target cell, in spite of their having been turned over by the activating enzyme. A labile intermediate form of activated C3 that was endowed with a metastable binding site through which it could bind to targets was therefore postulated; but failing binding to the target, metastable C3 would decay and accumulate in inactive form in the fluid phase (35). A similar mechanism of binding was proposed for activated C4 (36). This concept was entirely new in protein chemistry and envisaged unique properties for these two proteins that were without precedent. Later, Law and Levine (37) made the observation that C3b is bound to zymosan through a hydroxylamine-labile bond. They also found that hydroxamate was associated with the protein that was released from zymosan upon hydroxylamine treatment (38).

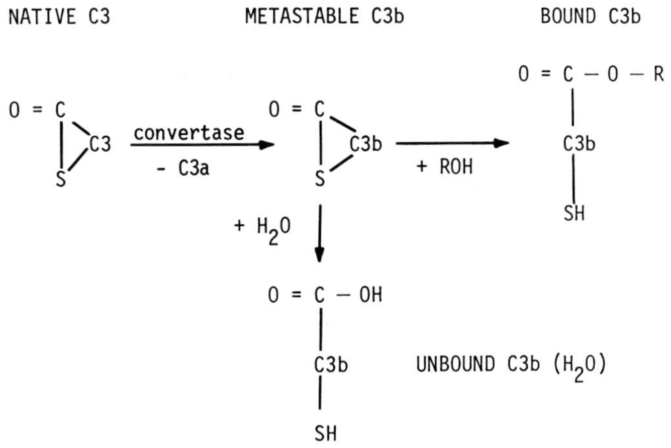

NATIVE C3 METASTABLE C3b BOUND C3b

O = C — O — R

O = C O = C

C3 convertase C3b + ROH C3b

S - C3a S SH

$+ H_2O$

O = C — OH

C3b UNBOUND C3b (H_2O)

SH

FIGURE 3. The binding reaction of C3. Formation of metastable C3b and transesterification of the carbonyl group in the thioester to an ester with a hydroxyl group on the receptive surface.

In current language, the enzymatically catalyzed binding of C3 to complement targets may be described as shown in Fig. 3. When native C3 is attacked by its activating enzymes and C3a is removed, the thioester of the d-domain of the α chain comes under stress. The reactive carbonyl in the thioester bond can now transfer to an ester bond formed with a hydroxyl group on the surface of the target (38). Alternatively, it may also form an amide bond with an amino group on the receptive surface (39, 40). C3b becomes thus covalently bound to a target and exhibits a free sulfhydryl group. Metastable C3b that fails to undergo transesterification of its thioester reacts with water and loses its binding site.

V. THE MULTIPLE FUNCTIONAL SITES OF C3b

Nothing expresses the versatility of C3 more than the occurrence of multiple functional sites on the C3b fragment. In addition to the metastable binding site, C3b possesses binding sites for Factor B, C5, properdin, Factor H, and Factor I. There are also the molecular regions that specifically bind to the C3b cell surface receptors and, as yet hidden in the C3b molecule, the sites that are specific for the cell surface C3bi and C3d receptors. Brief mention should be made also of the hypothetical recognition site on the target-bound C3b molecule (18, 41, 42). Depending on the microenvironment of bound C3b, it either binds preferentially Factor B to form the C3 convertase of the alternative pathway, or it binds Factor H and is subsequently degraded by Factor I. For instance, human C3b on human or sheep erythrocytes is rapidly degraded, whereas on rabbit erythrocytes or *E. coli* it is not (42-44). The diminished binding of Factor H to C3b in the latter two situations has been interpreted to suggest that C3b is endowed with a recognition site that can engage itself with a select variety of cell surface constituents and thereby weaken its Factor H binding (42). The various binding sites on C3b appear to be accessible to topological mapping using monoclonal antibodies to C3b that selectively inhibit individual binding sites (Tamerius, Pangburn, and Müller-Eberhard, unpublished observations) combined with high resolution electron microscopy (Smith, Pangburn, and Müller-Eberhard, unpublished observations).

VI. FUNCTIONALLY C3b-LIKE C3 GENERATED NONENZYMATICALLY BY HYDROLYSIS OF THE THIOESTER IN NATIVE C3

Native C3 expresses no detectable biological activity. Yet, when native C3, Factors B, D, and Mg^{2+} are admixed in physiological concentrations, C3 convertase activity rapidly appears (18, 45). It was hypothesized therefore that a C3 conformer, representing a very small proportion of native C3, might have C3b-like functional properties (18). Recent evidence strongly suggests that the postulated C3 conformer constitutes C3 that has lost the internal thioester by reacting with water. It was found that C3 with its thioester hydrolyzed [C3(H_2O)] exhibits all functional properties of C3b (46).

When studies of the effect of CH_3NH_2 on C3 made it likely that an internal thioester was opened up without any effect on the primary peptide structure of the protein, C3(CH_3NH_2) was subjected to functional and conformational analyses. It was found that C3(CH_3NH_2) can bind Factors B and H, can form a fluid phase C3 convertase with Factors B, D, and Mg^{2+}, and can be cleaved and inactivated by Factors H and I (26). Circular dichroism studies and fluorescence measurements of binding of 1-anilino-8-naphthalene sulfonate (ANS) detected the occurrence of marked spectral changes when C3 was converted to C3(CH_3NH_2) (47). The spectra of C3(CH_3NH_2) resembled those of C3b (48). The rate of conformational rearrangement was much slower than the rate of CH_3NH_2 uptake by C3 and the appearance of functional properties correlated with the conformational change rather than chemical modification. Also, the acquisition of Factor H binding capacity by CH_3NH_2-modified C3 was slower than the acquisition of Factor B binding sites. For instance, at a given CH_3NH_2 concentration and at 37°C the methylamine uptake was essentially complete at 5 min, whereas 50% Factor B and Factor H binding activity became expressed at 25 and 35 min, respectively (47). These kinetics suggest that C3, modified at the thioester site, has temporarily a slightly greater chance to form the fluid-phase C3 convertase than to become enzymatically degraded by Factors H and I.

The studies of C3(CH_3NH_2) prompted a reinvestigation of the spontaneous decay of C3 in aqueous solution (2) and of the effect of chaotropic agents on C3 (21). It was found (46) that the rate of spontaneous loss of the C3 binding site in

TABLE I. The C3b-Like Functions of C3(H_2O)

Properties	C3	C3b	C3(H_2O)
Binding of B	–	+	+
Formation of C3 convertase	–	+	+
Binding of H	–	+	+
Cleavage by I	–	+	+
Binding to cellular C3b receptors	–	+	+
Cleavage by C3 convertase	+	–	±
Metastable binding site	+	–	–

neutral buffer at 37°C was 0.005% per min. In the presence of 0.33 *M* KSCN the rate of inactivation was 1250-fold enhanced, or 6.25% per min. With progression of inactivation, a free sulfhydryl group appeared which is not present in native C3. The final product has been considered C3 with its thioester hydrolyzed [C3(H_2O)]. As listed in Table I, C3(H_2O) exhibits all functional properties of fluid-phase C3b. However, C3(H_2O) is structurally distinct from C3b in that it contains an intact α chain rather than the α' chain, which lacks the C3a domain. Although C3(H_2O) is structurally indistinguishable from native C3 by its appearance on SDS-polyacrylamide gel electrophoresis, unlike native C3, its α chain is susceptible to cleavage by Factor I. Factor I cleaves the α chain of C3(H_2O) into a 76,000 and a 40,000 molecular weight fragment. The 76,000-dalton fragment contains the 67,000-dalton piece of the α' chain of C3bi, plus covalently linked the 9,000-dalton C3a domain (46).

VII. THE ROLE OF $C3(H_2O)$, METASTABLE C3b, AND TARGET BOUND C3b IN THE INITIATION OF THE ALTERNATIVE PATHWAY

As schematically presented in Fig. 4, it is proposed (46) that the initial event in the alternative pathway is the spontaneous generation of $C3(H_2O)$ which is formed continuously at a slow rate. Due to the differential rate of appearance of binding sites during the transition of native C3 to the C3b-like form of the molecule, the fluid-phase C3 convertase $C3(H_2O)$,Bb may form and generate metastable C3b from native C3 before the enzyme becomes fully susceptible to control by Factors H and I. Metastable C3b so generated may randomly attach to surrounding receptive surfaces. Deposited C3b then exercises its discriminatory ability of distinguishing between different cells. On nonactivators of the alternative pathway it is rapidly degraded by Factors H and I to C3bi and subsequently by other enzymes to smaller fragments. On activators,

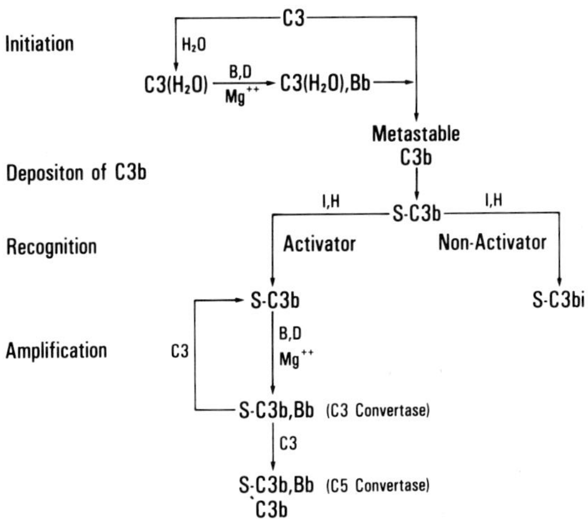

FIGURE 4. Proposed reaction mechanism of the alternative pathway of complement activation (46).

the affinity of C3b for Factor H is reduced and degradation is sufficiently retarded to allow C3 convertase formation on the target particle, amplification by the C3b-dependent positive feedback, and C5 convertase assembly with stabilization of the enzyme by properdin (18, 49).

The recognition of C3(H_2O) (26, 46) as a new functional form of C3 and the observation that C3(H_2O) arises spontaneously may resolve the long-standing question as to the manner in which the alternative pathway is initiated (18, 41, 45, 50, 51).

VIII. EVOLUTIONARY RELATIONSHIP AMONG C3, C4, AND C5

The three proteins exhibit many similarities and many differences. All three proteins are synthesized as a single polypeptide chain which is processed after translation into the respective chain structures (52). The α chain of each protein contributes one of the three anaphylatoxins in the form of the activation peptide. These peptides exhibit similar biological activities, 36-38% homology in primary structure and approximately 45% α-helical content (3, 11, 53). C4 contains the same type of metastable binding site as does C3 (36, 54, 55), but C5 does not. In fact, the sequence around the internal thioester is identical in C3 and C4 (28). C4 is genetically linked to the MHC, C3 and C5 are not (for references, see 4). C3 binds Factor B and C4 binds C2, which constitute two very similar serine proteases (56) genetically linked to the MHC and to each other [for references, see Raum *et al.* (4)].

IX. CONCLUSION

C3 fulfills many functions in host defense and inflammation. Whereas native C3 as such possesses no discernible biological activity, it harbors many distinct structures that constitute the precursors of functional sites. The internal thioester represents not only a novel chemical structure, but it is the strategic center that controls the expression of many functions of the molecule. Upon its spontaneous hydrolysis, native C3, without enzymatic modification, acquires the ability to form a fluid-phase C3 convertase together with Factors B, D, and Mg^{2+}. The reaction of native C3 with one molecule of water may therefore constitute the simple, nonspecific event that initiates perpetually the alternative pathway of complement activation which is regarded as one of the mechanisms of nonspecific resistance to infections. Enzymatic attack of native C3 by the C3 convertase of the classical or the alternative pathway generates metastable C3b. Whereas enzymatic cleavage of C3 occurs near the N-terminus of the α chain, it is the thioester in the d domain of the α chain, which is far removed from the cleavage site, that is affected. Within microseconds the reactive carbonyl group of the thioester in metastable C3b can undergo transesterification and form an ester bond with a hydroxyl group on the surface of biological particles. Thus, the transfer of C3 from solution to the solid phase of complement targets is effected. Deposited on a target by the classical pathway it becomes a subunit of its C5 convertase. Deposited via the alternative pathway it exercises a low specificity discriminatory function, furnishes two of the three subunits of the C3/C5 convertase, and ignites the unique amplification reaction which is the driving force of the alternative pathway. C3b also functions as an opsonin by serving as a ligand for specific cell surface receptors. Its degradation products, C3bi and C3d, fulfill similar ligand functions. The activation peptide C3a constitutes one of the three anaphylatoxins, which have inflammation-producing activity. The other two anaphylatoxins are derived from C4 and C5. These two proteins are considered evolutionary relatives of C3 because limited sequence analysis has revealed a degree of homology in primary structure.

The ultrastructural analysis of C3 and C3b in conjunction with the use of monoclonal antibodies is currently providing an initial topological map of functional C3b sites in relation to structural and immunochemical domains of C3b.

REFERENCES

1. Müller-Eberhard, H. J., Nilsson, U., and Aronsson, T. Isolation and characterization of two β_1-glycoproteins of human serum. *J. Exp. Med. 111*, 201 (1960).

2. Müller-Eberhard, H. J. and Nilsson, U. Relation of a β_1-glycoprotein of human serum to the complement system. *J. Exp. Med. 111*, 217 (1960).

3. Gorski, J. P., Hugli, T. E., and Müller-Eberhard, H. J. Characterization of human C4a anaphylatoxin. *J. Biol. Chem. 256*, 2707 (1981).

4. Raum, D., Donaldson, V. H., Alper, C. A., and Rosen, F. S. Genetics of complement and complement deficiencies. *In* "Immunology 80, Progress in Immunology" (M. Fougereau and J. Dausset, eds.), p. 1244. Academic Press, New York, 1980.

5. Dixon, F. J. and Wilson, C. B. Immunological renal injury produced by formation and deposition of immune complexes. *In* "Immunologic Mechanisms of Renal Disease" (C. B. Wilson, B. M. Brenner, and J. H. Stein, eds.), Contemporary Issues in Nephrology, Vol. 3, p. 1. Churchill Livingstone, New York, 1979.

6. Wilson, C. B. and Dixon, F. J. Renal injury from immune reactions involving antigens in or of the kidney. *In* "Immunologic Mechanisms of Renal Disease" (C. B. Wilson, B. M. Brenner, and J. H. Stein, eds.), Contemporary Issues in Nephrology, Vol. 3, p. 35. Churchill Livingstone, New York, 1979.

7. Cochrane, C. G. Mediation systems in neutrophil-independent immunologic injury of the glomerulus. *In* "Immunologic Mechanisms of Renal Disease" (C. B. Wilson, B. M. Brenner, and J. H. Stein, eds.), Contemporary Issues in Nephrology, Vol. 3, p. 106. Churchill Livingstone, New York, 1979.

8. Esser, A. F., Bartholomew, R. M., Jensen, F. C., and Müller-Eberhard, H. J. Disassembly of viral membranes by complement independent of channel formation. *Proc. Natl. Acad. Sci. U.S.A. 76*, 5843 (1979).

9. Schreiber, R. D., Morrison, D. C., Podack, E. R., and Müller-Eberhard, H. J. Bactericidal activity of the alternative complement pathway generated from eleven isolated plasma proteins. *J. Exp. Med. 149*, 870 (1979).

10. Schreiber, R. D., Pangburn, M. K., Medicus, R. G., and Müller-Eberhard, H. J. Raji cell injury and subsequent lysis by the purified cytolytic alternative pathway of human complement. *Clin. Immunol. Immunopathol. 15*, 384 (1980).

11. Hugli, T. E. and Müller-Eberhard, H. J. Anaphylatoxins: C3a and C5a. *Adv. Immunol. 26*, 1 (1978).

12. Chenoweth, D. E. and Hugli, T. E. Human C5a and C5a analogs as probes of the neutrophil C5a receptor. *Mol. Immunol. 17*, 151 (1980).

13. Stimler, N. P., Brocklehurst, W. E., Bloor, C. M., and Hugli, T. E. Complement anaphylatoxin C5a stimulates release of SRS-A-like activity from guinea-pig lung fragments. *J. Pharm. Pharmacol. 32*, 804 (1980).

14. Johnson, A. R., Hugli, T. E., and Müller-Eberhard, H. J. Release of histamine from rat mast cells by the complement peptides C3a and C5a. *Immunology 28*, 1067 (1975).

15. Gigli, I. and Nelson, R. A., Jr. Complement dependent immune phagocytosis. I. Requirements for C'1, C'4, C'2, C'3. *Exp. Cell Res. 51*, 45 (1968).

16. Huber, H., Polley, M. J., Linscott, W. D., Fudenberg, H. H., and Müller-Eberhard, H. J. Human monocytes: Distinct receptor B sites for the third component of complement and for immunoglobulin G. *Science 162*, 1281 (1968).

17. Porter, R. R. and Reid, K. B. Activation of the complement system by antibody-antigen complexes: The classical pathway. *Adv. Protein Chem. 33*, 1 (1979).

18. Müller-Eberhard, H. J. and Schreiber, R. D. Molecular biology and chemistry of the alternative pathway of complement. *Adv. Immunol. 29*, 1 (1980).

19. Podack, E. R., Esser, A. F., Biesecker, G., and Müller-Eberhard, H. J. Membrane attack complex of complement: A structural analysis of its assembly. *J. Exp. Med. 151*, 301 (1980).

20. Müller-Eberhard, H. J. Complement. *Annu. Rev. Biochem. 44*, 697 (1975).

21. Dalmasso, A. P. and Müller-Eberhard, H. J. Hemolytic activity of lipoprotein-depleted serum and the effect of certain anions on complement. *J. Immunol. 97*, 680 (1966).

22. Müller-Eberhard, H. J. Isolation and description of proteins related to the human complement system. *Acta Soc. Med. Ups. 66*, 152 (1961).

23. Müller-Eberhard, H. J. and Biro, C. E. Isolation and description of the fourth component of human complement. *J. Exp. Med. 118*, 447 (1963).

24. Tack, B. F., Harrison, R. A., Janatova, J., Thomas, M. L., and Prahl, J. W. Evidence for presence of an internal thiolester bond in third component of human complement. *Proc. Natl. Acad. Sci. U.S.A. 77*, 5764 (1980).

25. Law, S. K., Lichtenberg, N. A., and Levine, R. P. Covalent binding and hemolytic activity of complement proteins (inactivation by amines). *Proc. Natl. Acad. Sci. U.S.A. 77*, 7194 (1980).

26. Pangburn, M. K. and Müller-Eberhard, H. J. Relation of a putative thioester bond in C3 to activation of the alternative pathway and the binding of C3b to biological targets of complement. *J. Exp. Med. 152*, 1102 (1980).

27. Swenson, R. P. and Howard, J. B. Characterization of alkylamine-sensitive site in α_2-macroglobulin. *Proc. Natl. Acad. Sci. U.S.A. 76*, 4313 (1979).

28. Campbell, R. D., Gagnon, J., and Porter, R. R. Amino acid sequence around the proposed thiolester bond of human complement component C4 and comparison with the corresponding sequences from C3 and α_2-macroglobulin. *Biosci. Rep. 1*, 423 (1981).

29. Khan, S. A., Pangburn, M. K., Müller-Eberhard, H. J., and Erickson, B. W. The cyclic thioester form of a synthetic hexapeptide from human complement protein C3 resembles the C3b metastable binding site. *Fed. Proc., Fed. Am. Soc. Exp. Biol. 40*, 1679 (1981).

30. Sim, R. B. and Sim, E. Autolytic fragmentation of complement components C3 and C4 under denaturing conditions, a property shared with α_2-macroglobulin. *Biochem. J. 193*, 129 (1981).

31. Howard, J. B. Methylamine reaction and denaturation-dependent fragmentation of complement component 3: Comparison with α_2-macroglobulin. *J. Biol. Chem. 255*, 7082 (1980).

32. Pangburn, M. K., Schreiber, R. D., and Müller-Eberhard, H. J. Human complement C3b inactivator: Isolation, characterization and demonstration of an absolute requirement for the serum protein β1H for cleavage of C3b and C4b in solution. *J. Exp. Med. 146*, 257 (1977).

33. Lachmann, P. J. Complement. *In* "The Antigens" (M. Sela, ed.), Vol. 5, p. 284. Academic Press, New York, 1979.

34. Ghebrehiwet, B. and Müller-Eberhard, H. J. C3e: An acidic fragment of human C3 with leukocytosis inducing activity. *J. Immunol. 123*, 616 (1979).

35. Müller-Eberhard, H. J., Dalmasso, A. P., and Calcott, M. A. The reaction mechanism of β_{1C}-globulin (C'3) in immune hemolysis. *J. Exp. Med. 123*, 33 (1966).

36. Müller-Eberhard, H. J. and Lepow, I. H. C'1 esterase effect on activity and physicochemical properties of the fourth component of complement. *J. Exp. Med. 121*, 819 (1965).

37. Law, S. K. and Levine, R. P. Interaction between the third complement protein and cell surface. *Proc. Natl. Acad. Sci. U.S.A. 74*, 2701 (1977).

38. Law, S. K., Lichtenberg, N. A., and Levine, R. P. Evidence for an ester linkage between the labile binding site of C3b and receptive surfaces. *J. Immunol. 123*, 1388 (1979).

39. Campbell, R. D., Dodds, A. W., and Porter, R. R. The binding of human complement component C4 to antibody-antigen aggregates. *Biochem. J. 189*, 67 (1980).

40. Sim, R. B., Twose, T. M., Paterson, D. S., and Sim, E. The covalent-binding reaction of complement component C3. *Biochem. J. 193*, 115 (1981).

41. Schreiber, R. D., Pangburn, M. K., Lesavre, P., and Müller-Eberhard, H. J. Initiation of the alternative pathway of complement: Recognition of activators by bound C3b and assembly of the entire pathway from six isolated proteins. *Proc. Natl. Acad. Sci. U.S.A. 75*, 3948 (1978).

42. Pangburn, M. K., Morrison, D. C., Schreiber, R. D., and Müller-Eberhard, H. J. Activation of the alternative complement pathway: Recognition of surface structures on activators by bound C3b. *J. Immunol. 124*, 977 (1980).

43. Fearon, D. T. and Austen, K. F. Activation of the alternative complement pathway due to resistance of zymosan-bound amplification convertase to endogenous regulatory mechanisms. *Proc. Natl. Acad. Sci. U.S.A. 74*, 1683 (1977).

44. Pangburn, M. K. and Müller-Eberhard, H. J. Complement C3 convertase: Cell surface restriction of β1H control and generation of restriction on neuraminidase treated cells. *Proc. Natl. Acad. Sci. U.S.A. 75*, 2416 (1978).

45. Fearon, D. T. and Austen, K. F. Initiation of C3 cleavage in the alternative complement pathway. *J. Immunol. 115*, 1357 (1975).

46. Pangburn, M. K., Schreiber, R. D., and Müller-Eberhard, H. J. Formation of the initial C3 convertase of the alternative complement pathway: Acquisition of C3b-like activities by spontaneous hydrolysis of the putative thioester in native C3. *J. Exp. Med. 154*, 856 (1981).

47. Isenman, D. E., Kells, D. I. C., Cooper, N. R., Müller-Eberhard, H. J., and Pangburn, M. K. Nucleophilic modification of human complement protein C3: Correlation of conformational changes with acquisition of C3b-like functional properties. *Biochemistry 20*, 4458 (1981).

48. Isenman, D. E. and Cooper, N. R. The structure and function of the third component of human complement. I. The nature and extent of conformational changes accompanying C3 activation. *Mol. Immunol. 18*, 331 (1981).

49. Müller-Eberhard, H. J. Complement reaction pathways. *In* "Immunology 80, Progress in Immunology IV" (M. Fougereau and J. Dausset, eds.), p. 1001. Academic Press, New York, 1980.

50. Müller-Eberhard, H. J. and Götze, O. C3 proactivator convertase and its mode of action. *J. Exp. Med. 135*, 1003 (1972).

51. Nicol, P. A. E. and Lachmann, P. J. The alternate pathway of complement activation. The role of C3 and its inactivator (KAF). *Immunology 24*, 259 (1973).

52. Ooi, Y. M. and Colten, H. R. Genetic deficiency of C5 in mice: A defect in secretion. *J. Immunol. 124*, 1534 (1980).

53. Gorski, J. P., Hugli, T. E., and Müller-Eberhard, H. J. C4a: The third anaphylatoxin of the human complement system. *Proc. Natl. Acad. Sci. U.S.A. 76*, 5299 (1979).

54. Gorski, J. P. and Howard, J. B. Effect of methylamine on the structure and function of the fourth component of human complement, C4. *J. Biol. Chem. 255*, 10025 (1980).

55. Janatova, J. and Tack, B. F. The fourth component of human complement: Studies of an amine-sensitive site comprised of a thiol component. *Biochemistry 20*, 2394 (1981).

56. Medicus, R. G., Götze, O., and Müller-Eberhard, H. J. The serine protease nature of the C3 and C5 convertases of the classical and alternative complement pathways. *Scand. J. Immunol. 5*, 1049 (1976).

Immunopathology: VIIIth International Symposium, 1980

COMPLEMENT RECEPTORS: BIOLOGICAL AND BIOCHEMICAL CHARACTERIZATION

Manfred P. Dierich

Institut für Medizinische Mikrobiologie
der Johannes-Gutenberg-Universität,
Augustusplatz, D-6500 Mainz, FRG

The surface characteristics of cells are of absolute critical importance for cell biological behavior. Therefore, it is a central target of biomedical research to clarify the structure and function of cell membrane elements. Our efforts are directed toward elucidation of the biochemistry and biology of complement receptor activity. Cells endowed with this activity are capable of adhering to any cell whose surface is coated with fragments of certain complement components.

Since the original observation by Nelson in 1953 (33) that treatment of Trep. pallidum with serum enhanced its adherence to human erythrocytes (a phenomenon that Nelson termed "immune adherence") and the next step in 1968 by Lay and Nussenzweig (29) who found that mouse lymphocytes bound sensitized sheep erythrocytes coated with mouse complement, a large series of papers has appeared from various groups including our own describing complement receptor activity on a number of cells

ISBN 0-12-218320-7

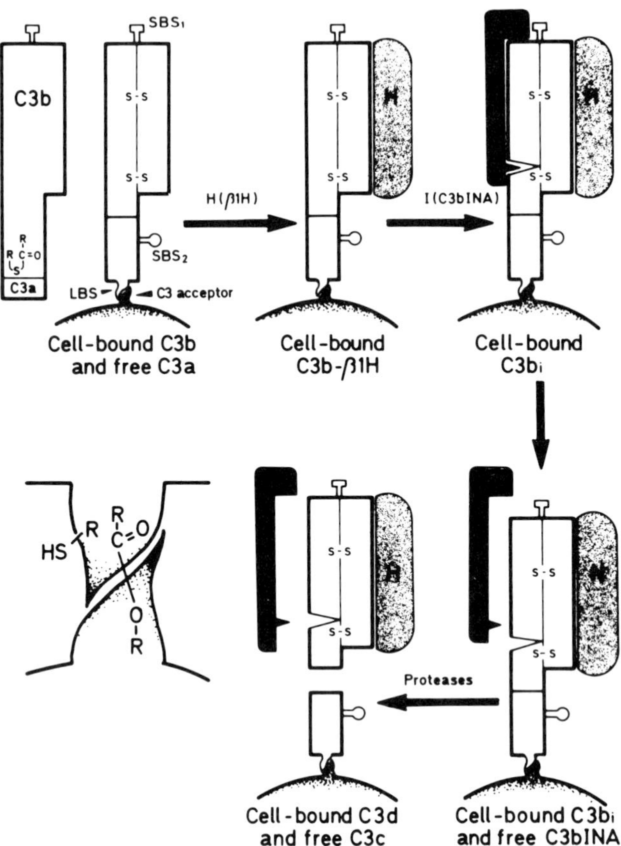

FIGURE 1. Schematic representation of the binding of nascent C3b to C3 acceptors and degradation of cell-bound C3b to cell-bound C3d by β1H (H) and C3b inactivator (C3bINA). Fixation of nascent C3b via a metastable site (LBS) in C3b results in a covalent binding between a carbonyl group in C3b and an OH group (C3b acceptors) on a cell surface. The location of factor H in this scheme is only to indicate that H binds to the C3c protein of C3b; whether this occurs in the α or β chain is not yet clarified. SBS_1 and SBS_2 indicate the capacity of C3b and C3d to interact with C3b and C3d receptors. Whether intact C3 carries these stable binding sites or they are expressed only on partially processed or denatured C3 is not yet decided.

(2, 4, 38, 48). It is the general consensus that it is primarily C3, the third component of the complement system, and its fragments that are inducing the binding of complement-coated particles to complement receptor positive cells (CR +C). However, contributions of C4 and C5 have been demonstrated (3, 28, 37).

With a better understanding of the activation of C3 and of the degradation of the biologically active fragments, our understanding of complement receptor reactivity has become more precise. In addition, our earlier statements have to be revised in part since in recent years we have had to realize that earlier C3 preparations were contaminated by traces of C5 and factor H of the alternate pathway.

Properly cleaved by proteases (C4b,2a of the classical pathway of complement activation; C3b,Bb of the alternate pathway; trypsin and others), C3 gives rise to C3a (9000 daltons) and C3b (180,000 daltons). If this activation of C3 occurs in the immediate vicinity of cell surfaces the nascent C3b becomes bound to membrane sites, termed "C3 acceptors." This binding appears to be a covalent interlinkage between a C3b carboxyl group liberated from a thioester and an hydroxyl group on the cell surface (for details see Müller-Eberhard earlier in this volume). Such C3 acceptors are distributed ubiquitously.

By the joint action of factor H of the alternate pathway (earlier termed $\beta 1H$) and I (C3b inactivator) C3bi is generated, characterized by a cleavage in the α chain of C3b. Factor H remains bound while factor I is probably released. Further cleavage of C3bi by proteases such as trysin results in generation of C3c and C3d; C3c is released, probably together with H, and C3d remains surface bound (Fig. 1).

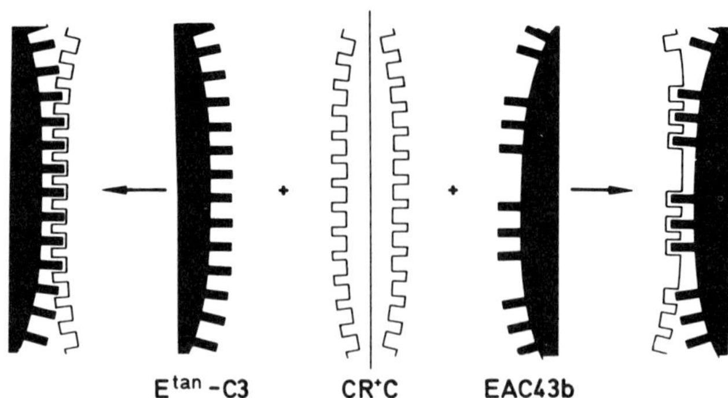

FIGURE 2. Scheme of the assumed arrangement of C3 receptors on complement receptor positive cells (CR^+C) during the reaction of CR^+C with EAC43b or E^{tan}-C3, respectively. For the interaction with EAC43b carrying C3b in clusters around the antibodies, the C3 receptors probably have to aggregate. For the reaction with E^{tan}-C3 carrying C3 randomly distributed, the C3 receptors can remain homogeneously distributed on CR^+C (28).

These C3b-, C3bi-, or C3d-carrying particles can be recognized by certain cells endowed with the proper "receptors," a phenomenon evidenced by rosette formation *in vitro*. This adherence to the complement receptor positive cells (CR^+C) is clearly dependent on the density of C3 molecules on the surface of the particle (41) and on their particular topographical distribution (28) (Fig. 2). If the C3 ligands are offered in clusters, then the receptors have to be arranged in the same way to allow an interaction to occur. From a detailed qualitative and quantitative study by Schmitt *et al.* (41) of human cells with intermediates prepared from purified complement components we know that the various cells have different receptor patterns (Figs. 3 and 4).

Using erythrocytes coated with 30,000 C3 molecules per cell, *peripheral blood leukocytes* formed 15% rosettes with EAC1-3b, 18% with EAC1-3bi, and 12% with EAC1-3d. Upon elimination of monocytes and most T cells by rosetting with sheep erythrocytes, the remaining cells formed 45% rosettes with

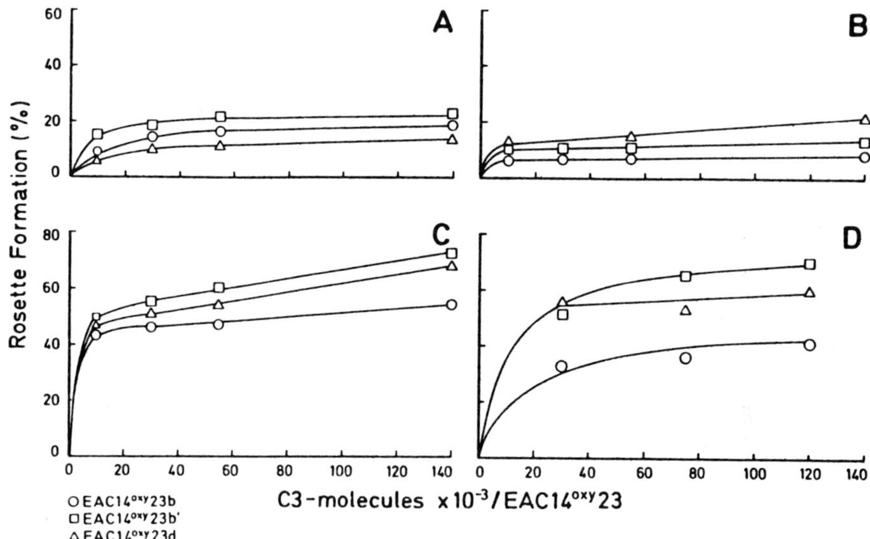

FIGURE 3. Dependence of the rosette formation among human peripheral blood leukocytes depleted of granulocytes (panel A), peripheral blood leukocytes depleted of adherent cells (panel B), peripheral blood lymphocytes enriched for B cells (panel C), tonsil lymphocytes (panel D), and EAC14^{oxy}23b, EAC1^{oxy}23b', EAC14^{oxy}23d on the amount of C3 molecules per EAC (41).

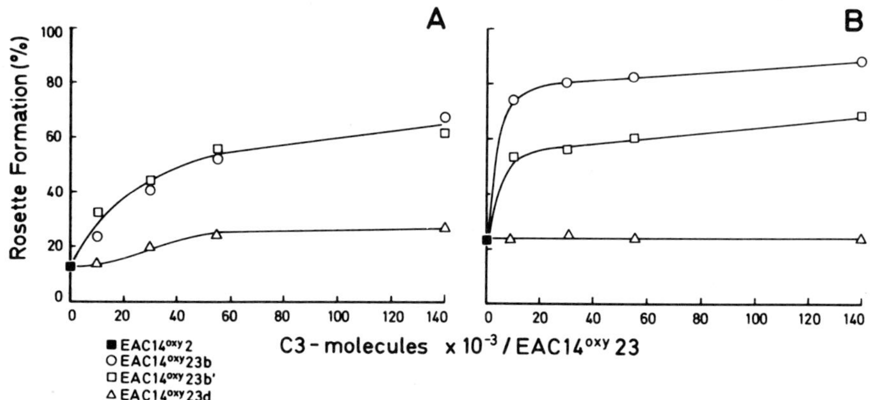

FIGURE 4. Dependence of the rosette formation between human granulocytes (panel A) and monocytes (panel B) and EAC14^{oxy}23b, EAC14^{oxy}23b', EAC14^{oxy}23d on the number of C3 molecules per EAC (41).

EACl-3b, 55% with EACl-3bi, and 50% with EACl-3d. *Tonsil lymphocytes* had a similar reaction pattern: 30, 50, and 55%, respectively. *Monocytes* (Fig. 4) from the peripheral blood showed reactivity with C3b, and to a lesser degree with C3bi intermediates, but not with C3d intermediates. The results concerning the behavior toward C3d intermediates have been controversial. It is our experience that the outcome clearly depends on the total conversion of C3bi to C3d.

TABLE I. Human Cells with Complement Receptors

Cells	C3b	C3bi	C3d	Reference
B Lymphocytes	++	++	++	
Monocytes	++	+	-	
Neutrophiles	++	++	-	
Erythrocytes	++	-	-	
Renal glomerulus (visceral epith. cells)	++ (+ with Salm. C^{m} or ^{hum})	?	-	(17a, 44)
Hepatocytes	(+ with human C3)			(23)
Langerhans skin cells	(+ with EAC^{m})			(45)
Peripheral nerve tissue (nerve fascicles)	(+ with EAC^{hum})			(34)
Synovial cells	(+ with EAC^{m} and fluid-$C3b^{hum}$)			(49)
Aortic valve	(+ with EAC^{m})			(26)
Raji cells	+	++	++	
Daudi cells	-	++	++	

Peripheral blood polymorphonuclear leukocytes (PMNL), like monocytes, recognized C3b and C3bi but not C3d (Fig. 4). But whereas granulocytes bound C3b and C3bi intermediates equally well, C3bi intermediates adhered to monocytes less well than did C3b intermediates. *Erythrocytes* bind C3b, but no C3bi or C3d intermediates. In other studies, receptors for complement have been described on the visceral epithelial cells of the glomeruli in human kidney (44), on hepatocytes (23), on Langerhans cells of the skin (45), in peripheral nerve tissue (34), on cells of the synovia (49), and on cells of the aortic valve (26) (Table I).

Lymphocytes from patients with acute lymphatic leukemia and chronic lymphatic leukemia have shown typical complement receptor patterns in that CLL lymphocytes showed reactivity for EAC1423d and not for EAC1423b whereas ALL lymphocytes were mostly CR negative (38). For detailed analysis, however, these studies await reevaluation with better defined intermediates.

B-lymphoblastoid cell lines have attracted great attention. They have been used as tools for elucidating the biochemistry of complement receptors and for detecting immune complexes carrying C3 fragments. [See the Raji cell assay described by Theofilopoulos *et al.* in 1974 (47).] For us, as for others, two cell lines derived from patients with Burkitt lymphoma have been of particular interest, namely, Raji and Daudi cells (41). Using erythrocytes with 30,000 C3 molecules per cell, Raji cells bind C3b (25% rosettes), and more intensively C3bi and C3d intermediates (90 and 95% rosettes, respectively). Particularly in the case of a C3 density of 30,000 molecules per E, it is obvious that binding of C3b intermediates is lower than that of C3bi or C3d intermediates. Daudi cells bind C3bi and C3d cells in a manner similar to Raji cells, but they do not bind C3b cells.

The fact that Daudi cells do not bind C3b intermediates but do bind others, while human erythrocytes bind C3b but not C3bi or C3d intermediates clearly suggests that the receptor activities for C3b on the one hand and C3bi and C3d on the other can be attributed to different entities, a notion supported by work with antisera (18, 37). Furthermore, C3bi and C3d are probably recognized by different sites since monocytes clearly show a reactivity for C3bi but not for C3d, whereas both C3bi and C3d are bound to B lymphocytes. The assumption that the receptors for C3b, C3bi, and C3d are different is also strengthened by our ongoing work with monoclonal antibodies directed against the various receptors (Dierich *et al.*, unpublished observations) (6a).

In the case of C3b and of C3d intermediates, it is very clear that the C3 fragment is the ligand for the corresponding receptor. In the case of C3bi intermediates the situation is less obvious since C3bi is actually at least a bimolecular complex consisting of C3bi itself and factor H (β1H) attached to it. Very recently, we compiled evidence (40) that factor H binds directly to complement receptor lymphocytes and is capable of mediating an H-dependent cytoadherence. This suggests that H itself is at least in part responsible for binding of C3bi to receptors. Whether in addition a new site in C3b itself is contributing is currently under investigation. Thus, we can now distinguish receptor reactivities for C3b, for C3d, for H (particularly when bound to C3b), and possibly for something else in C3bi. Whether receptors for these different ligands are also capable of binding other ligands is not finally established. Nevertheless, it seems very likely that the receptor for C3b (CR_1 or immune adherence receptor) can also act as the receptor for C4b (37) and possibly for C5b (27). The receptor for C3d (CR_2) is also probably the receptor for C5d, although present evidence for such an assumption is weak (7, 27). That part in C3b responsible for the interaction with the C3b receptor is not finally settled. Most likely it is the C3c protein (37). Whether C3d can be recognized in cell-bound C3b or is hidden below the C3c entity is not clear. It should be pointed out that C3b is a molecule with an enormous potential for interacting with other molecules. Thus, it binds C5, factors B, H, and I, properdin, and C3b receptor molecules. Clarification as to whether the latter has functions like the former is a particularly exciting research aim. Fearon's observation of a membrane-derived molecule with functions of a factor H-like molecule and determinants of C3b receptors is highly indicative (15).

The *functions of the C3 receptors* (Table II) are not conclusively established. There is no doubt that among all groups certain C3 receptors can bind certain C3-intermediates. C3-dependent adherence can be observed *in vitro*, e.g., by rosette formation. It may also be seen *in vivo*, e.g., in deposition of immune complexes carrying C3 fragments into the kidney (44), in deposition of C3-carrying antigens in the follicles of lymphatic tissue (13, 35), or by trapping of C3-intermediates in the spleen or the liver (see Frank *et al.*, this volume). But whether in addition to the passive adherence an active process can be triggered through C3-C3 receptor interaction remains inconclusive. Washout macrophages bind but do not ingest EA(IgM)C1423, whereas elicited macrophages bind and ingest (1). Obviously, cell status is of critical importance. In contrast to EA(IgM)C1423, EA(IgG)C1423 is both attached to and ingested by washout macrophages, suggesting that surface-bound IgG can act as a trigger whereas C3 cannot. This statement may, however, pertain only to complement-coated erythrocytes and not to bacteria, since it has recently been observed that *Legionella pneumophilia* or encapsulated *E. coli*, opsonized with IgM and complement, not only

TABLE II. Complement Receptor Function

Adherence (passive function)	
in vitro	- rosette formation of phagocytes and B lymphocytes
in vitro	- deposition of AgAbC in renal glomeruli
	- deposition of AgAbC in lymph nodes, spleen, liver
Stimulation (active function)	
phagocytes	- binding and ingestion of EA (IgM)C^{m} by elicited macrophages^{m}, no ingestion by washout cells (1)
	- enhanced intracellular killing by monocytes^{hum} (30)
	- modulation of C3 receptors on elicited macrophages^{m} by immobilized AgAbC^{m} (31)
	- C3b^{gp}-induced release of lysosomal enzymes from elicited macrophages^{gp} (42)
lymphocytes	- C3b^{gp}-induced secretion of lymphokines from spleen B lymphocytes (39)
	- C3b^{hum}-induced increased incorporation of thymidine into B lymphocytes^{m} (22)

adhered to macrophages but also were ingested (24). Although in conflict at the moment the erythrocyte data and the bacteria data might be totally compatible if it could be established that bacteria, once approximated to a phagocyte surface sufficiently closely by C3-dependent adherence, exert an extra trigger by a bacterial membrane constituent or some other factor as does IgG in the case of EA(IgG)C1423.

On the other hand, various experiments have been interpreted as suggesting that C3-C3 receptor interactions induce active processes: guinea pig C3b added to mouse macrophage cultures induces release of lysosomal enzymes within several hours (42). Complement (C3?) polymerized on plastic surfaces caused macrophages adherent to this surface to lose all

C3-receptor activity on the upper half of the cell, probably by moving all C3 receptors into those areas of the cell membrane facing the C3-coated plastic surface (31). It was suggested that binding of C3 to C3 receptors on macrophages enhanced killing of already phagocytosed bacteria (30). In the case of lymphocytes, addition of guinea pig C3b to guinea pig spleen lymphocytes induced secretion of factors chemotactic for macrophages (39). *Addition of human C3b or C3 to mouse spleen cells* caused increased incorporation of thymidine into B lymphocytes (22). With our earlier preparations of human C3 we were able to reproduce these latter results. But with our recent, certainly cleaner, preparations mouse spleen cells cannot be triggered any more directly, suggesting that the effect cannot be attributed to C3 but to other molecules.

In more recent experiments we identified factor H (β1H) of the alternate pathway of complement activation as the active principle (21a). Human factor H, if added to mouse spleen cells, induced increased thymidine incorporation into mouse spleen B lymphocytes, whereas neither human C3 nor C3b did (Fig. 5). On the other hand we observed that human C3, when added to mouse spleen cells stimulated by Con A, became bound to T-cell blasts (14). This effect was also expressed if CR^+C was eliminated first (21). On the basis of our present data we interpret this C3 effect as due to binding of C3b to C3 acceptors on T lymphocytes and not to C3 receptors. The relevance of these observations for those made earlier by Pepys (36), namely that depletion of C3 in a mouse by cobra venom affected only the antibody response to T-dependent antigens negatively whereas responses to T-independent antigens were unaltered, is not clear. In disucssing functional aspects I

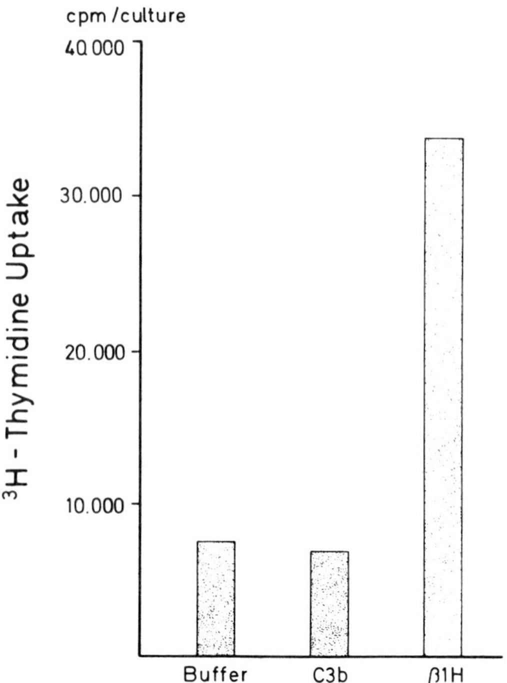

FIGURE 5. Increased thymidine incorporation by mouse spleen cells induced by human factor H (β1H) and not by human C3b. Factor H and C3b were both present during a 3-day culture at a concentration of 75 μg/ml. In the culture (300 μl) 1×10^6 BALB/c spleen cells were present.

also mention that experiments suggest that C3 receptors might be identical to the receptors for Epstein-Barr Virus (25); but the functional implications are unclear.

Enumeration of the various observations on the functional aspects of C3 receptors demonstrates that beyond the fact that C3 receptors serve as binding structures in cytoadherence we may not yet consider them sites of stimulation. This is even more so since *in vitro* observations were obtained in complex, often serum-containing systems. It is also complete speculation as to whether C3b, C3d, and C3bi receptors have different functions.

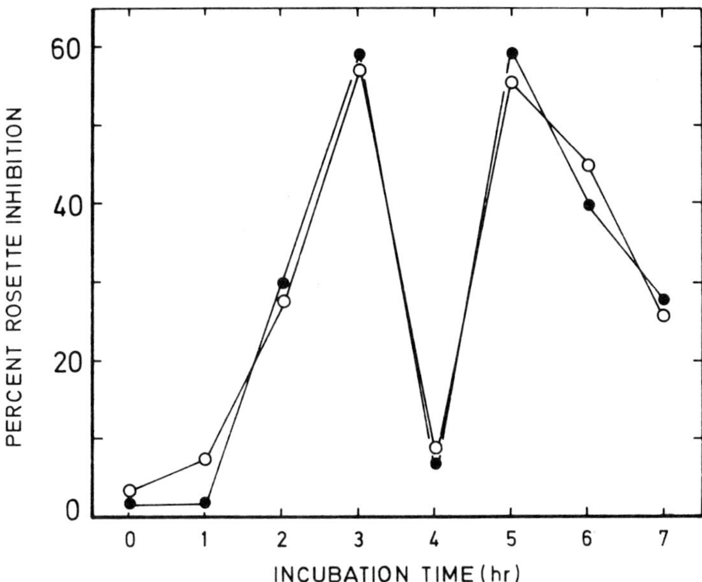

FIGURE 6. Shedding of complement receptor activity from Raji cells. Raji cells taken from mid-log-phase cultures when kept in serum-free medium shed receptor material in a rhythmic fashion capable of inhibiting C3-dependent rosette formation (% inhibition along the ordinate). This inhibiting material acts the same whether in the absence or presence of 1 m*M* diisopropyl fluorophosphate (two curves).

In spite of all this uncertainty we have every reason to consider the possibility that C3 receptor molecules shed from the surface in a functionally active state may have a regulatory impact. We could clearly show that *C3 receptor material shed from Raji cells* could inhibit C3-dependent rosette formation (Landen and Dierich, unpublished observations). Raji cells taken from cultures and suspended in serum-free medium released the receptors in a typical rhythmic fashion (Fig. 6). It has to be clarified as to whether C3 receptor oscillation is a peculiarity of Raji lymphoblastoid cells or if normal cells would show a similar phenomenon under appropriate test conditions.

Clarification of many questions will be facilitated if more light can be shed on *C3-receptor biochemistry*. We know that treatment of $CR^{+}C$ with trypsin, papain, or phospholipase C, with reduction and alkylation, or with sulfhydryl compounds such as AET resulted in loss of activity (4, 6), but more direct information is scarce. Using rosette inhibition as our test system, we were unable to detect any C3-receptor activity in detergent-solubilized membrane material of CR^{+} lymphocytes (11) and erythrocytes. But by applying 2 *M* KBr, solubilization of B-lymphoblastoid (Raji) cell membranes was achieved concomittant with preservation of C3 receptor activity (11). In KBr gradients the activity was like that of lipoprotein complexes. On Sepharose-4B columns run in the presence of KBr the rosette-inhibiting material had a molecular weight of about 1.2×10^{6}. In the absence of KBr such a material could be adsorbed onto EAC, from which, after washing, it could be desorbed by 0.5 *M* NaCl. When we introduced ^{125}I into the lymphocyte membrane by lactoperoxidase labeling before solubilization, the desorbed material was found on SDS-PAGE to be enriched in molecules of a molecular weight of 35,000 (4, 5, 11) (Fig. 7). Recently, a similar result was obtained by others using KBr solubilization of tonsil lymphocytes, adsorption onto EAC, immunization with the adsorbed material, and later immunoprecipitation by the antibody of detergent-solubilized tonsil lymphocyte membranes (19).

However, these results are in contrast to data by Fearon (15) who found that a factor H-like regulator protein of erythrocyte membranes obviously serves as a C3b-receptor molecule and has a molecular weight of 205,000. Yet another value was obtained when we recently solubilized human erythrocyte membranes by 2 *M* KBr and fractionated the 100,000-*g* supernatant of the KBr solute on a Sepharose-4B-C3 column. The receptor material thus isolated behaved, on Tris-PAGE and

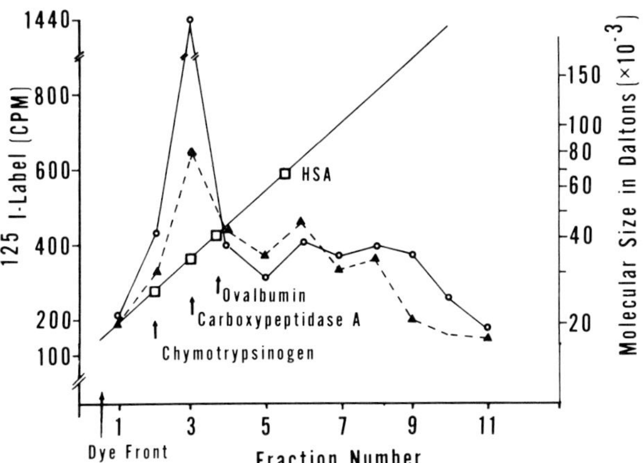

FIGURE 7. Analysis of C3 receptor material from Raji cells on SDS-PAGE. Intact Raji cells were labeled with ^{125}I using the lactoperoxidase technique. Membranes prepared by mitogen cavitation were solubilized by 2 *M* KBr. After ultracentrifugation, the supernate material was dialyzed against isotonic phosphate buffer and adsorbed onto $EAC14^{oxy}23$ (———) or $EAC14^{oxy}2$ (– – – –). After washing the material was desorbed by 0.5 *M* NaCl and analyzed on SDS-PAGE.

SDS-PAGE after Coomassie Blue and PAS-staining, as a glycoprotein of molecular weight about 55,000 (32). A reconciliation of such divergent results is now a prime target. The carbohydrate moiety of the erythrocyte C3 receptor material is clearly of critical importance to its biological function (32). This matches our earlier observation that the carbohydrate entity of α_1-antitrypsin can interfere with C3b-dependent rosette formation (9). We are now in the process of characterizing biochemically the C3d and C3bi receptors.

No discussion of C3 receptors and of C3-dependent cell interactions is complete without at least briefly touching on an additional aspect of C3 dependent cytoadherence. We have compiled evidence in favor of the following concept: membrane-associated complement components on one cell and membrane-associated proteases on other cells can cooperate to form

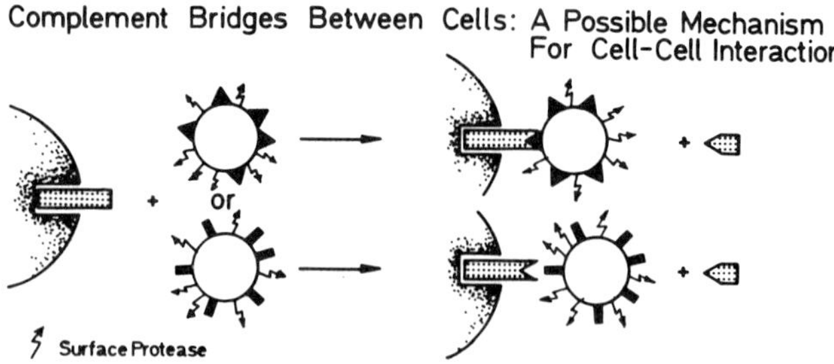

FIGURE 8. Bridge formation between a cell carrying uncleaved complement components and a cell endowed with membrane-associated proteases. The assumed mechanism is generation of new binding sites on the membrane-associated complement components by the action of membrane-associated proteases. This concept is based on the need for unfragmented complement components and on the inhibition of this mechanism by protease inhibitors.

"complement bridges" between cells (Fig. 8) (7, 8). The presence of complement components in membranes, of lymphocytes for instance, has now been demonstrated by various groups (16, 17, 20, 46) including our own (Dierich *et al.*, unpublished observations). Proteases present on tumor cells (12), cells infected with Herpes simplex virus (10), cells transformed with Epstein-Barr viruses (43), and T lymphocytes in a blast state (21) can all utilize complement components on adjacent cells. The proteases obviously generate new binding sites on the membrane-associated complement components, possibly as it happens during cleavage of fluid phase C3, C4, or C5. The cooperation of membrane-associated proteases and membrane-associated complement components in the interaction still has to be proven to be not only a complement-related *in vitro* model. Nevertheless, I consider this model of such potential general importance that it should be extensively explored.

REFERENCES

1. Bianco, C., Griffin, F. M., and Silverstein, S. C. Studies of the macrophage complement receptor. Alteration of receptor function upon macrophage activation. *J. Exp. Med. 141*, 1278-1290 (1975).

2. Bianco, C. and Nussenzweig, V. Complement receptors. *Contemp. Top. Mol. Immunol. 6*, 145-175 (1977).

3. Bokisch, V. A. and Sobel, A. T. Receptor for the fourth component of complement on human B lymphocytes and cultured human lymphoblastoid cells. *J. Exp. Med. 140*, 1336-1342 (1974).

4. Dierich, M. P. Receptors for C3 and its fragments: Attempts toward a biological and biochemical characterization. *Behring Inst. Mitt.* No. 59, 11-21 (1976).

5. Dierich, M. P. C3 receptors on lymphoid cells: solubilization by KBr and partial purification by immunadsorption. *Fed. Proc., Fed. Am. Soc. Exp. Biol. 35*, 1700 (1976).

6. Dierich, M. P., Ferrone, S., Pellegrino, M. A., and Reisfeld, R. A. Chemical modulation of cell surfaces by sulfhydryl compounds: effect on C3b receptors. *J. Immunol. 113*, 940-947 (1974).

6a. Dierich, M. P., Mussel, H. H., Scheiner, O., Ehlen, T., Burger, R., Peters, H., Schmitt, M., Trepke, S., and Zimmer, G. Differentiation of C3 receptors on human lymphocytes, phagocytes, erythrocytes and renal glomerulus cells by monoclonal antibodies. *Immunology 45*, 85-96 (1982).

7. Dierich, M. P. and Landen, B. Complement bridges between cells. Analysis of a possible cell-cell interaction mechanism. *J. Exp. Med. 146*, 1484-1499 (1977).

8. Dierich, M. P. and Landen, B. Involvement of proteases in the binding of $EAC14^{oxy}23b$ to complement receptor cells. *J. Immunol. 122*, 1686-1690 (1979).

9. Dierich, M. P., Landen, B., and Schmitt, M. Complement receptor analogous factors in human serum: I. Isolation of a molecule inhibitory for complement dependent rosette formation, its identification as α_1-antitrypsin and its functional characterization. *Immunobiology 156*, 153-167 (1979).

10. Dierich, M. P., Landen, B., Schulz, T., and Falke, D. Protease activity on the surface of HSV-infected cells. *J. Gen. Virol. 45*, 241-244 (1979).

11. Dierich, M. P. and Reisfeld, R. A. C3 receptors on lymphoid cells: isolation of active membrane fragments and solubilization of receptor complexes. *J. Immunol. 114*, 1676-1682 (1975).

12. Dierich, M. P., Schulz, T., Yefenof, E., and Klein, G. Detection of proteolytic (C3-cleaving) activity on mouse mastocytoma (P815) cells and other mouse cell lines by formation of cell contact with C3-carrying mouse lymphocytes. *Eur. J. Immunol. 9*, 928-932 (1979).

13. Dukor, P., Bianco, C., and Nussenzweig, V. Tissue localization of lymphocytes bearing a membrane receptor for antigen-antibody-complement complexes. *Proc. Natl. Acad. Sci. U.S.A. 67*, 991-997 (1970).

14. Erdei, A., Hammann, K. P., Gergely, J., and Dierich, M. P. Modulation of the mitogen response of mouse spleen cells by the third complement component (C3). I. Effect of human C3 on the LPS- and ConA-response of mouse spleen cells. *4th Intern. Congress Immunol., abstract* 15.3.07 (1980).

15. Fearon, D. T. Identification of the membrane glycoprotein that is the C3b receptor of the human erythrocyte, polymorphonuclear leukocyte, B-lymphocyte and monocyte. *J. Exp. Med. 152*, 20-30 (1980).

16. Ferrone, S., Pellegrino, M. A., and Cooper, N. R. Expression of C4 on human lymphoid cells and possible involvement in immune recognition phenomena. *Science 193*, 53-55 (1976).

17. Fuest, G., Erdei, A., S'Armay, G., Medgyesi, G. A., and Gergely, J. Functionally active Cl on the surface of human peripheral lymphocytes: Its role in the complement mediated inhibition of the Fc-receptor of B-lymphocytes. *Clin. Immunol. Immunopathol. 5*, 377-387 (1976).

17a. Gelfand, M. C., Frank, M. M., and Green, I. A receptor for the third component of complement in the human renal glomerulus. *J. Exp. Med. 142*, 1029-1039 (1975).

18. Gerdes, J., Klatt, U., and Stein, H. Xenoantiserum to human C3 receptors: its preparation and effect on the C3b and C3d receptors of tonsil cells and the C3b receptors of erythrocytes and neutrophils. *Immunology 39*, 75-84 (1980).

19. Gerdes, J. and Stein, H. Human membrane-bound C3 receptors. VI. Physicochemical properties of the C3b and C3d receptors isolated from tonsil cells by immunoprecipitation. *Scand. J. Immunol. 12*, (1980).

20. Halbwachs, L. and Lachmann, P. J. Factor B of the alternative complement pathway on human lymphocytes. *Scand. J. Immunol. 5*, 697-704 (1976).

21. Hammann, K. P., Erdei, A., Gergely, J., and Dierich, M. P. Binding of human and mouse C3 to ConA-induced mouse T blasts. *Immunobiology 157*, 225-226 (1980).

21a. Hammann, K. P., Raile, A., Schmitt, M., Mussel, H. H., Peters, H., Scheiner, O., and Dierich, M. P. β1H stimulates mouse-spleen B lymphocytes as demonstrated by increased thymidine incorporation and formation of B cell blasts. *Immunobiol. 160*, 289-301 (1981).

22. Hartmann, K. U. and Bokisch, V. A. Stimulation of murine B lymphocytes by isolated C3b. *J. Exp. Med. 142*, 600-610 (1975).

23. Hopf, U., Meyer zum Büschenfelde, K.-H., and Dierich, M. P. Demonstration of binding sites for IgG Fc and the third complement component (C3) on isolated hepatocytes. *J. Immunol. 117*, 639-645 (1976).

24. Horwitz, M. A. and Silverstein, S. C. Influence of the Escherichia coli capsule on complement fixation and on phagocytosis and killing by human phagocytes. *J. Clin. Invest. 65*, 82-94 (1980).

25. Jondal, M., Klein, G., Oldstone, M. B. A., Bokisch, V. A., and Yefenof, E. Surface markers on human B and T lymphocytes. VIII. Association between complement and Epstein-Barr virus (EBV) receptors on human lymphoid cells. *Scand. J. Immunol. 5*, 401-410 (1976).

26. Kasukawa, R., Okada, M., and Igari, S. Receptors for IgG Fc and complement in the mammalian aorta. *Int. Arch. Allergy Appl. Immunol. 61*, 175-182 (1980).

27. Landen, B. and Dierich, M. P. Identity of C3- and C5-receptors on lymphoid cells. *J. Immunol. 122*, 1015-1017 (1979).

28. Landen, B., Strunkheide, K., and Dierich, M. P. C3-mediated cytoadherence. II. Dependence of cell attachment on similar topographical distribution of the receptors (for C3) and of the ligands (C3/C3b). *J. Immunol. 121*, 2539-2541 (1978).

29. Lay, W. H. and Nussenzweig, V. Receptors for complement on leucocytes. *J. Exp. Med. 128*, 991-1007 (1968).

30. Leigh, P. C. J., von den Barselaar, M. T., van Zwet, T. L., Daha, M. R., and van Furth, R. Requirement for extracellular complement and immunoglobulin for intracellular killing of micro-organisms by human monocytes. *J. Clin. Invest. 63*, 772-784 (1979).

31. Michl, J., Pieczonka, M. M., Unkeless, J. C., and Silverstein, S. C. Effects of immobilized immune complexes on Fc- and complement-receptor-function in resident and thioglycollate-elicited mouse peritoneal macrophages. *J. Exp. Med. 150*, 607-621 (1979).

32. Mussel, H. H., Ehlen, T., Schmitt, M., Kazatchkine, M. D., Neyses, L., and Dierich, M. P. Isolation and characterization of the C3b-binding entity of C3b-receptor from human erythrocytes. *Immunology Letters 4*, 1-6 (1982).

33. Nelson, R. A. The immune-adherence phenomenon. An immunologic specific reaction between microorganisms and erythrocytes leading to enhanced phagocytosis. *Science 118*, 733-737 (1953).

34. Nyland, H., Matre, R., and Fönder, O. Complement receptors in human peripheral nerve tissue. *Acta Pathol. Microbiol. Scand., Sect. C 87*, 7-10 (1979).

35. Papamichail, M., Gutierrez, C., Embling, P., Johnson, P., Holborrow, E. J., and Pepys, M. P. Complement dependence of localization of aggregated IgG in germinal centres. *Scand. J. Immunol. 4*, 343-347 (1975).

36. Pepys, M. P. Role of complement in induction of the allergic response. *Nature (London), New Biol. 237*, 157-159 (1972).

37. Ross, G. D. and Polley, M. J. Specificity of lymphocyte complement receptors. *J. Exp. Med. 141*, 1163-1178 (1975).

38. Ross, G. D. Identification of human lymphocyte subpopulations by surface marker analysis. *Blood 53*, 799-811 (1979).

39. Sandberg, A. L., Wahl, M. S., and Mergenhagen, St. E. Lymphokine production by C3b-stimulated B cells. *J. Immunol. 115*, 139-143 (1975).

40. Schmitt, M. and Dierich, M. P. Complement-dependent cell-cell interaction: Evidence for β1H-binding reactivities on Raji cells. *Immunobiology 157*, 276 (1980).

41. Schmitt, M., Mussel, H.-H., and Dierich, M. P. Qualitative and quantitative assessment of C3-receptor-reactivities on lymphoid and phagocytic cells. *J. Immunol. 126*, 2042-2047 (1981).

42. Schorlemmer, H. U., Davies, P., and Allison, A. C. Ability of activated complement components to induce lysosomal enzyme release from macrophages. *Nature (London) 261*, 48 (1976).

43. Schulz, T., Dierich, M. P., Yefenof, E., and Klein, G. C3-activating proteases on human lymphoblastoid cells superinfected with Epstein-Barr Virus. *Cell. Immunol. 51*, 168-172 (1980).

44. Shin, M. L., Gelfand, M. C., Nagle, R. B., Carlo, J. R., Green, J., and Frank, M. M. Localization of receptors for activated complement on visceral epithelial cells of the human renal glomerulus. *J. Immunol. 118*, 869-873 (1977).

45. Stingl, G., Wolff-Schreiner, E. C., Pichler, W. J., Gschnait, F., Knapp, W., and Wolff, K. Epidermal Langerhans cells bear Fc and C3 receptors. *Nature (London) 268*, 245-246 (1977).

46. Sundsmo, J. S., Curd, J. G., Kolb, W. P., and Müller-Eberhard, H. J. Leukocyte complement: Assembly of the membrane attack complex of complement by human peripheral blood leukocytes in the presence and absence of serum. *J. Immunol. 120*, 855-860 (1978).

47. Theofilopoulos, A. N., Wilson, C. G., Bokisch, V. A., and Dixon, F. J. Binding of soluble immune complexes to human lymphoblastoid cells. II. Use of Raji cells to detect circulating immune complexes in animal and human sera. *J. Exp. Med. 140*, 1230-1244 (1974).

48. Theofilopoulos, A. N. and Dixon, F. J. The biology and and detection of immune complexes.*Adv. Immunol. 28*, 89-220 (1979).

49. Theofilopoulos, A. N., Larson, D. A., Favanoli, M., Slovin, S. F., Speers, W. C., Jensen, F. B., and Vaughan, J. H. Evidence for the presence of receptors for C3 and IgG Fc on human synovial cells. *Arthritis Rheum. 23*, 1-9 (1980).

Immunopathology: VIIIth International Symposium, 1980

BIOCHEMISTRY AND PATHOPHYSIOLOGIC EFFECTS OF THE HAGEMAN FACTOR SYSTEM[1]

Charles G. Cochrane

Department of Immunopathology,
Scripps Clinic and Research Foundation,
La Jolla, California

I. INTRODUCTION

In attempts to gain a greater understanding of the biochemistry of the inflammatory process, attention has been directed to interactions between humoral components of the plasma and cells. One of the plasma systems of interest for its potential role in the development of inflammation is the contact system or Hageman factor (HF) system. When plasma comes in contact with negatively charged surfaces, a burst of enzymatic events follow, leading to the generation of bradykinin, coagulation, and under certain conditions, to the

[1]*This publication is No. 2329 from the Department of Immunopathology, Scripps Clinic and Research Foundation, La Jolla, California. This work was supported in part by National Institutes of Health grants AI-07007, HL-16411, Office of Naval Research Contract N00014, and the Council for Tobacco Research*

ISBN 0-12-218320-7

formation of plasmin and C5a activity. In this chapter, the biochemistry of activation of this system will be reviewed briefly, and then recent studies into the potential role of components of the system in the inflammatory process will be presented.

The components of the HF system are presented in Fig. 1. The physical characteristics and biochemistry of activation of the components in solution and on a negatively charged surface are the subject of a recent review from this laboratory (2). In brief, when plasma contacts a negatively charged surface, a group of proteins interacts on the surface to produce a sequence of conversions of proenzymes to enzymes. This occurs as a burst of activity within seconds. Hageman factor, prekallikrein, high MW kininogen, and clotting Factor XI are the principal molecules that undergo initial proteolytic cleavage as activation occurs. This cleavage appears to be essential for the rapid activation of each component. Hageman factor binds rapidly to the surface in whole plasma, and the peptide

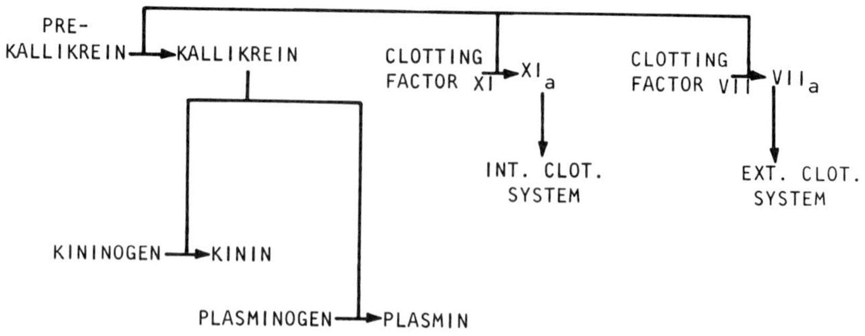

FIGURE 1. Diagram of the sequences of activation of components of the Hageman factor system.

chain is cleaved so as to produce chains of 28,000 and 52,000 MW which are held together by a small disulfide bridge. Cleavage then occurs on the N-terminal site of the disulfide bridge, allowing the smaller chain which bears the enzymatic site of Hageman factor to dissociate into the fluid phase (15). The larger fragment remains surface bound.

The enzyme in plasma responsible for the rapid cleavage of Hageman factor is kallikrein. Its precursor, prekallikrein is itself cleaved into heavy and light chains and activated by Hageman factor. Thus, a reciprocal activation by these two molecules was proposed as a control mechanism of activation of the contact system (1). The reciprocal enzymatic cleavage and activation of HF and prekallikrein is augmented by the fact that when bound to the surface, Hageman factor is more than 100-fold more susceptible to enzymatic cleavage (7). In the absence of prekallikrein, Hageman factor is cleaved and activated slowly, suggesting other enzymes may play a secondary role. However, in the absence of prekallikrein, the clotting and kinin-generating activities are markedly retarded (23).

Prekallikrein and Factor XI exist in plasma as a complex with high MW kininogen (11, 17). The high MW kininogen, acting stoichiometrically with Hageman factor (5), brings prekallikrein and Factor XI to the surface where they are able to interact with Hageman factor (20). The light chain of high MW kininogen bears a domain extremely rich in histidine residues which is apparently responsible for the adherence of the molecule to negatively charged surfaces (8). A portion of the light chain is also responsible for the complexing of high MW kininogen with prekallikrein and Factor XI (18, 19). Thus, high MW kininogen acts as a cofactor, in a stoichiometric relation with Hageman factor, to promote the receeiprocal activation of prekallikrein and Hageman factor (5, 13) and the cleavage and activation of Factor XI by Hageman factor.

Kallikrein rapidly dissociates from high MW kininogen on the surface and cleaves and activates other surface-bound Hageman factor molecules (3). The dissociating kallikrein also rapidly cleaves high MW kininogen both on the surface and in fluid phase.

The initial event that triggers the activation of Hageman factor and prekallikrein is not precisely understood. And although it has long been thought that Hageman factor is activated upon binding to a surface, this has recently been questioned. In the absence of prekallikrein or high MW kininogen, Hageman factor still becomes surface bound, but does not activate and does not undergo cleavage for several minutes (well after the burst of activity seen in normal plasma) (16). Single chain, zymogen Hageman factor binds [^{3}H]DFP extremely slowly, and this is not influenced by contact with a surface (4, 6). Data supporting surface activation have been presented in which zymogen or activated Hageman factor were found to activate prekallikrein at the same rate (9). The prekallikrein was present in great excess (more than 60-fold higher concentration than that of normal plasma relative to the amount of Hageman factor used), and the possibility remained that rapid reciprocal cleavage and activation of the two molecules took place. This is especially true in view of the speed of reciprocal activation by kallikrein (3). The possibility exists that an undetected exogenous enzyme could activate either prekallikrein or Hageman factor, although no evidence for this has been obtained. And finally, the possibility that Hageman factor and prekallikrein are "active zymogens" has been raised (2). In support of this theory are the findings that both Hageman factor and prekallikrein slowly take up [^{3}H]DFP in a manner similar to that of trypsinogen (2). A summary of the molecular assembly leading to the activation of HF is given in Fig. 2. At the upper left portion of the

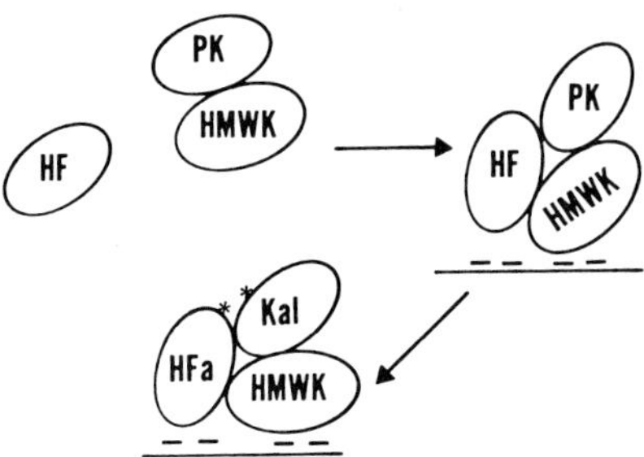

FIGURE 2. Proposed mechanism of activation of Hageman factor (HF) and prekallikrein (PK), the cofactor, high MW kininogen (HMWK). The proteins are seen in solution in the upper left. Upon contact with a negatively charged surface (right), the proteins are assembled, leading to activation of HF and PK. HMWK is cleaved in the process. See text for details. * = active site.

figure, HF and the complex of PK and high MW kininogen (HMWK) are depicted in the plasma. It should be noted that Factor XI and HMWK also exist in plasma as a complex. When presented with a negatively charged surface (right side of the figure), HF and the complex of PK and HMWK become bound to the surface. This occurs by virtue of positively charged residues on the heavy chain of HF and a histidine-rich portion (termed fragment 1-2) of the light chain of HMWK. The HF and PK are thus brought into apposition and activation of each takes place. This is aided by apparent conformational changes occurring in the HF upon surface contact in that the surface-bound molecule is approximately 500-fold more sensitive to enzymatic cleavage than the unbound HF. The initial event in triggering activation could be from an as yet undetected extraneous enzyme which could cleave and activate either HF or PK. However, HF and PK slowly take up [^{3}H]DFP into the active site of their light chains over a period of 24 hr, thereby rendering the molecules nonactivatable; and zymogen HF, when brought onto a negatively charged surface in apposition with other zymogen HF molecules, leads to cleavage and "autoactivation" of the population of surface-bound HF. This latter event fails to occur when the HF molecules are less densely dispersed on the surface. We thus propose that HF and prekallikrein are "active zymogens" which, when brought into contact with each other, can induce a triggering event leading to proteolytic cleavage and activation. The kallikrein binds to high MW kininogen with relatively low affinity and rapidly dissociates, leading to cleavage of HF molecules bound elsewhere on the surface. This movement of kallikrein in fluid phase probably accounts for a great majority of activation of the HF. The kallikrein at the same time cleaves high MW kininogen in both the fluid phase and on the surface.

II. BIOLOGY AND PATHOPHYSIOLOGY OF THE CONTACT SYSTEM

I will review here our studies on the interactions between these components and various cells of the tissues and blood that are commonly involved in inflammation and our studies on the participation of these proteins in the development of inflammation injury.

III. ACTIVATION OF PROTEINS OF THE CONTACT SYSTEM BY CELLULAR ENZYMES

Several cells are now known to contain enzymes capable of cleaving and activating components of the HF system. Endothelial cells contain an enzyme(s) capable of cleaving HF into 52,000 and 28,000 MW fragments. When assessed for activity, the cleaved HF was found, in turn, to cleave and activate both prekallikrein and Factor XI when bound to a negatively charged surface (21). The presence of the cofactor, high MW kininogen, greatly enhanced the reaction with Factor XI, presumably by bringing the Factor XI to the surface where it encountered the cell enzyme-activated HF. The endothelial cell enzyme was associated with the 100,000 *g* pellet of the cell, containing cytoplasmic and microsomal membranes, and was inhibited by diisopropylphosphofluoridate (DFP) (2 m*M*) but not soy bean trypsin inhibitor (50 μg/ml), hirudin (8 mg/ml), or purified antibodies to prekallikrein or plasmin. Thus, this cell located at the focal point of the initial inflammatory damage contains an activator of the HF system.

Recent studies have revealed another pathway by which cellular constituents react with components of the HF system. In collaboration with Drs. Newball, Meier, Lichtenstein, and Kaplan, washed fragments of normal human lung were submitted to anaphylactic challenge and the supernatant fluid examined for the presence of histamine and enzymes capable of cleaving and activating components of the HF system. Following such challenge it was possible to isolate enzymes that cleaved HF, prekallikrein, Factor XI and high MW kininogen, but not components of the complement system (C3, C5, C4, Factor B) or plasminogen (14). The high MW kininogen released kinin during the interaction with enzyme as revealed by contraction of the estrus rat uterus. The HF was cleaved in disulfide-linked fragments of 52,000 and approximately 28,000 MW which cleaved the HF substrate D-Pro-Phe-Arg-*p*-nitroanalide. Prekallikrein was cleaved by an enzyme separable from the above enzymes on SP-Sephadex and DEAE-Sephacel and was found in turn to cleave its peptide substrate Bz-Pro-Phe-Arg-*p*-nitroanalide (which is not cleaved by activated HF). Other assays on prekallikrein activity have not been performed. Thus, during the anaphylactic response, enzymes are released that generate activity of the HF system and release kinin. The role played by these components in anaphylaxis or similar IgE-initiated reactions, remains to be determined.

Another interaction, proposed by Kaplan and Austen (10), was that kallikrein induces chemotaxis of neutrophils, but not eosinophils, whereas prekallikrein or DFP-inactivated kallikrein did not possess activity. We have attempted to repeat these observations several times using peripheral blood neutrophils and kallikrein from both rabbit and human origin without success. A wide dosage range of kallikrein was employed, and kallikrein neither augmented nor inhibited chemotaxis induced by zymosan-treated serum (unpublished observations). Recently, Dr. R. C. Wiggins in our laboratory, together with Dr. P. Giclas, found that an intermediate component of plasma was essential for the chemotactic stimulation of rabbit neutrophils by rabbit kallikrein (22). Kallikrein, HF, and HMW kininogen, either alone or in combination over a wide dosage range failed to stimulate chemotactic movement of neutrophils. However, in the presence of C5, kallikrein induced chemotaxis and release of β-glucuronidase. An anodally migrating species of C5 was generated by the interaction of kallikrein and C5. Thus, a novel activity of kallikrein on C5 was observed which generated a factor capable of stimulating both chemotaxis and exocytosis of neutrophils. Its relationship with C4A is not clear at present. In addition, a relationship of the C5-related chemotactic factor to the factor generated in the studies of Kaplan is uncertain.

IV. PARTICIPATION OF THE CONTACT SYSTEM IN PULMONARY INFLAMMATORY INJURY

We have extended these studies on the biological activities of the HF and complement system proteins to certain inflammatory conditions. I will report on one condition in which evidence suggests a participation of these proteins during the development of disease. The studies were initiated in order to examine fluids emanating from areas of inflammation of the lung for the presence of factors that mediate the injury. Accordingly, bronchoalveolar lavage fluids were obtained from patients with acute and chronic pulmonary inflammatory disease and with noninflammatory conditions such as may be found with small solitary tumors. Among the inflammatory diseases studied have been adult respiratory distress syndrome (ARDS) and both active and inactive pulmonary fibrosis. Lavage fluid obtained from such patients was incubated with approximately 0.1 μg of ^{125}I-labeled HF, prekallikrein, plasminogen, high MW kininogen, and C3, C4, C5, and Factor B of the complement system. After 20-min incubation, the ^{125}I-labeled proteins were assessed for proteolytic cleavage in reduced SDS-polyacrylamide electrophoresis (SDS-PAGE). Of 21 cases of ARDS examined, 16 have shown the presence of free enzyme capable of cleaving each of the above-mentioned ^{125}I-labeled proteins. HF was cleaved in into heavy and light chains along with prekallikrein and high MW kininogen. A fragment of about 10,000 MW was cleaved from the α chain of C3. Plasminogen and the other complement components were cleaved into small fragments with the amounts of lavage fluid employed. The cleavage fragments of HF and high MW kininogen differed in size from those produced by kallikrein. When the lavage fluid-treated HF was tested for activity, using cleavage of prekallikrein into heavy and light chains as an indication of HF activation, activity was observed. The activity was not as great as that produced by HF activated by kallikrein (and then separated from the kallikrein). Activity of the other components has not yet been assessed.

In seven of the patients, several lavage samples were obtained during the course of the illness. Of these at least one, and often three or four, of the samples did not contain active enzyme. Several that were negative on the day that ARDS was suspected, became positive on subsequent days, and several that were positive during the illness became negative as the patient recovered. In still others, fluids that contained detectable enzyme were intermixed with negative fluids on subsequent daily lavage samples.

In attempts to identify the enzyme(s), inhibitors of proteases were employed. DFP at 10^{-4} *M* was inhibitory but C1 inh was not, suggesting that plasmin, C1r, C1s and kallikrein were not involved. IgG antikallikrein also failed to inhibit the lavage fluid enzyme. When 30 μl of the fluid was exposed to 10 μl normal human plasma, the activity was blocked, but when homozygous α_1-antitrypsin (A_1AT)-deficient plasma was employed, inhibition was not observed. Addition of highly purified A_1AT to the A_1AT-deficient plasma allowed inactivation of the enzyme to occur in a manner identical to that of normal plasma.

These data suggested that cellular enzymes were involved. Antibodies to neutrophil elastase were obtained from Dr. Aaron Janoff, and the fluids containing enzyme activity were also found to contain elastase antigen. In collaboration with Dr. Alan Cohen, elastin plates were employed to assess elastase activity, and elastin-cleaving activity was observed in each fluid that contained HF-cleaving activity. In addition, the pattern of HF-cleavage by the lavage fluid could be produced with purified neutrophil elastase. Thus, the major enzyme appeared similar to, if not identical with leukocytic elastase.

The bronchoalveolar lavage fluids that did not contain free enzyme were examined in immunoelectrophoresis for the presence of elastase and A_1AT. Several of these were found to exhibit both proteins simultaneously, and rather than showing the normal electrophoretic migration of the protein (α-globulin position for the A_1AT and γ-globulin position for the elastase), an identical position of electrophoretic migration was observed for each, midway between the α and γ positions. This suggested that complex existed in these fluids between elastase and its inhibitor. In most of these free A_1AT was also observed, migrating in the α-globulin position. Such fluids along with enzyme-free fluids that contained only A_1AT, when added to fluids containing free enzyme, inhibited the enzyme. In each patient recovering from ARDS, enzyme inhibitor was found.

It was of note that several fluids were found to contain free, active enzyme and yet displayed free A_1AT in immunoelectrophoresis. The A_1AT in these cases was assessed for its ability to interact with [^{125}I]trypsin and found not to possess this capacity. Fluids from patients recovering from ARDS readily bound the [^{125}I]trypsin. Thus, the A_1AT present during the disease was found in certain cases to be inactive. The possibility is raised that oxidizing radicals, generated by leukocytes in the inflammatory reaction, might inhibit the A_1AT, as described by Janoff. Recent data have confirmed that the inactive A_1AT was oxidized.

Lavage fluid from over 100 patients with noninflammatory lung disease has been assessed and did not contain enzyme. Lavage fluid of patients with bronchopneumonia contained free enzyme in about 20% of samples. Since large numbers of neutrophils were present, it was not clear whether the enzyme was present in solution prior to lavage and subsequent handling. These data have appeared in abstract (12).

V. SUMMARY

The biochemistry of the components of the contact (Hageman factor) system of plasma and its activation upon surface contact have been presented (Figs. 1 and 2). In addition, data have been presented showing that components of the HF system may interact with enzymes of endothelial cells, enzymes derived from the anaphylactic challenge of human lung, and that kallikrein may act on C5 of the complement system to induce directional movement of neutrophils. Although some or all of these interactions may take place in the inflammatory process, it became apparent in one disease of man, the adult respiratory distress syndrome, that enzymes are released from leukocytes capable of cleaving components of both the HF and complement systems and that HF is activated in the process. The possible significance of this in the pathogenesis of ARDS, which is marked by edema in the lung, was underscored by the recent observation (Yamamoto and Cochrane, unpublished observations) that as little as 3-5 ng HFa can induce edema in the skin of guinea pigs or rhesus monkeys. This represents one ten thousandth of the availbable HF in 1.0 ml plasma. Thus, activation of the HF system, together with components of the complement system, may play a role in the pathogenesis of ARDS, although definitive evidence is lacking. Of greater importance, an enzyme, leukocytic elastase, has been identified in the lavage fluid of patients with ARDS that may be of significance in the pathogenesis of this disease.

REFERENCES

1. Cochrane, C. G., Revak, S. D., and Wuepper, K. D. The activation of Hageman factor in solid and fluid phases. A critical role. *J. Exp. Med. 138*, 1564 (1973).

2. Cochrane, C. G. and Griffin, J. H. Molecular assembly in the contact phase of the Hageman factor system. *Am. J. Med. 67*, 657 (1979).

3. Cochrane, C. G. and Revak, S. D. Dissemination of contact activation in plasma by plasma kallikrein. *J. Exp. Med. 152*, 608 (1980).

4. Fujikawa, K., Walsh, K. A., and Davie, E. W. Isolation and characterization of bovine Factor XII (Hageman factor). *Biochemistry 16*, 2270 (1977).

5. Griffin, J. H. and Cochrane, C. G. Mechanisms for the involvement of high molecular weight kininogen in surface-dependent reactions of Hageman factor. *Proc. Natl. Acad. Sci. U.S.A. 73*, 2554 (1976).

6. Griffin, J. H. Molecular mechanism of surface-dependent activation of Hageman factor (coagulation Factor XII). *Fed. Proc., Fed. Am. Soc. Exp. Biol. 36*, 324 (1977).

7. Griffin, J. H. The role of surface in the surface-dependent activation of Hageman factor (Factor XII). *Proc. Natl. Acad. Sci. U.S.A. 75*, 1998 (1978).

8. Han, Y. N., Komiya, M., Iwanaga, S., and Suzuki, T. Studies on the primary structure of bovine high molecular weight kininogen. *J. Biochem. (Tokyo) 77*, 55 (1975).

9. Heimark, R. L., Kurachi, K., Fujikawa, K., and Davie, E. W. Surface activation of blood coagulation, fibrinolysis and kinin formation. *Nature (London) 208*, 456 (1980).

10. Kaplan, A. P. and Austen, K. F. A prealbumin activator of prekallikrein. III. Appearance of chemotactic activity by the conversion of prekallikrein to kallikrein. *J. Exp. Med. 135*, 81 (1972).

11. Mandle, R., Colman, R. W., and Kaplan, A. P. Identification of prekallikrein and high molecular weight kininogen as a complex in human plasma. *Proc. Natl. Acad. Sci. U.S.A. 11*, 4179 (1976).

12. McGuire, W. W., Cochrane, C. G., and Spragg, R. G. Analysis of enzymes cleaving components of the Hageman factor (HF) system in adult respiratory distress syndrome (ARDS). *Am. Rev. Respir. Dis. 121*, 275 (1980).

13. Meier, H. K., Webster, M. E., Mandle, R., Colman, R. W., and Kaplan, A. P. Enhancement of surface dependent Hageman factor activation by high molecular weight kininogen. *J. Clin. Invest. 60,* 18 (1977).

14. Newball, H. H., Meier, H. L., Kaplan, A. P., Revak, S. D., Cochrane, C. G., and Lichtenstein, L. M. Anaphylactic release of human lung kinin-generating activities. *Fed. Proc., Fed. Am. Soc. Exp. Biol. 39,* 906 (1980).

15. Revak, S. D. and Cochrane, C. G. The relationship of structure and function in human Hageman factor. The association of enzymatic and binding activities with separate regions of the molecule. *J. Clin. Invest. 57,* 852 (1976).

16. Revak, S. D., Cochrane, C. G., and Griffin, J. H. The binding and cleavage characteristics of human Hageman factor during contact activation. A comparison of normal plasma with plasmas deficient in Factor XI, prekallikrein, or high molecular weight kininogen. *J. Clin. Invest. 59,* 1167 (1977).

17. Thompson, E., Mandle, R., and Kaplan, A. P. Association of Factor XI and high molecular weight kininogen in human plasma. *J. Clin. Invest. 60,* 1376 (1977).

18. Thompson, R. E., Mandle, R., and Kaplan, A. P. Characterization of human HMW kininogen: Procoagulant activity associated with the light chain of kinin-free HMW-kininogen. *J. Exp. Med. 147,* 488 (1978).

19. Waldman, R., Scicli, A. G., Scicli, G. M., Guimaraes, J. A., Carretero, O. A., Kato, H., Han, Y. N., and Iwanaga, S. Significant role of fragment 1-2 plus light chain of bovine high molecular weight kininogen in contact mediated coagulation. *Thromb. Haemostasis 38,* 14 (1977).

20. Wiggins, R. C., Bouma, B. N., Cochrane, C. G., and Griffin, J. H. Role of high molecular weight kininogen in surface-binding and activation of coagulation Factor XI and prekallikrein (Hageman factor, contact activation, fibrinolysis). *Proc. Natl. Acad. Sci. U.S.A. 74,* 4636 (1977).

21. Wiggins, R. C., Loskutoff, D. J., Cochrane, C. G., Griffin, J. H., and Edgington, T. S. Activation of rabbit Hageman factor by homogenates of cultured rabbit endothelial cells. *J. Clin. Invest. 65,* 197 (1980).

22. Wiggins, R. C. and Giclas, P. C. Plasma kallikrein requires C5 for neutrophil chemotaxis in rabbits. *Fed. Proc., Fed. Am. Soc. Exp. Biol. 39*, 1049 (1980).

23. Wuepper, K. D. Prekallikrein deficiency in man. *J. Exp. Med. 138*, 1345 (1973).

LUNG INJURY PRODUCED BY OXYGEN METABOLITES

Peter A. Ward
Joseph C. Fantone
Kent J. Johnson

Department of Pathology,
The University of Michigan, Medical School,
Ann Arbor, Michigan

I. INTRODUCTION

Since the initial studies of Klebanoff and others [reviewed in Babior (1) and Klebanoff (14)] which have directly implicated the role of oxygen-derived products in the bactericidal action of neutrophils, abundant evidence has accumulated suggesting a broader potential for these metabolites. Recent investigations suggest that free radicals and metabolites derived from molecular oxygen or other sources represent a common mechanism of cell and tissue injury produced by toxic levels of oxygen (16, 20), herbicides such as paraquat and diquat (3, 24), antineoplastic drugs (9), and leukocyte-dependent reactions (5, 11, 17, 28-30).

In vitro, specific oxygen radicals and other metabolites may be generated enzymatically by xanthine oxidase and myeloperoxidase. The concentrations of individual metabolites are

ISBN 0-12-218320-7

modulated by enzymes (e.g., superoxide dismutase, glutathione peroxidase, catalase) and by specific radical scavengers (e.g., mannitol, histidine, thiourea, xanthine). Under certain conditions these metabolites are directly capable of causing cell and tissue injury (1, 13-15, 22). Additional studies have shown that neutrophils and macrophages have the ability to generate many different oxygen metabolites (including O_2^-, H_2O_2, $^1O_2$, OH•, and HOCl) during phagocytosis (7, 21) and after stimulation with chemotactic factors (2, 10) and phorbol myristate acetate (8, 31). Under these conditions, neutrophils have been shown to injure a variety of cell targets including red blood cells (13, 29), endothelial cells (23), and tumor cells (11). However, in the presence of specific inhibitors of oxygen metabolites (described above), the cytotoxic effects of neutrophils (5, 11, 29) as well as activated macrophages (17) and T-lymphocytes (25) can be blocked. Our own studies (reviewed below) also suggest that similar oxygen products may play a role in immune complex-mediated lung injury.

Recent data have presented contrasting roles for oxygen metabolites in modulating neutrophil chemotactic activity. Petrone *et al.* (19) have demonstrated the generation of a heat-labile chemotactic activity from human plasma after incubation with the superoxide generating system, xanthine-xanthine oxidase. Their preliminary evidence suggests that this chemotactically active material may be a lipid bound to albumin. Additional investigations by Perez and Goldstein (18) have demonstrated the generation of a chemotactic lipid from the interaction of arachadonic acid with an O_2^- generating system. However, Clark *et al.* (6) present contrasting evidence showing the *in vitro* inactivation of chemotactic peptides [C5a and *N*-Formylmethionylleucylphenylalanine (F-Met-Leu-Phe)] by a myeloperoxidase-H_2O_2-halide system. The inactivation of these chemotactic peptides is thought to be the result of oxidation of methionyl residues. Thus, through their production of oxygen products, neutrophils may potentially have either enhancing or inhibiting effects on the inflammatory system. Finally, Carp and Janoff (4) have reported the *in vitro* inactivation by neutrophil-derived oxygen metabolites of serum α_1-proteinase inhibitor, indicating that oxygen products of neutrophils may also indirectly modulate the inflammatory response in a manner that leads to intensification of tissue injury. Clarification of the precise regulatory role of neutrophil-derived oxygen metabolites in the inflammatory system awaits further study.

II. POSSIBLE ROLE OF O_2^- IN ACUTE IMMUNE COMPLEX-INDUCED TISSUE INJURY

Since it has been demonstrated that leukocytes activated by contact either with immune complexes or with chemotactic factors produce substantial quantities of superoxide anion (O_2^-) and H_2O_2 as well as other oxygen products (OH•, $^1O_2$, etc.), we have investigated the role of oxygen metabolites in acute immune complex-induced vasculitis and alveolitis. The acute vasculitis developing over a 2-hr period was produced by the intradermal injection of 100 μg antibody N (using rabbit IgG rich in antibody to bovine serum albumin, anti-BSA) followed by the intravenous injection of 10 mg BSA. Quantitation of the tissue injury was accomplished by measuring the amount of extravasation from blood of ^{125}I-labeled homologous (rat) IgG (12). These inflammatory reactions with their attendant tissue injury are well known to be dependent on the availability of both the complement system, which serves as the source of the generation of C5-derived chemotactic peptides (27), as well as circulating neutrophils (26). The latter requirement is presumably related to the release of lysosomal proteases

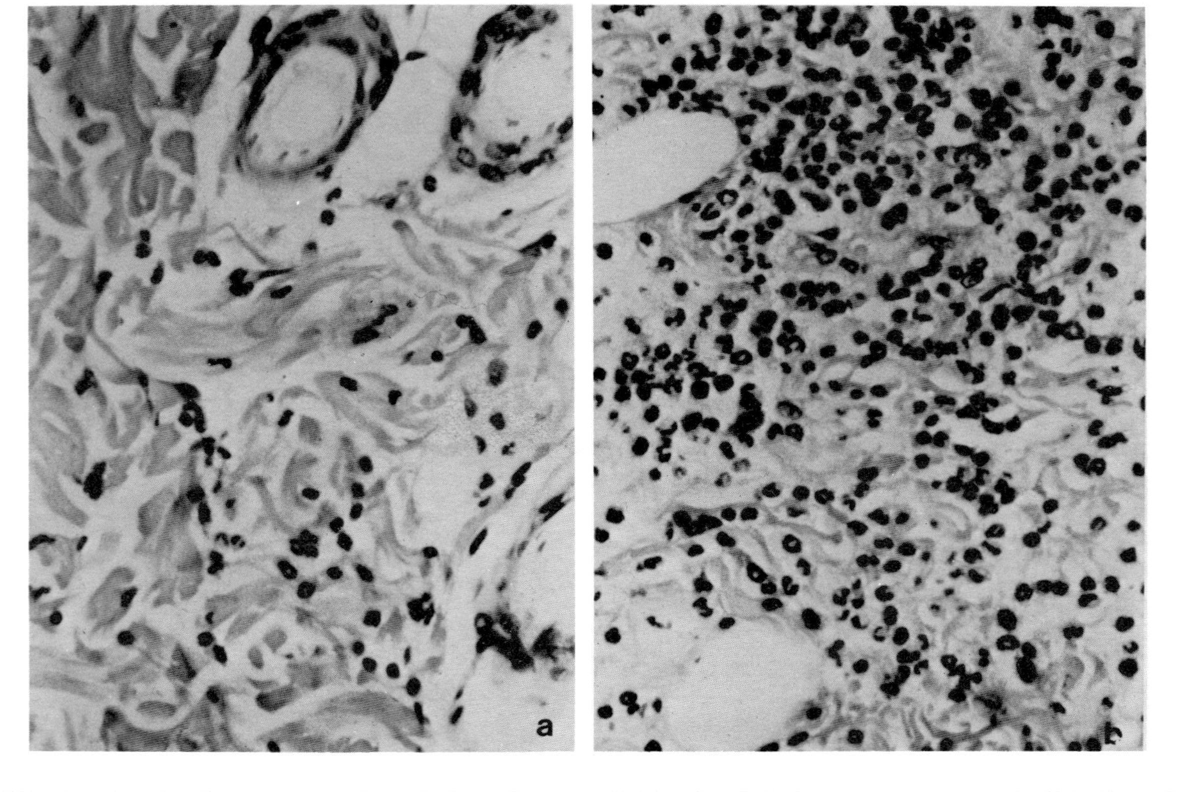

FIGURE 1. Acute immune complex induced vasculitis in (*a*) the presence and (*b*) the absence of superoxide dismutase, SOD. When SOD is mixed with the intradermally injected antibody, the extent of the inflammatory reaction is markedly suppressed (hematoxylin and eosin × 65).

and perhaps also due to the generation of oxygen metabolites which directly or indirectly (through amplification of the inflammatory response) produce acute tissue injury. In the usual course of the immune complex-induced vasculitis in rat skin, an intense perivascular and interstitial accumulation of neutrophils associated with hemorrhage develops within the first 2 hr. In companion skin sites of the same animals in which the injected antibody was mixed with 500 μg (1800 units) superoxide dismutase (SOD), there was marked suppression (Table I, 68% inhibition) of the inflammatory reaction and the related tissue injury (Fig. 1a,b). By the application of immunofluorescent techniques, it was possible to demonstrate that, in spite of the suppressed reactions, antigen (BSA) and the third component of complement (C3) were present in the typical perivascular and interstitial locations, suggesting that SOD did not interfere with formation and deposition of the complexes and their subsequent fixation of complement.

TABLE I. Suppression of Immune Complex Vasculitis and Alveolitis

Reaction	Treatment animals*	Number of animals	Suppression of tissue injury** (%)
Immune complex vasculitis	None	10	
	SOD	12	68
Immune complex alveolitis	None	10	
	SOD	10	75

*See text for dose and treatment schedule.

**The extent of leakage of radioactivity (^{125}I-labeled rat IgG) into the tissues was compared to that measured in non-SOD treated rats. Background values (leakage of I^{125}-labeled rat IgG) were obtained in rats in which antibody was employed in the absence of antigen.

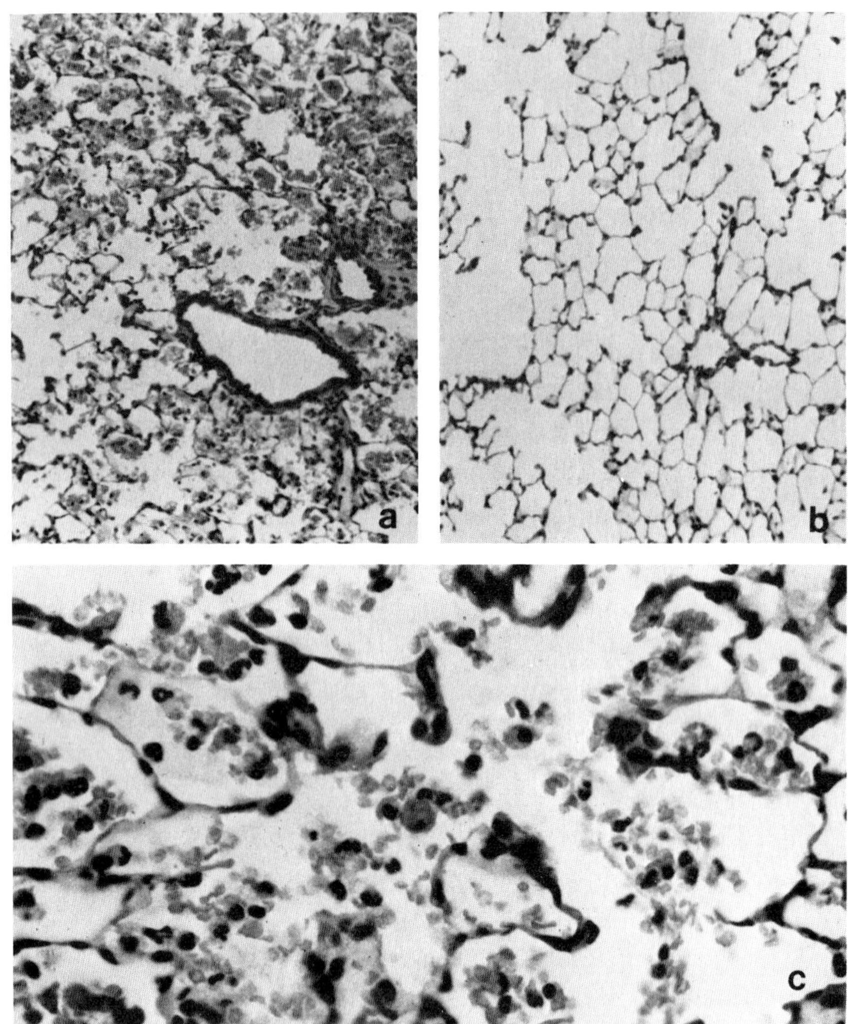

FIGURE 2. Acute immune complex-induced alveolitis in the (*b*) presence and (*a,c*) absence of SOD. In animals pretreated systemically with SOD, there is an intense intraalveolar accumulation of neutrophils and hemorrhage (*a,c*) whereas in the SOD-treated animals there is virtually complete protection, with little or no evidence of pulmonary inflammation or hemorrhage (*b*) (hematoxylin and eosin, *a* and *b* × 20, *c* × 65).

Similar experiments were performed with the lung model of acute immune complex-induced alveolitis in the rat. Here, 100 µg N anti-BSA was instilled into the airways using a tracheostomy approach. Antigen (10 mg BSA) was then injected intravenously along with 0.5 µCi ^{125}I-labeled IgG (approximately 1.0 µg). When the animals were sacrificed 2 hr later, the pulmonary vasculature was perfused with saline to remove blood-associated radioactivity and the amount of intraparenchymal leakage of radioactivity into the lung tissue (which reflects injury) measured. Morphologically, the reactions within the lung were characterized by intraalveolar hemorrhage and the accumulation of large numbers of neutrophils (Fig. 2-a,c). In a companion series of experiments, rats were systemically pretreated with SOD. This protocol involved the intraperitoneal injection of 5 mg of SOD 2 hr before the intrapulmonary instillation of antibody (which was injected at time 0 and 2 hr). The intraperitoneal instillation of SOD has been shown to achieve persistent blood levels of SOD as compared to the intravenous route (25). In animals treated in this fashion the morphological studies revealed a sharp reduction in the intensity of the lung inflammatory reaction (Fig. 1b) and the extent of injury to the lung (Table I, 75% inhibition of lung damage). By immunofluorescence, antigen (BSA) was readily detected in lung tissue from these suppressed animals, suggesting that SOD did not interfere with immune complex formation and deposition. These studies have indicated that, in the very early course of developing immune complex vasculitis and alveolitis, tissue injury can be suppressed by SOD, suggesting that O_2^- plays a direct or an indirect role in the tissue injury.

III. ABILITY OF GLUCOSE OXIDASE AND LACTOPEROXIDASE TO PRODUCE ACUTE AND PROGRESSIVE LUNG INJURY

The data described above have suggested that the generation of O_2^- by leukocytes (neutrophils) may be relevant to the early injury developing in the course of immune complex-induced inflammatory reactions. Since it has been shown that activated leukocytes generate large amounts of H_2O_2, which can be converted by myeloperoxidase (on other peroxidases) to halide-dependent toxic products, we undertook to investigate the

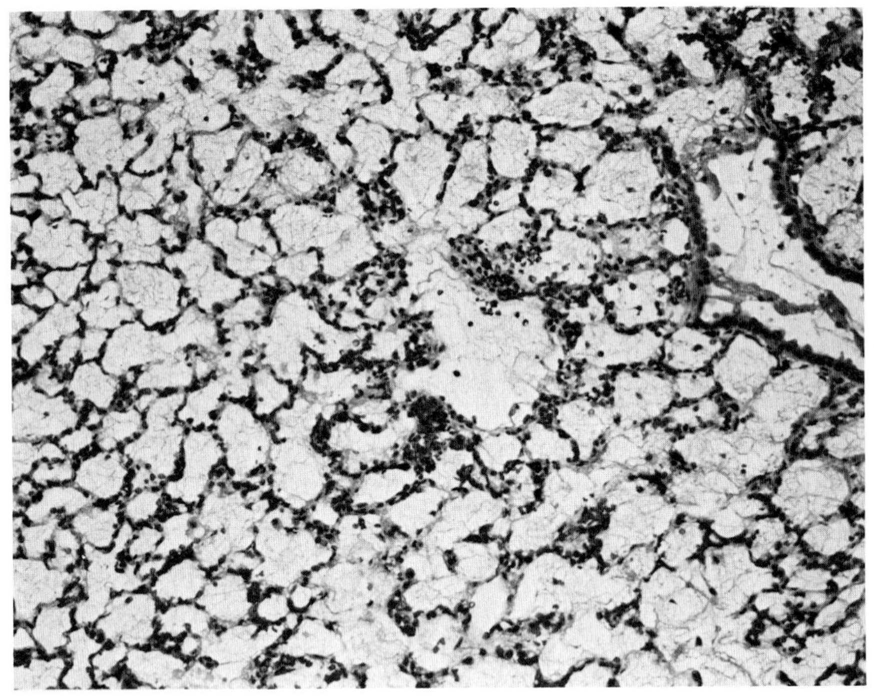

FIGURE 3. Acute lung injury in rat induced 4 hr earlier by the airway instillation of glucose (1 mg), glucose oxidase (30 units), and lactoperoxidase (0.7 units). There are neutrophil accumulations in and around alveolar septae as well as extensive intraalveolar depostis of fibrin (hematoxylin and eosin × 33).

effects of instilling into the rat lung a mixture that would generate H_2O_2 and peroxidase-related products. Glucose (1 mg), glucose oxidase (30 units), and lactoperoxidase (1.7 units) were mixed at neutral pH (7.4) and immediately instilled into the airways of rats. In earlier experiments it was shown that the intrapulmonary instillation of individual enzymes failed to produce significant injury (12a). When the combination described above was instilled into airways of rats, acute pulmonary injury resulted. Morphologically at 4 hr this was associated with clusters of neutrophils in alveolar septal walls and spaces, together with heavy intraalveolar accumulations of fibrin and evidence of intraalveolar hemorrhage (Fig. 3). By

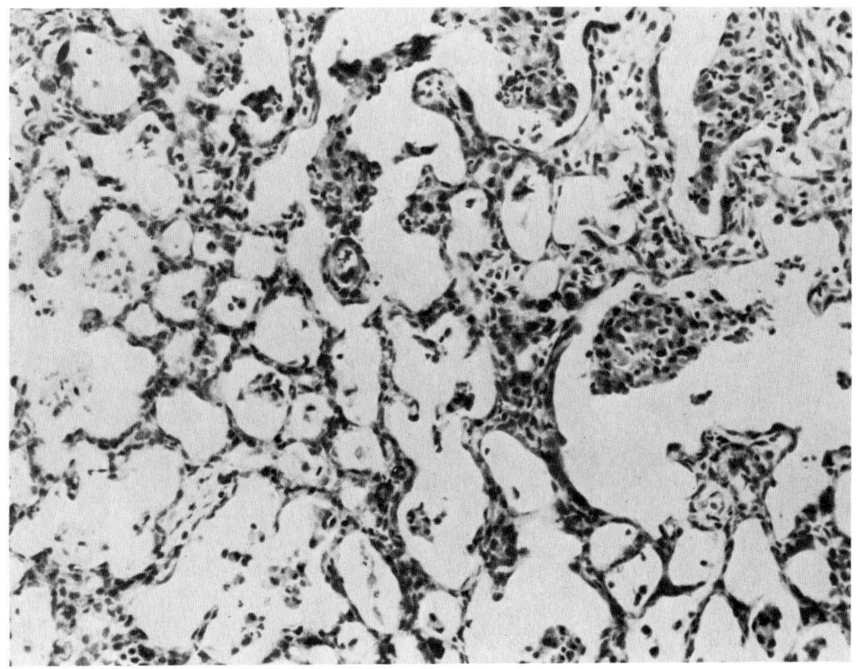

FIGURE 4. Lung from rats treated similar to that in Fig. 3, at 5 days. The interstitium is thickened and is hypercellular. Special stains indicate the presence of greatly increased amounts of collagen in the interstitium (hematoxylin and eosin × 33).

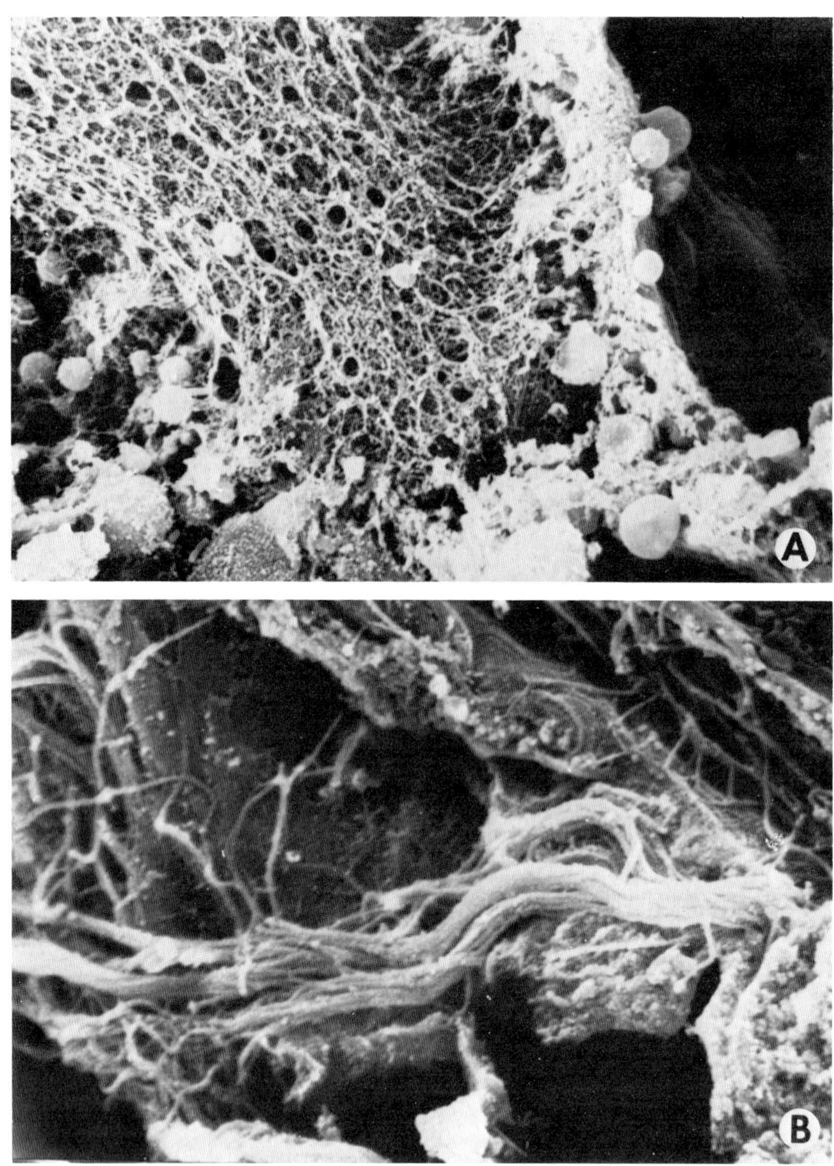

FIGURE 5. Scanning electron microscopy of lungs from animals treated similarily to those described in Figs. 3 and 4. (A) At 4 hr, there is extensive intraalveolar deposition of fibrin. Red cells and leukocytes are present along the alveolar walls (× 1560). (B) At 1 week, thick bands of collagen are present, coursing through the interstitial network (× 10,000).

5 days it was evident that there was a marked interstitial reaction consisting of hypercellularity due to increased numbers of spindled (fibroblast-like) cells and round cells, with a relative clearing of the intraalveolar exudate (Fig. 4). Trichrome stains revealed marked increases in the amounts of collagen in the pulmonary interstitium. By scanning electron microscopy the changes at 4 hr were accentuated by heavy intraalveolar deposits of fibrin together with red cells and leukocytes along the alveolar walls (Fig. 5A); at 1 week, the alveolar spaces were relatively clear, while the interstitium was moderately thickened and contained wide bands of collagen bundles (Fig. 5B). These studies have suggested that generation in the lung of H_2O_2 in the presence of lactoperoxidase will produce acute injury that evolves to chronic and progressive interstitial changes. Since immune complexes and chemotactic factors will trigger leukocytes to produce products similar to those generated by glucose oxidase and lactoperoxidase, the potential exists that immune injury may be related to leukocyte-generated O_2^-, H_2O_2 and other oxygen metabolites.

In Table II we have shown that exposure of rat red cells to glucose, glucose oxidase, and lactoperoxidase results in significant red cell injury as demonstrated by a six-fold increase in the release of hemoglobin into the supernatant fluid. Neither glucose oxidase nor lactoperoxidase alone caused red cell damage. That a halide-independent peroxidase is ineffective in producing red cell injury is shown by the inability of horse radish peroxidase to produce red cell lysis when mixed with glucose oxidase and glucose. The pattern of red cell injury in these experiments is similar to the damage of red cells by neutrophils activated with phorbol myristate acetate (29).

TABLE II. Damage of Rat Red Cells by Oxygen Metabolites

Material added to rat red cells*	Red cell damage (O.D. at 500 nm)
Saline	0.025, 0.026
Glucose oxidase	0.023, 0.031
Glucose oxidase + lactoperoxidase	0.162, 0.173
Glucose oxidase + horseradish peroxidase	0.027, 0.014
Lactoperoxidase	0.031, 0.028

**Rat red blood cells (10^8 cells in 0.2 ml) were incubated in phosphate buffered saline (pH 7.4) containing 1.0 mg glucose, and where indicated, glucose oxidase (10 units), and lactoperoxidase (1.0 unit). Cell suspensions were incubated at 37°C for 15 min, 1.0 ml saline added, and the cells removed by centrifugation. The concentration of soluble hemoglobin was determined at O.D. 500 nm.*

These studies suggest that oxygen-derived free radicals have the ability to produce tissue injury directly. The evidence suggests that a variety of oxygen metabolites, including O_2^-, H_2O_2, and myeloperoxidase derivatives, may play an important role in leukocyte-dependent tissue injury, such as that induced by immune complexes. In addition, progression of acute lung injury to interstitial pulmonary fibrosis resulting from the intratracheal instillation of glucose, glucose oxidase, and a halide-dependent peroxidase suggests that these active products of oxygen may directly or indirectly represent an important factor in the pathogenesis of pulmonary fibrosis. Future investigation is necessary to identify more precisely the specific site of tissue injury caused by oxygen metabolites and to define the role which oxygen products may play in initiating the fibrotic response.

REFERENCES

1. Babior, B. M. Oxygen-dependent microbial killing by phagocytes (Part I). *N. Engl. J. Med. 298*, 659 (1978).

2. Becker, E. L., Sigman, M., and Oliver, J. M. Superoxide production induced in rabbit polymorphonuclear leukocytes by synthetic chemotactic peptides and A23187. *Am. J. Pathol. 95*, 81 (1979).

3. Burls, R. E., Lawrence, R. A., and Love, M. M. Liver necrosis and lipid peroxidation in the rat as a result of paraquat and diquat adminstration. Effect of selenium deficiency. *J. Clin. Invest. 65*, 1024 (1980).

4. Carp, H. and Janoff, A. A. *In vitro* suppression of serum elastase inhibitory capacity by reactive oxygen species generated by phagocytosing polymorphonuclear leukocytes. *J. Clin. Invest. 63*, 793 (1979).

5. Clark, R. A. and Klebanoff, S. J. Neutrophil-mediated tumor cell cytotoxicity: Role of the peroxidase system. *J. Exp. Med. 141*, 1442 (1975).

6. Clark, R. A., Szot, S., Venkatasubramanian, K., and Schiffman, E. Chemotactic factor inactivation by myeloperoxidase mediated oxydation of methionine. *J. Immunol. 124*, 2020 (1980).

7. Curnutte, J. T. and Babior, B. M. Biologic defense mechanisms. The effects of bacteria and serum on superoxide production by granulocytes. *J. Clin. Invest. 53*, 1662 (1974).

8. De Chatelet, L. R., Shirley, P. S., and Johnston, R. B. Effect of phorbol myristate acetate on the oxidative metabolism of human polymorphonuclear leukocytes. *Blood 47*, 545 (1976).

9. Doroshow, J. H., Locker, G. Y., and Myers, C. E. Enzymatic defenses of the mouse heart against reactive oxygen metabolites. Alterations produced by doxorubicin. *J. Clin. Invest. 65*, 128 (1980).

10. Goldstein, I. M., Roos, D., Kaplan, H. B., and Weissman, G. Complement and immunoglobulin stimulate superoxide production by human leukocytes independently of phagocytosis. *J. Clin. Invest. 56*, 1155 (1975).

11. Hafeman, D. D. and Lucas, Z. J. Polymorphonuclear leukocyte mediated antibody dependent cellular cytotoxicity against tumor cells. Dependence on oxygen and the respiratory burst. *J. Immunol. 123*, 55 (1979).

12. Johnson, K. J. and Ward, P. A. Acute immunologic pulmonary alveolitis. *J. Clin. Invest. 54*, 349 (1974).

12a. Johnson, K. J., Fantone, J. C., Kaplan, J., and Ward, P. A. *In vivo* damage of rat lungs by oxygen metabolites. *J. Clin. Invest. 67*, 983 (1981).

13. Kellogg, E. W. and Fridovich, I. Liposome oxidation and erythrocyte lysis by enzymatically generated superoxide and hydrogen peroxide. *J. Biol. Chem. 252*, 6721 (1977).

14. Klebanoff, S. J. Antimicrobial mechanism in neutrophil polymorphonuclear leukocytes. *Semin. Hematol. 12*, 117 (1975).

15. Lynch, R. F. and Fridovich, I. Effects of superoxide on the erythrocyte membrane. *J. Biol. Chem. 253*, 1838 (1978).

16. Mustafa, M. G. and Tierny, D. F. Biochemical and metabolic changes in the lung with oxygen, ozone, and nitrogen dioxide toxicity. *Am. Rev. Respir. Dis. 118*, 1061 (1978).

17. Nathan, C. E., Brukner, L., Silverstein, S. C., and Cohn, Z. A. Extracellular cytolysis by activated macrophages and granulocytes. *J. Exp. Med. 149*, 100 (1979).

18. Perez, H. D. and Goldstein, I. M. Generation of a chemotactic lipid from arachadonic acid by exposure to a superoxide generating system. *Fed. Proc., Fed. Am. Soc. Exp. Biol. 39*, 1170 (1980). Abstr.

19. Petrone, W. E., English, D. K., Wong, K., and McCord, J. M. Free radicals and inflammation: The superoxide dependent activation of a neutrophil chemotactic factor in plasma. *Proc. Natl. Acad. Sci. U.S.A. 77*, 1159 (1980).

20. Rister, M. and Baehner, R. L. The alteration of superoxide dismutase, catalase, glutathione peroxidase, NAD(P)H, cytochrome C reductase in guinea pig polymorphonuclear leukocytes and alveolar macrophages during hyperoxia. *J. Clin. Invest. 58*, 1174 (1976).

21. Root, R. K., Metcalf, J., Oshino, W., and Chance, B. H_2O_2 release from human granulocytes during phagocytosis. I. Documentation, quantitation, and some regulating factors. *J. Clin. Invest. 55*, 945 (1975).

22. Rosen, H. and Klebanoff, S. J. Bacterial activity of a superoxide-anion generating system. *J. Exp. Med. 149*, 27 (1979).

23. Sachs, T., Moldow, C. E., Craddock, P. R., Bowers, J. K., and Jacob, H. S. Oxygen radical mediated endothelial cell damage by complement-stimulated granulocytes. An *in vitro* model of immune vascular damage. *J. Clin. Inves Invest. 61*, 1161 (1978).

24. Smith, L. L., Rose, M. S., and Wyatt, I. The pathology and biochemistry of paraquat. *Ciba Found. Symp. 65*, 321 (1979).

25. Thorne, K. J., Svvensen, R. J., and Franko, D. Role of hydrogen peroxide in the cytotoxic reaction of T-lymphocytes. *Clin. Exp. Immunol. 39*, 486 (1980).

26. Ward, P. A. and Cochran, C. G. Bound complement and immunologic injury of blood vessels. *J. Exp. Med. 122*, 215 (1965).

27. Ward, P. A. and Hill, J. H. Complement derived leukotactic activity extractable from lesions of immunologic vasculitis. *J. Immunol. 108*, 1137 (1972).

28. Weiss, S. J. Neutrophil generated hydroxyl radicals destroy RBC targets. *Clin. Res. 27*, 466A (1979). Abstr.

29. Weiss, S. J. The role of superoxide in the destruction of erythrocyte targets by human neutrophils. *J. Biol. Chem. 255*, 9912 (1980).

30. Weiss, S. J. and LoBuglio, A. F. An oxygen dependent mechanism of neutrophil-mediated cytotoxicity. *Blood 55*, 1020 (1980).

31. Weiss, S. J., Rustagi, P. K., and LoBuglio, A. F. Human granulocyte generation of the hydroxyl radical. *J. Exp. Med. 147*, 316 (1978).

EXTENSIVE MUTATIONAL CHANGES DURING LONG-TERM PERSISTENT INFECTION BY RNA VIRUSES: IMPLICATIONS FOR THE IMMUNE RESPONSE[1]

John J. Holland
Katherine Spindler
Frank Horodyski
Charlotte Jones
Elizabeth Grabau

Department of Biology,
University of California at San Diego,
La Jolla, California

Lola Reid
Nagahiro Minato
Barry Bloom

Departments of Immunology, Microbiology,
and Molecular Pharmacology,
Albert Einstein College of Medicine,
Bronx, New York

I. INTRODUCTION

For the past 8 years we have been studying the persistence of vesicular stomatitis virus (VSV), a negative strand, enveloped rhabdovirus *in vitro* in BHK_{21} hamster cells. This persistent infection was initiated (11) by coinfection of BHK_{21}

[1]*Supported by U.S.P.H.S. Grant No. Al-14627.*

ISBN 0-12-218320-7

baby hamster kidney cells with the tsG31 matrix protein mutant of Pringle (23) in addition to its homologous defective interfering (DI) particles. The presence of DI particles was required to attenuate the cell lethality of both wild-type and temperature-sensitive (ts) mutants in order to prevent 100% cell death (11). After a period of recurrent cytopathic crises during the first months of persistence, the carrier cells (designated CAR4) resumed normal growth rates despite the continuing presence in all, or nearly all, cells of large amounts of viral antigen. By employing similar procedures we have established long-term carrier states in BHK_{21} cells with measles virus, mumps virus, influenza virus, rabies virus, and Sendai (parainfluenza) virus. In every case, approximately 100% of the cells are virus antigen-positive most of the time; they are specifically resistant to superinfection by homologous, but not heterologous virus, and they shed only very low levels of mature infectious virus. These have been extensively covered in several recent reviews (9, 10) and publications (8, 12, 16, 27, 28) and their back references. It should be noted that the types of persistent infection described herein in BHK_{21} cells is rather different from the type described by Youngner and colleagues (33, 34) and others (20, 21, 24); the latter involve interferon rather than DI particles as the major mechanism preventing cell lethality, and in these interferon-regulated carrier cultures, persistence is at the cell population level with most of the cells in the culture remaining uninfected at most times due to the protective effects of interferon. Youngner and Preble (35) have recently reviewed this type of RNA virus persistence in which temperature-sensitive mutants and interferon mediate a population-level carrier state. In this chapter we will cite our recent studies with particle-mediated persistence of VSV in BHK_{21} cells with emphasis on our recent evidence that the genome of the original tsG31 virus continuously accumulates mutational changes over many years of persistence. Some examples of altered interaction with the immune system resulting from this mutational change will be presented and its implications for persistent virus disease discussed.

II. OLIGONUCLEOTIDE AND PEPTIDE MAPPING SHOW THAT THE VSV GENOME ACCUMULATES EXTENSIVE MUTATIONAL CHANGE DURING YEARS OF PERSISTENT INFECTION OF BHK_{21} CELLS

Multiply-cloned tsG31 virus and purified virus-free DI particles were originally employed to establish the CAR4 carrier, so all virus later recovered from this carrier represents progeny from a single virus particle. Oligonucleotide maps of this original clone were compared to maps of virus recovered at various intervals over more than 7 years of persistence. A gradual progression was observed in which more and more mutations accumulated in the viral genome (8) with each year of persistence. This technique is capable of observing only the larger 10% (unique) T_1 ribonuclease fragments of RNA so only about 10% of all mutations can be detected. Nevertheless, it can be estimated that over 250 mutations have accumulated after 8 years and more mutations continue to accumulate beyond the sixth and seventh years. These mutations occur in different carrier cultures. The mutants recovered after more than 5 years of persistence are all ts, small plaque mutants that grow slowly at any temperature. They are rather stable mutants which retain their biological characteristics and their altered oligonucleotide maps after repeated lytic passages in cell culture or multiple lethal passages in mice (8).

Peptide mapping demonstrates that these mutations are not all silent mutations since all 5 of the viral proteins showed multiple peptide map changes after 5 years (28).

III. EXTENSIVELY MUTATED VIRUS FROM PERSISTENT INFECTION CHANGES ITS VIRULENCE PROPERTIES AND MAY ESTABLISH NEW PERSISTENT INFECTIONS IN THE ABSENCE OF DI PARTICLES

Since the VSV mutants recovered after more than 5.5 years of persistent infection are ts, slowly replicating mutants, we examined their virulence for mice by the intracerebral route of inoculation. All mutants recovered after 5.5 years had completely lost the ability to cause obvious disease or death in young adult outbred Levin mice. This was true even when millions of pfu were injected intracerebrally. In contrast, wild-type VSV Indiana kills nearly 100% of mice when more than 10 pfu are injected intracerebrally. This decreased virulence is seen also at the cellular level *in vitro* since virus mutants recovered beyond 5.5 years of persistence exhibit such reduced cytopathology that they can establish persistent infections in BHK_{21} cells without added DI particles (although DI particles quickly appear in the newly established carrier cells) (28). An interesting mutation in the opposite direction was observed in one of our BHK_{21} rabies carriers. These carriers were established using HEP Flury rabies vaccine virus and their DI particles. During the first year of persistence virulent mutants were recovered, and these caused typical rabies upon intracerebral inoculation into adult mice (in contrast to the parental HEP vaccine virus which causes no disease in adult mice). However, virus subsequently recovered from this HEP rabies BHK_{21} carrier after 2 years has regularly been avirulent, causing no disease in adult mice (10).

Obviously, mutations during rabies virus persistence may either increase or decrease virulence. However, since the selective pressures in persistent infections favor virus that causes less cell damage (due to selection of the more rapidly growing infected cells) the trend in viral mutants should generally tend toward loss of virulence, and this is what we observe (10, 28).

IV. VIRAL MUTANTS SHOWING ALTERED INDUCTION AND RESPONSE TO NATURAL KILLER CELLS

In a series of collaborative studies among three laboratories (16, 18, 25, 26) we have employed a number of our RNA virus carrier cells for *in vivo* studies of persistence in athymic nude mice. We were surprised to find that all of our virus carrier cells (VSV-BHK, rabies-BHK, mumps-BHK, measles-BHK, influenza-BHK, mumps-HeLa, measles-HeLa, and Sendai-BHK do not usually form tumors when injected subcutaneously into nude mice, although the parental (and virus-cured) BHK_{21} and HeLa cells rapidly form large tumors (25). The carrier cells are restricted (or rejected) by NK cells in the nude mice so that only small nodules (or nothing) appear at the site of injection. When a tumor is produced by carrier cells, the cells comprising the tumor are generally found to be "cured" of persistent infection (i.e., to have eliminated the virus). A more interesting type of tumor has been observed very rarely after the carrier cells have been restricted for many months as a nodule at the site of injection. One such tumor arose from a nodule between 7 and 8 months after carrier cell injection, then formed a serially transplantable, rapidly growing tumor which metastasized (16). Large amounts of mature virus and of viral surface antigen are produced by these cells (designated CAR4-P), so their failure to be controlled or rejected by NK cells was puzzling. *In vitro* NK cell cytolytic assays (18) demonstrated that CAR4-P cells are extremely potent inducers of interferon and of NK activity in recipient nude mice. In contrast, they are extremely refractory to the killing activity of NK cells which they induce (or which are induced by other means). This explains why they form tumors despite strong expression of viral antigens. We next investigated whether this escape from NK cell sensitivity was due to viral or cellular mutation. Virus shed by CAR4-P tumors was isolated, cloned replicated at high moi to produce DI particles, then used to establish new carriers. These new VSV carriers exhibited the same characteristics as CAR4-P. They regularly formed large tumors with metastases and expressed large amounts of surface antigen and mature virus, and they were refractory to NK cell killing *in vitro* (16).

Although it is not known how viruses convert infected cells into targets for NK cell killing, it presumably involves viral alterations of the cell plasma membrane, regardless of whether viral antigens participate directly as part of the NK cell target, or indirectly by altering cell surface configurations. It seems clear that among the many mutations occuring during persistent infection we have selected *in vivo* a mutant virus that does not present an efficient target for NK cell killing. This should prove useful in studying NK cell target specificity. Another, less surprising type of virus mutant showing altered interactions with NK cells was derived *in vitro* without selection. The CAR4 carrier between 5 years and 6.5 years of persistence shed only very small amounts of infectious virus (less than 10^{-4} pfu/cell/day). Throughout this period it regularly produced invasive tumors and metastases (although these progressed more slowly *in vivo* than do tumors of the parental BHK_{21} cells). This late carrier state is a very poor inducer of interferon and of NK cells, probably in part because it sheds so few mature infectious virus particles or DI particles. Also, differences in cell surface expression may play a role in this poor NK cell induction and interferon induction.

Since it is known that interferon is the major regulatory molecule operating in the induction of at least certain subsets of NK cells (4, 31), antiserum to interferon has been examined (26) for its effects on the tumorigenicity of our carrier cells in nude mice. Sheep antimouse interferon prepared by Gressor and colleagues (4) when injected intravenously at the time of carrier cell injection into nude mice completely prevented NK cell rejection of the carrier cells. Carrier cells that would otherwise have been rejected formed rapidly growing invasive tumors with a high incidence of metastases. It appears that interferon-mediated NK cell activity is a critical determinant in NK cell response to virus-infected cells. Our findings indicated that at least several different kinds of virus mutants can escape this interferon-activated NK cell killing of virus-infected cells. Such mutants might be biologically significant during some acute virus infections, and they could be expected to occur more frequently during long-term persistent infections *in vivo*.

V. ALTERED ANTIBODY REACTIVITY OF MUTANT VIRUS RECOVERED AFTER YEARS OF PERSISTENCE *IN VITRO*

Since oligonucleotide maps and peptide maps showed extensive accumulation of mutations during VSV persistence (including mutations in the G and M membrane-associated antigens) it was of interest to determine whether antigenic changes occurred as a result of these mutations. Antigenic drift is well known among influenza viruses but it is also more common than is generally recognized in other viruses. Visna virus undergoes

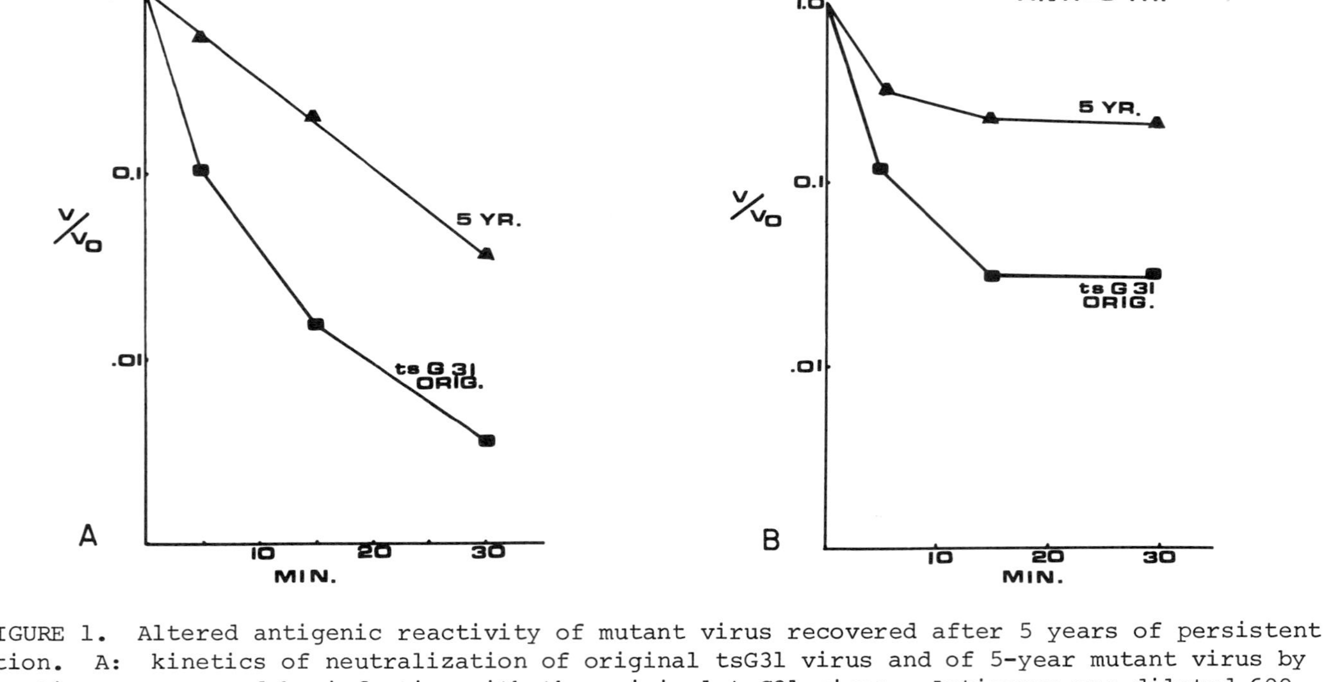

FIGURE 1. Altered antigenic reactivity of mutant virus recovered after 5 years of persistent infection. A: kinetics of neutralization of original tsG31 virus and of 5-year mutant virus by mouse antiserum prepared by infection with the original tsG31 virus. Antiserum was diluted 600-fold in Eagles minimum essential medium, 1/10th volume of a dilute virus suspension was added, and virus was incubated for the indicated number of minutes at 37°C, diluted 1/100 at each time point and replicate plaque assays were performed immediately. B: conditions are as for A except that antiserum was prepared by infection of mice with virus recovered after 5 years of persistent infection. This antiserum was diluted 1/320 before use, as in A.

regular antigenic shifts during persistent infection (5, 19, 29) as does equine infectious anemia virus (2), and these give rise to a series of antigenically distinct mutants in a rather regular pattern. Swine vesicular disease virus, and human coxsackie B5 viruses show considerable antigenic relatedness and both undergo considerable antigenic variation in nature (7), suggesting that they have recently evolved from a common progenitor strain. Herpes simplex virus type 1 has been shown to evolve some antigenic changes during persistent infections in humans (1) and without antibody selection in cell cultures (6). Foot and mouth disease virus serotypes also drift antigenically in nature (15). Monoclonal antibody selection *in vitro* leads to rapid appearance of antigenic variants in VSV, Sendai and influenza A viruses (22), and rabies virus (32).

We have examined the serological reactivity of one of our mutants isolated after 5 years of persistence using antibody prepared by infection of mice with original tsG31 mutant used to establish persistence and with the 5-year mutant. The results presented in Fig. 1A show that antibody against tsG31 original virus neutralized tsG31 with more rapid kinetics than it neutralizes the 5-year mutant virus. The converse experiment using antiserum against the 5-year mutant virus (Fig. 1B) shows unexpectedly that homologous 5-year mutant virus is neutralized more slowly than the tsG31 virus. This could be due to strange antigenic characteristics, to structural differences in the mutant virus, to the much higher particle to pfu ratio in the mutant virus, or to other factors, but it is clear that the serological reactivity of the mutant virus has become altered during persistence in the absence of immunoselection. We are carrying out further studies with mutants derived with and without antibody selection *in vivo* and *in vitro* to assess the significance and extent of antigenic drift during VSV persistence. Persistent and acute infections may select for significant antigenic drift in many enveloped RNA viruses. Monoclonal antibody analysis by Koprowski and co-workers shows that different rabies strains can differ significantly in their antigenic determinants, although they resemble each other much more closely than Mokola or other rabies related viruses (3).

VI. FACTORS FAVORING EXTENSIVE ACCUMULATION OF MUTATIONS DURING RNA VIRUS PERSISTENCE

Studies in progress by Spindler and Holland (10, 30) suggest that mutations can also accumulate at a high rate during lytic passages of VSV *in vitro* but that they are much more marked if virus is passaged undiluted rather than diluted at each passage. The strain of virus also influences these results. Since DI particles are present much more regularly and in larger numbers during undiluted passages they may influence mutational changes. Intergenic complementation during high moi passages may also be important and we are investigating these effects. We recently observed that during persistent VSV infection, DI particles are selecting for virus mutants able to escape the homologous interfering effect of the first DI particles used to establish persistence (13). This was first observed during rabies persistence by Kawai *et al.* (17), and our findings with VSV parallel theirs exactly. Furthermore, we have found that this selective process is continuous during persistence so that the virus and DI particle interactions must be very complex and constantly evolving (14). The role of DI particles in helping to drive the evolution of DI particle requires more extensive investigation. It has been known for decades that RNA viruses have a high mutation rate, but the very large number of mutant forms able to compete and remain viable has not until recently been realized. This mutational plasticity may provide for RNA viruses the degree of biological adaptability afforded the DNA viruses by recombination. In both RNA and DNA virus chronic infections, mutational changes affecting interactions with immunocytes and antibodies may be much more common and more important in the disease process than is currently believed, especially whenever a mutant arises that might exploit a specific immunological blind spot in any individual. This process might also lead to generation of new serotypes in virus evolution.

VII. SUMMARY

Persistent infection of BHK_{21} cells by VSV for over 7 years has led to extensive and continuing mutational change in the virus genome. Numerous recovered mutant clones are viable and stable in phenotype and by oligonucleotide map analysis. Among these are mutants altered in their antigenic reactivity and mutants that fail to induce interferon and NK cell activity or which fail to render infected cells susceptible to the cytolytic activity of NK cells. DI particles play a complex role in selecting populations of virus mutants during persistence. Virus mutants capable of escaping even partially from NK cell, antibody, T cells, etc. may be very important in diseases resulting from persistent infection, since specific immunological "blind spots" in any individual might be exploited to cause recurrence, exacerbation, or fatal progression of pathology.

ACKNOWLEDGMENT

We thank E. Bussey for excellent technical assistance.

REFERENCES

1. Ashe, W. K., and Scherp, H. W. Antigenic variations in herpes simplex virus isolants from successive recurrences in herpes Dabialis. *J. Immunol. 94*, 385-394 (1965).

2. Crawford, T. B., Cheevers, W. P., Klevjer-Anderson, P., and McGuire, T. C. Equine infectious anemia: Virion characteristics, virus-cell interaction and host responses. *In* "Persistent Viruses" (J. G. Stevens, G. J. Todaro, and C. F. Fox, eds.), pp. 727-749. Academic Press, New York, 1978.

3. Flamand, A., Wiktor, T. J., and Koprowski, H. Use of hybridoma monoclonal antibodies in the detection of antigenic differences between rabies and rabies-related virus proteins. II. The glycoproteins. *J. Gen. Virol. 48*, 105-109 (1980).

4. Gidlund, M., Orn, A., Wigzell, J., Senik, A., and Gresser, I. Enhanced NK activity in mice injected with interferon and interferon inducers. *Nature (London) 273*, 759-761 (1978).

5. Haase, A. T., Brahic, M., Carroll, D., Scott, J., Stowring, L., Traynor, B., and Ventura, P. Visna: An animal model for studies of virus persistence. *In* "Persistent Viruses" (J. G. Stevens, G. J. Todaro, and C. F. Fox, eds.), pp. 643-654. Academic Press, New York, 1978.

6. Hampar, B. and Keehn, M. A. Cumulative changes in the antigenic properties of herpes simples virus from persistently infected cell cultures. *J. Immunol. 99*, 554-557 (1967).

7. Harris, T. J. R. and Brown, F. Correlation of polypeptide composition with antigenic variation in the swine vesicular disease and Coxsackie B5 viruses. *Nature (London) 258*, 758-760 (1975).

8. Holland, J. J., Grabau, E. A., Jones, C. L., and Semler, B. L. Evolution of multiple genome mutations during long-term persistent infection by VSV. *Cell 16*, 495-504 (1979).

9. Holland, J. J., Kennedy, S. I. T., Smeler, B. L., Jones, C. L., Roux, L., and Grabau, E. A. Defective interfering RNA viruses and the host cell response. *Compr. Virol. 16*, 137-192 (1980).

10. Holland, J., Spindler, K., Grabau, E., Semler, B., Jones, C., Horodyski, F., Rowlands, D., Janis, B., Reid, L., Minato, N., and Bloom, B. Viral mutation in persistent infection. *In* "Animal Virus Genetics" (B. Fields, R. Jaenisch, and C. F. Fox, eds.), pp. 695-709. Academic Press, New York, 1980.

11. Holland, J. J. and Villarreal, L. P. Persistent non-cytocidal VSV infections mediated by defective T particles that suppress virion transcriptase. *Proc. Natl. Acad. Sci. U.S.A. 71*, 2956-2960 (1974).

12. Holland, J. J., Villarreal, L. P., Welch, R. M., Oldstone, M. B. A., Kohne, D., Lazzarini, R., and Scolnick, E. Long term persistent VSV and rabies virus infection of cells *in vitro*. *J. Gen. Virol. 33*, 193-211 (1976).

13. Horodyski, F. M. and Holland, J. J. Viruses isolated from cells persistently infected with VSV show altered interactions with defective interfering particles. *J. Virol. 36*, 627-631 (1980).

14. Horodyski, F. M. and Holland, J. J. Continuing evolution of virus-DI particle interaction resulting during VSV persistent infection. *In* "Negative Strand Viruses" (D. H. L. Bishop and R. Compans, eds.), Elsevier/North Holland, New York, pp. 887-892. 1981.

15. Hyslop, N. S. G. Isolation of variant strains from foot and mouth disease virus propagated in cell cultures containing antiviral sera. *J. Gen. Microbiol. 41*, 135-142 (1965).

16. Jones, C., Spindler, K. R., and Holland, J. J. Studies on tumorigenicity of cells persistently infected with VSV in nude mice. *Virology 103*, 158-166 (1980).

17. Kawai, A., Matsumoto, S., and Tanabe, K. Characterization of rabies viruses recovered from persistently infected BHK cells. *Virology 67*, 520-533 (1975).

18. Minato, N., Bloom, B. R., Jones, C., Holland, J., and Reid, L. M. Mechanism of rejection of virus persistently infected tumor cells by athymic nude mice. *J. Exp. Med. 149*, 1117-1133 (1979).

19. Narayan, O., Griffin, D. E., and Chase, J. Antigenic shift of visna virus in persistently infected sheep. *Science 197*, 376-378 (1977).

20. Nishiyama, Y. Studies of L cells persistently infected with VSV: Factors involved in the regulation of persistent infection. *J. Gen. Virol. 35*, 265-279 (1977).

21. Nishiyama, Y., Ito, Y., and Shimokata, K. Properties of viruses selected during persistent infection of L cells with VSV. *J. Gen. Virol. 40*, 481-484 (1978).

22. Portner, A., Webster, R. G., and Bean, W. Similar frequencies of antigenic variants in Sendai, VSV and influenza A viruses. *Virology 104*, 235-238 (1980).

23. Pringle, C. R. Genetic characteristics of conditional lethal mutants of VSV induced by 5-fluorouracil, 5-azacytidine and ethyl methane sulfonate. *J. Virol. 5*, 559-567 (1970).

24. Ramseur, J. M. and Friedman, R. M. Prolonged infection of interferon-treated cells by VSV: Possible role of ts mutants and interferon. *J. Gen. Virol. 37*, 523-533 (1977).

25. Reid, L. M., Jones, C. L., and Holland, J. Virus carrier state suppresses tumorigenicity of tumor cells in athymic (nude) mice. *J. Gen. Virol. 42*, 609-614 (1979).

26. Reid, L. M., Minato, N., Gresser, I., Holland, J., Kadish, A., and Bloom, B. Influence of antimouse interferon on the growth and metastases of virus persistently infected tumor cells, and of human prostatic tumors in athymic nude mice. *Proc. Natl. Acad. Sci. U.S.A. 78*, 1171-1175 (1980).

27. Roux, L. and Holland, J. J. Viral genome synthesis in BHK_{21} cells persistently infected with Sendai virus. *Virology 100*, 53-64 (1980).

28. Rowlands, D., Grabau, E., Spindler, K., Jones, C., Semler, B., and Holland, J. J. Virus protein changes and RNA termini alterations evolving during persistent infection. *Cell 19*, 871-880 (1980).

29. Scott, J. V., Stowring, L., Haase, A. T., Narayan, O., and Vigne, R. Antigenic variation in visna virus. *Cell 18*, 321-327 (1979).

30. Spindler, K. and Holland, J. J. High multiplicities of infection favor rapid and random evolution of VSV. *Virology*, in press.

31. Welsh, R. M. Cytotoxic cells induced during lymphocytic choriomeningitis virus infection of mice. I. Characterization of natural killer cell induction. *J. Exp. Med.* *148*, 163-181 (1978).

32. Wiktor, T. J. and Koprowski, H. Monoclonal antibodies against rabies virus produced by somatic cell hybridization: Detection of antigenic variants. *Proc. Natl. Acad. Sci. U.S.A.* *75*, 3938-3942 (1978).

33. Youngner, J. S., Preble, O. T., Jones, E. V., and Creager, R. S. Evolution of virus populations in persistent infections of L cells with VSV. *In* "Persistent Viruses" (J. G. Stevens, G. J. Todaro, and C. F. Fox, eds.), pp. 417-429. Academic Press, New York, 1978.

34. Youngner, J. S., Dubovi, E. J., Quogliana, D. O., Kelly, M., and Preble, O. T. Role of temperature-sensitive mutants in persistent infections initiated with VSV. *J. Virol.* *19*, 90-101 (1976).

35. Youngner, J. S. and Preble, O. T. Viral persistence: evolution of viral populations. *Compr. Virol.* *16*, 73-135 (1980).

DISCUSSION

Dr. Choppin commented that viral serotypes (such as measles) may be stable because certain antigenic determinants are essential for virus infectivity, and therefore must be conserved.

Dr. Oldstone commented that evolution of one serotype to another may be more common and rapid then most virologists suspect. He cited Hilary Koprowski's monoclonal antibody which reacts with an antigenic determinant of both VSV and rabies virus as evidence for relatedness of quite distinct viruses.

Immunopathology: VIIIth International Symposium, 1980

MECHANISMS OF VIRUS PERSISTENCE AND ESCAPE FROM IMMUNE SURVEILLANCE: ANTIBODY-INDUCED MODULATION AS A MODE OF INITIATING MEASLES VIRUS PERSISTENCE

Michael B. A. Oldstone
Robert S. Fujinami

Department of Immunopathology[1]
Scripps Clinic and Research Foundation,
La Jolla, California

I. INTRODUCTION

Because several kinds of viruses persist in man despite his mounting a vigorous immune response, we have evaluated such responses and their roles in initiating and maintaining virus infection. Of the various naturally occurring infections of this type, my colleagues and I have chosen to analyze measles virus infection in detail because of its medical importance, effects on immune function, clearcut connection with chronic disease, and severe aftermath.

[1]*This is publication No. 2310. This research was supported by U.S.P.H.S. grants NS-12428 and AI-07007.*

ISBN 0-12-218320-7

A. *Measles Virus Infection: Acute and Persistent*

Measles virus infection in man usually follows an acute, self-limiting course, during which the subject mounts an immune response that clears the virus from his tissues. Convalescence is marked by immunity to the virus, and throughout life the patient continues to produce low titers of antibody and immune lymphocytes to measles virus [reviewed in Perrin *et al.* (22) and ter Meulen *et al.* (26)]. In contrast to this usual situation, measles virus infrequently causes a chronic infection termed subacute sclerosing panencephalitis (SSPE). During this chronic measles virus infection, patients develop extraordinarily high titers of antimeasles virus antibody, yet the virus persists in both their central nervous system and lymphoid tissues. Antibody titers in their sera and other body fluids are at least 10-fold and usually 100- to 1000-fold higher than in the acutely infected or newly convalescent patients (26). In addition to these high levels of cytotoxic and neutralizing antibodies, the immune system's main humoral effector and amplifier, the complement system, is functionally active and cytotoxic immune lymphocytes are present in the peripheral blood of the patient (14, 16, 22).

B. *Rationale for the Theory that Persistent Measles Virus Infection Is Initiated by Antiviral Antibody*

We have postulated that the events intrinsic to SSPE begin when antibody to measles virus strips or modulates measles virus antigen off the surfaces of virus-infected cells (13, 18). This hypothesis is based on a series of observations in which specific measles virus antibodies added to cultured infected cells strip viral antigens from the cell surface, preventing such cells from expressing sufficient antigens for recognition and subsequent lysis by either humoral or cell mediated immune constituents (13, 19). Thus, infected cells denuded of surface viral antigens escape immunologic assault, yet retain viral genetic information. It is important to note that the morphologic picture of virus-infected cells cultured in the presence of antibody closely resembles that of cells obtained by biopsy from patients with SSPE (11, 17). That is, the surfaces of infected cells are devoid of antigen, or relatively so, whereas numbers of viral nucleocapsids increase dramatically inside the cell in random arrangements (Fig. 1).

Further evidence to support the hypothesis of antibody-induced modulation comes from studies of ours and others indicating that patients with chronic measles virus infection have sufficient amounts of effective cytotoxic lymphocytes, cytotoxic antibody, and complement in their circulations to clear the virus (14, 16, 19, 22, 26). We have also noted that 50-fold less antibody is needed to strip viral antigens off the surfaces of infected cells than is required for lysing such cells in the presence of complement (13, 14, 18). Hence, enough antibody to strip measles virus antigens from the surfaces of infected cells is available before cytotoxic lymphocytes (22) or cytotoxic antibody can act to lyse such cells. Thus, quantitatively, the local production of antibody by plasma cells favors modulation over immune lysis. If plasma cells make antibody in such compartments as the central nervous system where there is little or no hemolytic complement activity, then lysis does not occur until the blood-brain barrier becomes sufficiently damaged to allow plasma proteins access to this site. Furthermore, a significant number of patients with acute measles virus infections experience transient depletion of complement components, including most notably in the alternative activation pathway (5).

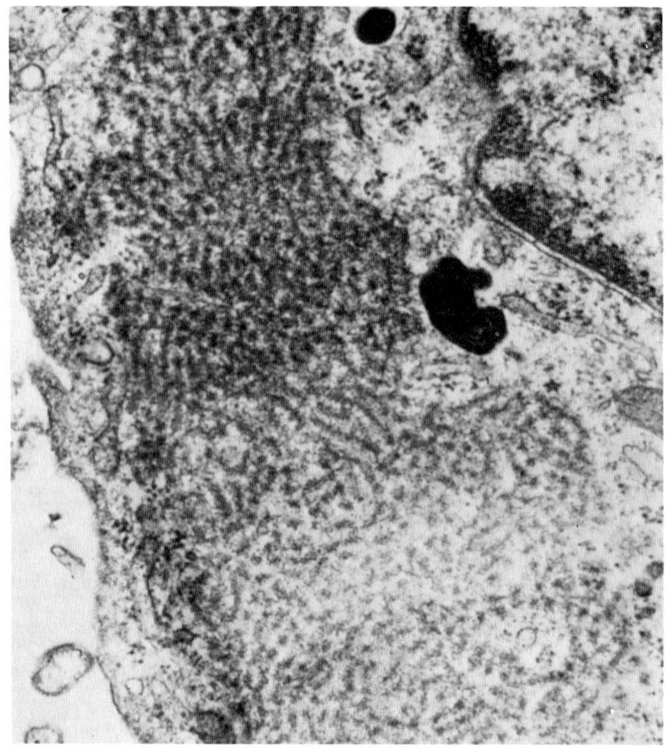

FIGURE 1. Electron micrograph showing packed measles virus nucleocapsids arranged at random in the cytoplasm of a HeLa cell infected with measles virus. This cell was cultured in the presence of antibodies to measles virus. Note the absence of measles virus on the cell surface. This picture, the result of antibody-induced modulation of measles virus antigens off the cell surface *in vitro*, closely resembles the biopsies of patients with subacute sclerosing panencephalitis in which nucleocapsids are distributed and arranged similarly in the cytoplasm and no viral antigens appear on the surfaces of cells. This lack of viral antigen expression on the cell surface allows such cells to escape ordinarily effective antibody and cell-mediated killing (see Fig. 3).

In addition to the above-stated evidence documented *in vitro*, antibody-induced antigenic modulation is likely to occur *in vivo*. Albrecht and colleagues showed that measles virus (SSPE virus) inoculated into monkeys produces significant subacute or persistent infection only when the monkeys had preexisting antibodies to measles virus (1). Results were similar in newborn hamsters infected with measles virus and suckling on mothers having antibodies to measles virus, as noted by Wear and Rapp (27).

II. MECHANISM OF ANTIBODY-INDUCED MODULATION OF MEASLES VIRUS ANTIGENS

A. *Background*

When antibody reacts with viral antigens expressed on the infected cell's plasma membrane, among the biological and molecular events that follow is redistribution of antigens [reviewed in Oldstone *et al.* (20)]. Frequently, the result is aggregation, capping, and/or shedding (12, 21). This occurs not only on virus-infected cells but in other biological models as well (20). For example, binding of a ligand induces specific cell surface macromolecules (to which the ligand reacts) to disappear in studies with paramecium (6) and mycoplasm (24). Other studies show that a variety of cells infected by a wide assortment of infectious agents can be capped (20). An additional and increasing body of information indicates that self regulation of membrane receptors is frequently controlled by antibody-induced redistribution. For example, acetylcholine receptor turnover and modulation occur in part from interactions between the corresponding antibody and the receptor (10). Moreover, the importance of aggregation, cross-linking, capping, and/or endocytosis of receptors for insulin (15) and antigen receptors on lymphocytes (23) is also clear relative to the effectiveness or disruption of their functions.

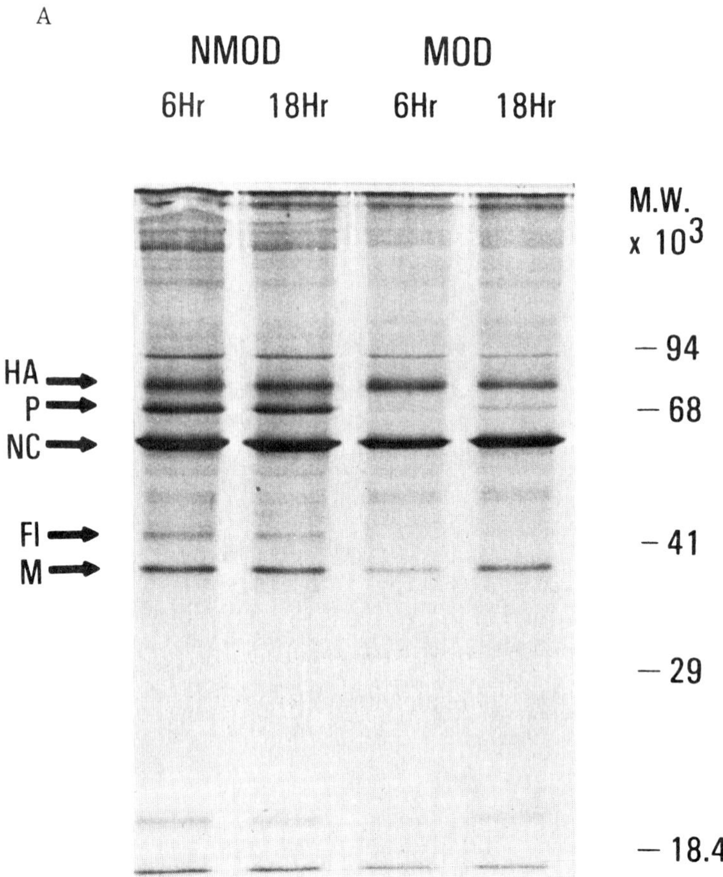

FIGURE 2A. Autoradiogram of measles virus polypeptides from nonmodulated (NMod) or modulated (Mod) infected HeLa cells. Panel A: cells were incubated in the absence or presence of measles virus antibody for 6 or 18 hr and then pulse-labeled with $[^{35}S]$methionine for 2 hr. P protein and F are reduced in antibody-treated cells. Viral polypeptides are HA, hemagglutinin; P, phosphoprotein; NC, nucleocapsid; F, fusion or hemolysin; and M, matrix or membrane protein. Note the internal control in the NMod preparation demonstrating the experimental consistence of F and P proteins (i.e., free from proteolytic degradation due to technical aspects of the protocol used).

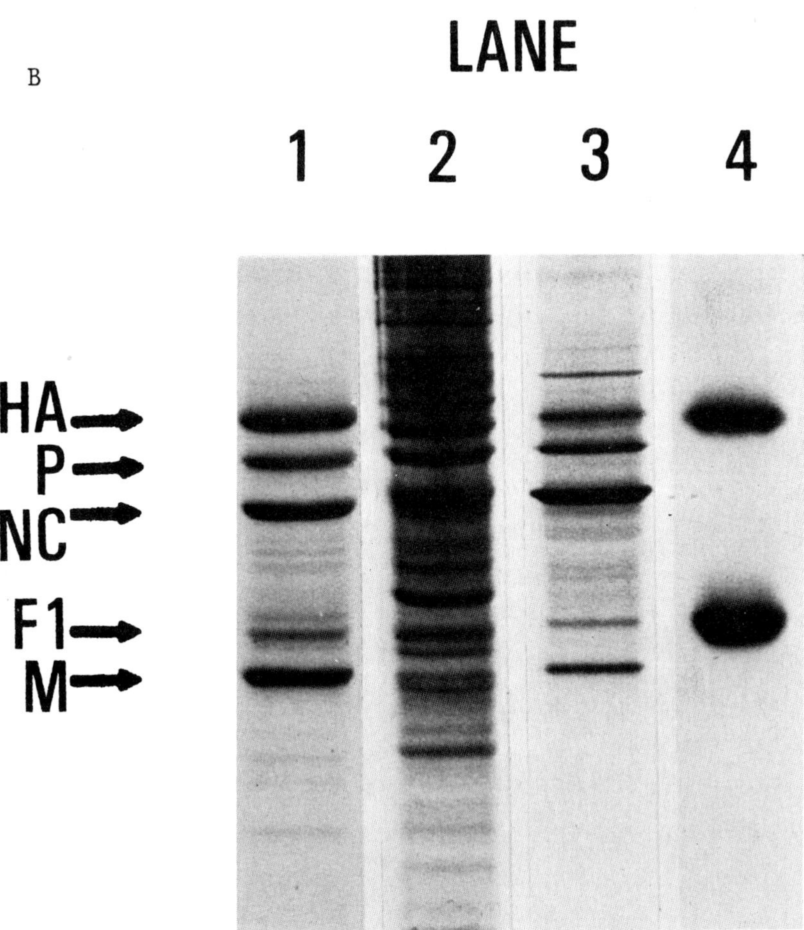

FIGURE 2B. Panel B demonstrates measles virus polypeptides in the virion (Lane 1), infected cell cytoplasm-nonimmune precipitated with antibody to all measles virus polypeptides (Lane 2). Lane 3 is the same as Lane 2 but immunoprecipitated with antibody to measles virus polypeptides. The viral polypeptides expressed on the cell surface (HA and F) and shown in Lane 4. [For experimental details, see Fujinami and Oldstone (7-8a).]

B. Description of Antibody-Induced Modulation

In culture, measles virus antigens can be removed from surfaces of infected HeLa cells when the medium is supplemented with heat-inactivated human or rabbit serum containing antibodies to measles virus, the whole IgG, or its Fab fragments (7, 8, 13). The number of measles virus antigens usually expressed on the cell surface decreases markedly in both acutely (Fig. 2) and persistently infected cells within 6 hr of addition of antimeasles virus antibodies. The effect of antimeasles virus antibody is specific in that antibodies directed against an unrelated virus (VSV) or against nonviral cell surface antigens (HeLa cell surface, HLA) do not modulate measles virus antigens. Stripping of measles virus antigens on the cell surface is reversible; that is, measles virus antigens are reexpressed on the cell surface within 24 hr of removing antibody from the media (13). However, when cells are cultured for long periods with serum containing antimeasles virus antibody, modulation results in a population of cells devoid of surface measles virus antigens. As exposure to antiviral antibody lengthens, the rate at which viral antigens return to the cell surface progressively slows, once antibody is removed (13). Thus, after only one day's incubation with antiviral antibody, viral antigens reappear on 50% of the cells within 24 hr. However, after five days of incubation, an additional six days are required before surface viral antigens become detectable on 50% of the cells. After six weeks of culture with antibody, it is difficult to detect any reexpression of measles virus antigens on the surfaces of infected HeLa cells.

C. *Biological Consequences of Antibody-Induced Modulation: Escape from Immune Surveillance and Maintenance of Measles Virus Persistence*

A direct relationship exists between stripping of measles virus antigens from cell surfaces and lysis of virus-infected cells by either antibody and complement or cytotoxic lymphocytes. As seen in Fig. 3, the ability of either antibody and complement or of cytotoxic immune lymphocytes to kill measles virus-infected cells directly parallels the quantity of viral antigens expressed on the cell surface. Under modulating conditions, as measles virus antigens depart from the cell surface, infected cells resist immune lysis. Upon removal of

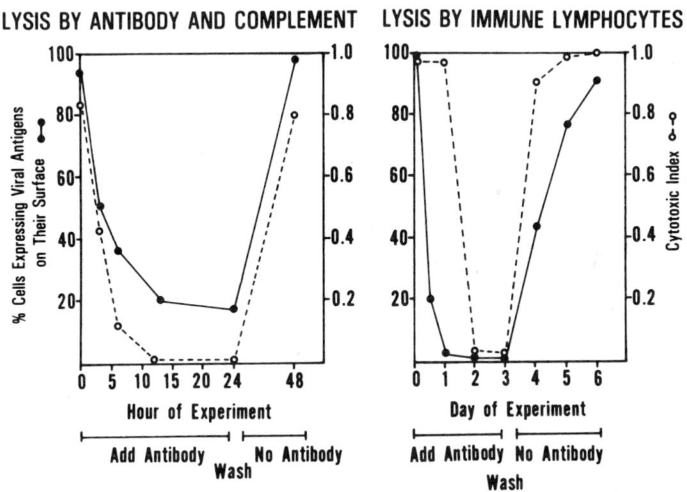

FIGURE 3. Antibody-induced stripping of measles virus antigens off the surfaces of infected cells allows such infected cells to escape immune mediated attack by cytotoxic antibody and cytotoxic lymphocytes. Left Panel: alteration of surface expression of measles virus antigens (●———) and the ability of measles virus antibody and complement (○----) to specifically lyse infected HeLa cells. Right panel: alteration of surface expression of measles virus antigens (●———) and the ability of immune lymphocytes (○----) to specifically lyse infected HeLa cells. [For experimental details, see Joseph and Oldstone (13) and Oldstone and Tishon (19)].

these modulating antibodies from the media, cells reexpress their viral antigens and become subject to immune destruction.

D. *Molecular Events Associated with Antibody-Induced Modulation*

Recently, we have begun to delineate the molecular events that occur during antibody-induced modulation. Of particular interest is the observation that the expression of measles virus polypeptides on the cell surface as well as inside the cell alters significantly when virus-infected cells are cultured with antimeasles virus antibodies (Fig. 2). HeLa cells acutely infected with measles virus during a 24-hr incubation express the following measles virus polypeptides: the large (L) protein with a molecular weight of 160,000; hemagglutinin (HA) with a molecular weight of 80,000; phosphoprotein (P) with a molecular weight of 70,000; nucleocapsid (NC) with a molecular weight of 60,000; fusion protein (F) with a molecular weight of 42,000; and the membrane or matrix protein (M) with a molecular weight of 36,000. When infected cells are cultured for at least 6 hr and for as long as 24 hr in the presence of antimeasles virus antibody and labeled with either [^{35}S]methionine or [^{32}P]orthophosphate, the radioactive counts representing externally expressed measles virus polypeptide F and internally expressed polypeptide P are markedly reduced. Thus, of the two viral polypeptides destined for the cell surface, HA and F, during the first 24 hr of antibody-induced modulation HA remains relatively unaffected, whereas the number of F molecules diminishes markedly. However, when antibody is kept in the culture medium for 72 hr or longer, the HA is efficiently removed from the cell surface, as evaluated by radioimmune and immunofluorescence binding assays (13, 19).

In the quantitative experiment shown in Fig. 2, over 80% of the P protein and 70% of the F protein disappeared or were not made during antibody-induced modulation (7, 8).

E. Specificity of Molecular Events in Antibody-Induced Modulation

The results indicating the decrease in F and P proteins were observed consistently in multiple experiments, under varied gel conditions with and without urea. Although P protein is susceptible to proteolytic digestion, this kind of laboratory artifact did not cause the diminished amounts of P we saw, considering that P protein was analyzed in the presence of proteolytic enzyme inhibitors and in the cold. Furthermore, in the control cytosol preparation run concurrently (Fig. 2: NMod), no proteolytic digestion of P protein was noted. Because P protein seems to form complexes with NC and L proteins, possibly P is a rate-limiting element in the synthesis of measles virus polypeptides. Thus, the increased numbers of NC proteins found in the cytoplasms of virus-infected cells may be related to disturbances of this P protein. Whether the failure to detect P protein is a consequence of a transcriptional or translational block or results from the rapid degradation of P is unknown at present. Additional experimentation with the incorporation of ^{32}P into viral polypeptides during antibody modulation indicates that the M polypeptide, which is also a phosphoprotein, is enhanced in ^{32}P residues (7, 8). These changes in the phosphorylation of M protein might alter nucleocapsid recognition and alignment at the plasma membrane, thereby interfering with viral maturation.

F. Consequence of Modulating Fusion (F) Protein

Although the biological consequences of the foregoing findings in relation to P and M proteins are perhaps still unclear, the loss of F protein from the surface of virus-infected cells has a clear functional outcome: the prevention of cell-cell fusion. Cell fusion ordinarily results in giant cell and syncytia formation leading to cell death. Infected cells lacking F molecules on their surfaces are relatively normal in cytomorphology, continue to live and yet retain viral genetic information.

In summary, the antibody-induced antigenic modulation described here is specific, inasmuch as the aberrations in measles virus polypeptides (F, P, and M) are associated only with antibodies binding to measles virus antigens on the cell surface. Antibodies to nonviral structural antigens expressed on the surface of infected cells do not cause this activity. The phenotypes seen with antibody induced modulation *in vitro* are reminiscent of the picture of the virus-infected cells seen *in vivo*.

G. Antibody-Induced Modulation in Other Virus Infections

The loss of a particular type of antigen on the surface of cells cultured with the specific antibody was first observed by Boyse and colleagues and was termed antigenic modulation (3). Working with the TL differentiation antigen normally present on thymus cells and on leukemia cells, these workers found that the phenotypic expression of TL antigen was suppressed by TL antibodies both *in vivo* and *in vitro*.

Thereafter, several workers demonstrated that antibody-induced antigenic modulation occurred with several retrovirus infections [reviewed in Oldstone *et al*. (20)]. Aoki and

Johnson (2) studied Gross virus-induced leukemia and Genovesi *et al.* (9) studied Friend leukemia virus-infected cells with immune serum against Friend leukemia virus; in both experiments, antibody induced antigenic modulation. Calafat *et al.* (4) showed that murine mammary tumor virus antigens could undergo redistribution and modulation. With a different murine tumor cell line, Yagi *et al.* (28) obtained similar results and suggested that the polypeptide profile of the mammary tumor viral antigens changed when antibody was added to cultured cells. Recently, Stevens and Cook (25) and Alberghetti and associates (personal communication) suggested that antibody-induced modulation may also play a role in herpes simplex virus infections and chronic hepatitis B virus infection.

III. CONCLUSIONS

Antibody-induced redistribution of antigens expressed on the plasma membrane occurs frequently in the field of biology. Studies of antimeasles viral antibody-induced modulation of measles virus antigens on the surfaces of infected cells provides a model for understanding the biological and molecular events by which an ordinarily acute virus infection may be changed to a persistent virus infection. The future will test the strength of these observations in explaining not only the persistence of viruses like measles but also cytomegalovirus, herpes simplex, hepatitis B, etc., all infections occurring with a vigorous host immune response. In these instances antibody may initiate the process of virus persistence by modulating antigens and may maintain the process by immune selection of virus variants that favor persistence. Virus mutants, by a variety of mechanisms including formation of defective interfering particles or temperature-sensitive mutants, could also code for fewer virus antigens on the cell surface, thereby evading immune reactants and initiating or maintaining persistent infection. In SSPE, the diminished expression of viral antigens on the cell surface leads to escape from immune surveillance, whereas the associated accumulation of viral polypeptides inside the cell leads to dysfunction of the infected cell. These points are common features in this hypothesis, explaining measles virus persistence and mechanism(s) of tissue injury.

ACKNOWLEDGMENTS

The author acknowledges the contributions of several colleagues in this Viral-Immunobiology Laboratory over the last several years working on this and related studies with measles virus. Included are Professor Peter Lampert (University of California, San Diego) continuing collaborator; Antoinette Tishon; and the following post-doctoral fellows: Patrick Sissons, Martin Haspel, Luc Perrin, and Barry Joseph.

REFERENCES

1. Albrecht, P., Burnstein, T., Klutch, M., Hicks, J., and Ennis, F. Subacute sclerosing panencephalitis: Experimental infection in primates. *Science 195*, 64-66 (1977).

2. Aoki, T. and Johnson, P. A. Suppression of Gross leukemia cell-surface antigens: A kind of antigenic modulation. *J. Natl. Cancer Inst. 49*, 183-189 (1972).

3. Boyse, E. A., Stockert, E., and Old, L. J. Modification of the antigenic structure of the cell by thymus-leukemia (TL) antibody. *Proc. Natl. Acad. Sci. U.S.A. 58*, 954-957 (1967).

4. Calafat, J., Hilgers, J., van Bitterswijk, W., Verbeet, M., and Hageman, P. Antibody induced antigenic modulation and shedding of mammary tumor virus antigens on the surfaces of G-2 ascites leukemia cells as compared with normal antigens. *J. Natl. Cancer Inst. 56*, 1019-1029 (1976).

5. Charlesworth, J., Pussell, B., Roy, L., Robeston, M., and Beveridge, J. Measles infection: Involvement of the complement system. *Clin. Exp. Immunol. 24*, 401-406 (1976).

6. Dwyer, D. Antibody-induced modulation of Leishmania donovani surface membrane antigens. *J. Immunol. 117*, 2081-2091 (1976).

7. Fujinami, R. S. and Oldstone, M. B. A. Antiviral antibody reacting on the plasma membrane alters measles virus expression inside the cell. *Nature (London) 279*, 529-530 (1979).

8. Fujinami, R. S. and Oldstone, M. B. A. Alterations in expression of measles virus polypeptides by antibody: Molecular events in antibody-induced antigenic modulation. *J. Immunol. 125*, 78-85 (1980).

8a. Fujinami, R. S., Sissons, J. G. P., and Oldstone, M. B. A. Immune reactive measles virus polypeptides on the cell's surface: Turnover and relationship of the glycoprotein to each other and to HLA determinants. *J. Immunol. 127*, 935-1092 (1981).

9. Genovesi, E., Marx, P., and Wheelock, F. Antigenic modulation of Friend virus erythroleukemia cells *in vitro* by serum from mice with dormant erythroleukemia. *J. Exp. Med. 146*, 520-534 (1977).

10. Heineman, S., Merlie, J., and Lindstrom, J. Modulation of acetylcholine receptors in rat diaphragm by antireceptor sera. *Nature (London) 274*, 65-67 (1978).

11. Iwasaki, Y. and Koprowski, H. Cell to cell transmission of virus in the central nervous system. I. Subacute sclerosing panencephalitis. *Lab. Invest. 31*, 187-196 (1974).

12. Joseph, B. S. and Oldstone, M. B. A. Antibody-induced redistribution of measles virus antigens on the cell surface. *J. Immunol. 113*, 1205-1209 (1974).

13. Joseph, B. S. and Oldstone, M. B. A. Immunologic injury in measles virus infection. II. Suppression of immune injury through antigenic modulation. *J. Exp. Med. 142*, 864-876 (1975).

14. Joseph, B. S., Cooper, N. R., and Oldstone, M. B. A. Immunologic injury of cultured cells infected with measles virus. I. Role of IgG antibody and the alternative complement pathway. *J. Exp. Med. 141*, 761-774 (1975).

15. Kahn, C., Baird, K., Jarrett, B., and Flier, J. Direct demonstration that receptor crosslinking or aggregation is important in insulin action. *Proc. Natl. Acad. Sci. U.S.A. 75*, 4209-4213 (1978).

16. Kreth, H. W. and ter Meulen, V. Cell-mediated cytotoxicity against measles virus in SSPE. I. Enhancement by antibody. *J. Immunol. 118*, 291-295 (1977).

17. Lampert, P. W., Joseph, B. S., and Oldstone, M. B. A. Morphologic changes in cells infected with measles or related viruses. *Prog. Neuropathol. 3*, 51-68 (1976).

18. Oldstone, M. B. A. Role of antibody in regulating virus persistence: Modulation of viral antigens expressed on the cell's plasma membrane and analyses of cell lysis. *In* "Development of Host Defenses" (M. D. Cooper and D. H. Dayton, eds.), pp. 223-235. Raven, New York, 1977.

19. Oldstone, M. B. A. and Tishon, A. Immunologic injury in measles virus infection. IV. Antigen modulation and abrogation of lymphocyte lysis of virus-infected cells. *Clin. Immunol. Immunopathol. 9*, 55-62 (1978).

20. Oldstone, M. B. A., Fujinami, R. S., and Lampert, P. W. Membrane and cytoplasmic changes in virus infected cells induced by interactions of antiviral antibody with surface viral antigen. *Prog. Med. Virol. 26*, 45-93 (1980).

21. Perrin, L. and Oldstone, M. B. A. The formation and fate of virus antigen-antibody complexes. *J. Immunol. 118*, 316-322 (1977).

22. Perrin, L. H., Tishon, A., and Oldstone, M. B. A. Immunologic injury in measles virus infection. III. Presence and characterization of human cytotoxic lymphocytes. *J. Immunol. 118*, 282-290 (1977).

23. Sidman, C. and Unanue, E. Receptor-mediated inactivation of early B lymphocytes. *Nature (London) 257*, 149-151 (1975).

24. Stanbridge, E. and Weiss, R. L. Mycoplasma capping on lymphocytes. *Nature (London) 276*, 583-587 (1978).

25. Stevens, J. G. and Cook, M. L. Maintenance of latent herpetic infection: An apparent role for antiviral IgG. *J. Immunol. 113*, 1685-1693 (1974).

26. ter Meulen, V., Katz, M., and Muller, D. Subacute sclerosing panencephalitis: A review. *Curr. Top. Microbiol. 57*, 1-38 (1972).

27. Wear, D. and Rapp, F. Latent measles virus infection of the hamster central nervous system. *J. Immunol 107*, 1593-1598 (1971).

28. Yagi, M. J., Blair, P. B., and Lane, M. Modulation of mouse mammary tumor virus production in the MJY-alpha cell line. *J. Virol. 28*, 611-623 (1978).

Immunopathology: VIIIth International Symposium, 1980

ANTIBODIES AGAINST MEASLES VIRUS POLYPEPTIDES IN DIFFERENT DISEASE CONDITIONS

Erling Norrby
Claes Örvell

Department of Virology,
Karolinska Institute, School of Medicine,
Stockholm, Sweden

I. INTRODUCTION

Measles virus can cause both acute and persistent infections. The most extensively studied form of persistent infection is the rare disease subacute sclerosing panencephalitis (SSPE). One important feature of this disease is the occurrence of an accentuated humoral immune response (16). Serum antibody titers are 10-100 times higher than in normal late convalescent sera and in cerebrospinal fluid measles virus-specific oligoclonal IgG, which is locally produced in the central nervous system, can be demonstrated.

Furthermore, an accentuated humoral immune response has been found in studies of sera from patients with atypical measles. This form of measles occurs in individuals who have received inactivated measles vaccine. Because of an antigen

ISBN 0-12-218320-7

defect of the vaccine it does not give long-term protection but does provide conditions for development of immune pathological reactions (13).

Increased measles virus antibody titers have also been encountered in certain other disease conditions. Patients with systemic lupus erythematosus and chronic active hepatitis frequently have high serum antibody levels (6). However, this phenomenon concerns not only measles virus antibodies but also antibodies to some other viruses, for example, rubella. An increase in measles virus serum antibody titers, although less pronounced, is also seen in patients with multiple sclerosis (11). In addition, about 60% of these patients produce oligoclonal measles virus-specific IgG in the central nervous system. It was also found that in patients with multiple sclerosis the changes in antibody production are not unique to measles virus antibodies, and it has therefore been proposed that the phenomena observed reflect a more general disturbance of immune regulation.

Antibodies to viral antigens can be studied by nonselective techniques such as complement fixation (CF) tests with whole virus antigen or by other techniques demonstrating antibodies to certain structural components, as for example in neutralization or hemagglutination-inhibition (HI) tests. Recently, the radioimmune precipitation assay (RIPA) has been employed to demonstrate selectively the occurrence of antibodies reacting with different structural components. In several studies the RIPA test was used to characterize the antibody response to measles virus polypeptides in different groups of patients. Special interest has been focused on the antibody response to the matrix (M) antigen since it was found that in patients with SSPE the antibody response to this polypeptide is very weak or undetectable, despite an accentuated antibody response to other polypeptides (3, 9, 22). It has been proposed that the poor antibody response is attributable to a defect in production of M antigen or a rapid degradation of this antigen in infected cells. However, later studies (15) have shown that the antibody response to M antigen in connection with a regular infection is weak and that the titers of antibodies rapidly decline to undetectable levels. Thus, M antigen antibodies were found only in sera from patients with symptoms of measles, either in connection with natural disease or in atypical measles (8), whereas sera from patients with multiple sclerosis did not contain matrix antigen antibodies (5).

The purpose of the present study was to compare the antibody response to the nucleoprotein [NP antigen, which dominates the antibody response in connection with a regular measles infection (12)] and the M antigen in different disease conditions. Antibodies to the two components were determined not only by the RIPA test, but also by CF tests in which purified preparations of NP and M components (19) were used as antigens. The groups of sera studied were collected about 2 weeks and more than 10 years after regular measles and from patients with atypical measles, SSPE, multiple sclerosis, and chronic active hepatitis. In order to improve possibilities for detection of M antigen antibodies both late convalescent sera and sera from patients with chronic active hepatitis were screened for HI antibodies, and samples of the 25% in each group with the highest titers were selected for further analysis.

TABLE I. The Antibody Response to Measles Virus NP and M Antigens in Different Sets of Sera as Determined by RIPA Tests*

Set of serum samples	No. of sera	Range of HI serum titers**	Range of ratios of NP/M antibody titers in RIPA tests***
Measles early convalescent	10	160- 2,560	25 - > 125 (8)
Measles late convalescent	14	320- 2,560	125 - > 625 (3)
Multiple sclerosis	6	20- 640	125 - 3125 (2)
SSPE	6	160- 5,120	>125 - >3125 (1)
Chronic active hepatitis	6	1,280-20,480	>125 - > 625 (1)
Atypical measles	5	2,560-10,240	25 - > 125 (5)

* *Number of sera in each group with detectable antibodies to M antigen and the ratio of NP/M antibody titers are given. The range of HI serum titers in each set of serum samples is also presented.*

** *HI tests performed as described in Norrby and Gollmar (12).*

*** *Number of sera with detectable antibodies to M antigen are given in parentheses.*

II. CHARACTERIZATION BY RIPA TESTS OF ANTIBODIES TO NP AND M ANTIGENS IN DIFFERENT GROUPS OF PATIENTS AND IN HEALTHY INDIVIDUALS

SDS polyacrylamide gel electrophoresis has demonstrated six different structural components in measles virions: large (L), hemagglutinin (H), polymerase (P), NP, fusion (F_1), and M polypeptides (10, 18). Under the conditions of the RIPA test (14, 17, 19) H, NP, F_1, and M polypeptide antibodies were readily detectable. However, antibodies against L and P components were not demonstrable due to the relatively small quantity of the L component and the breakdown of the P polypeptide under the conditions of labeling for a longer time (4). The use of long-term (3 days) labeled cell-associated antigens also caused the appearance in the antigen preparation of some proteolytic breakdown products of the NP polypeptide, predominantly of a size of about 45,000.

Table I gives a summary of the range of ratios of antibody titers against NP and M antigen in RIPA tests. This form of relative expression is used since inherent technical qualities do not allow absolute titer determinations in RIPA tests. Factors such as the varying degree of labeling of different antigen preparations and the time of autoradiography exposure influence antibody titers. Antibodies to the NP antigen always predominate over antibodies to other structural proteins. However, whereas NP antigen antibodies occur in all samples there is a markedly varying presence of M antigen antibodies. In many cases, therefore, it was necessary to describe the ratio of antibodies to NP and M antigens as larger than a certain value.

Of 10 early convalescent sera (collected 10-20 days after appearance of rash) 5 contained antibodies detectable to M antigen. In one case the ratio of NP to M antibodies was 25,

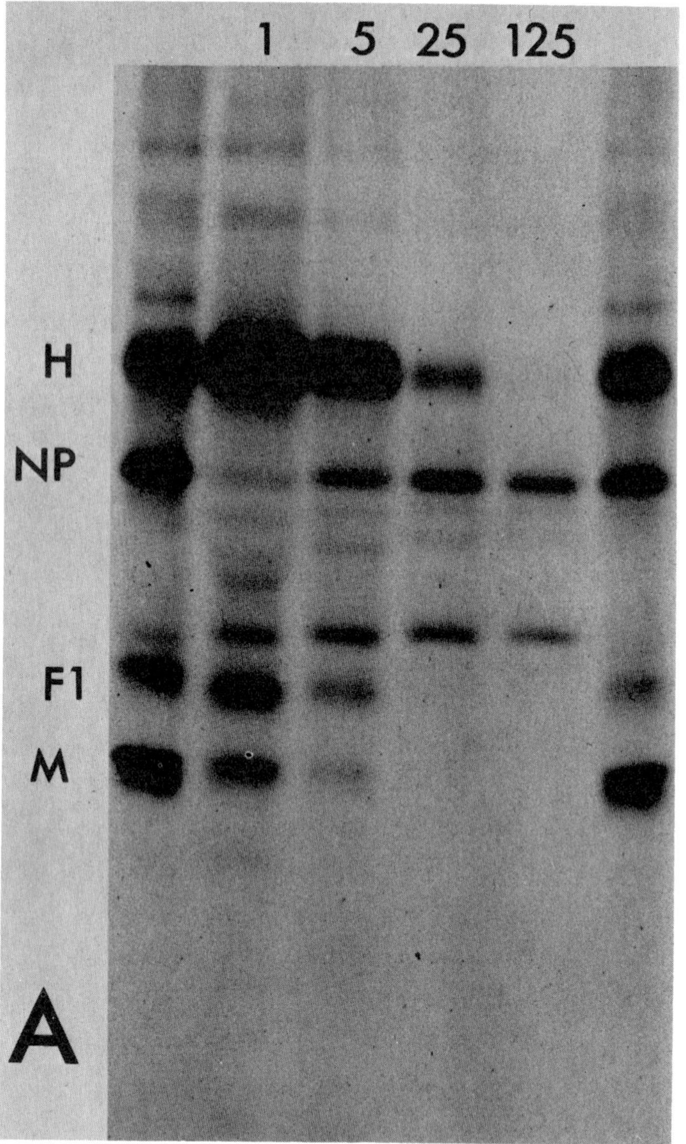

FIGURE 1. Radioimmune precipitation of measles virus polypeptides in sera collected 10 days after regular measles (A), more than 10 years after regular measles from a healthy individual (B), and from a patient with definite MS (C). The following polypeptides can be identified: hemagglutinin (H, 79K), nucleoprotein (NP, 60K), hemolysin-fusion factor (F_1, 41K), and matrix protein (M, 37K). Serial five-fold dilutions of 20 μl of serum in a final reagent volume of 0.5 ml were tested. Lanes not labeled with dilution factors contain reference virus preparations.

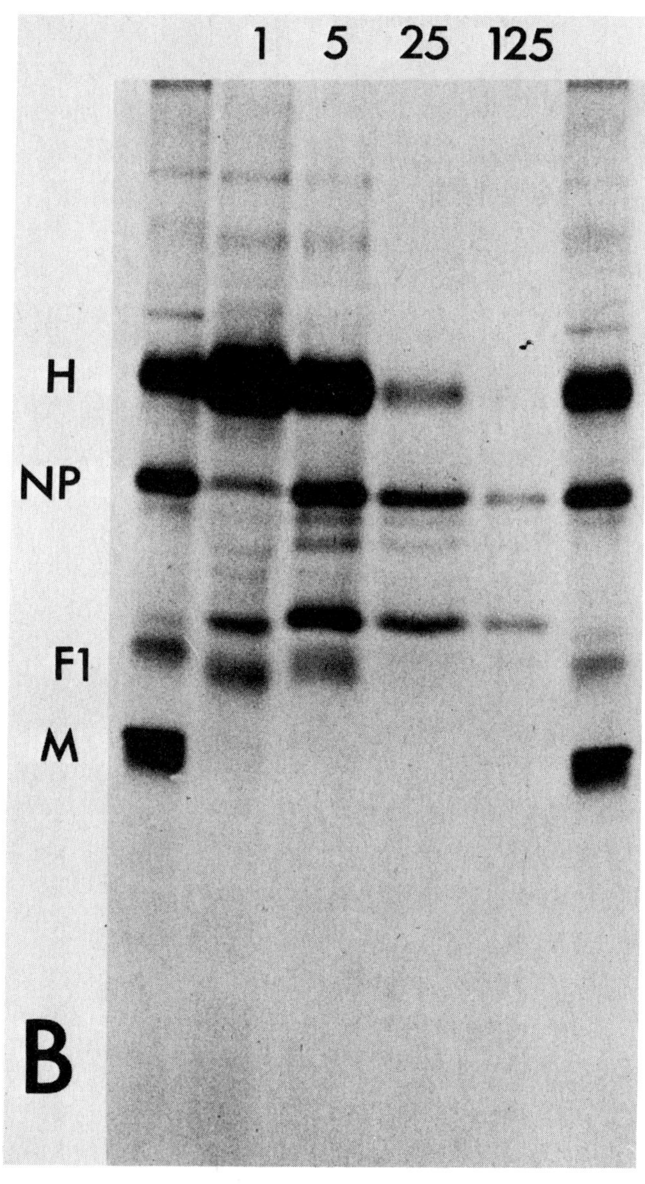

FIGURE 1 (*Continued*)

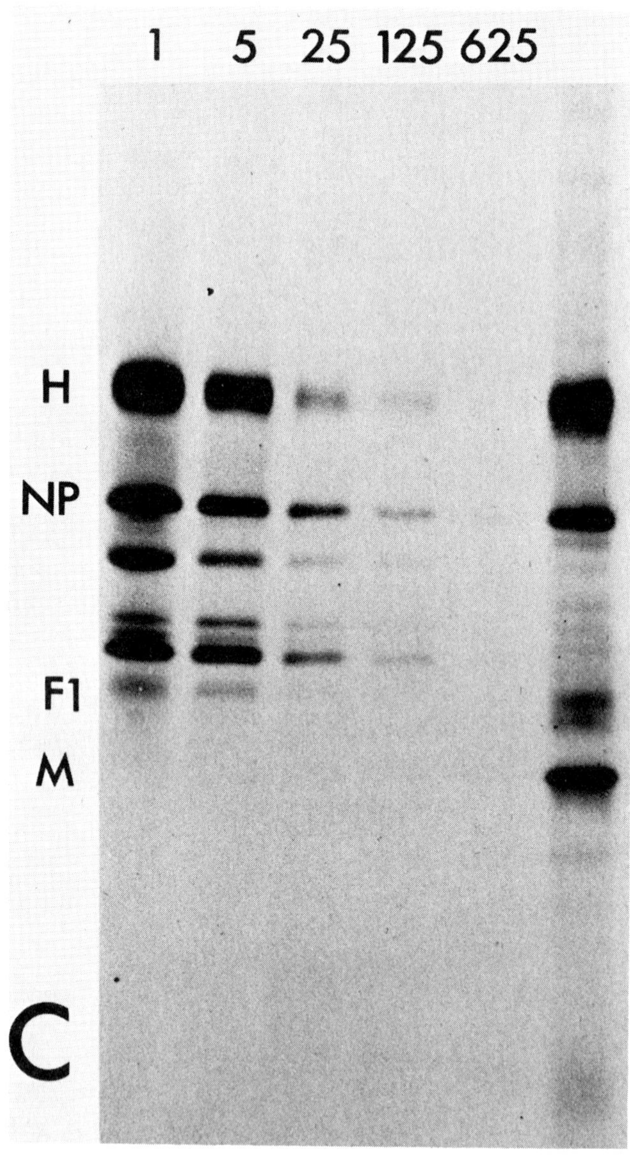

FIGURE 1 (*Continued*)

but in the other cases it was 125 or higher. The antibody response to M antigen appeared both weak and transient (cf. Fig. 1). Only 2 out of the 10 selected high titer late convalescent sera [more than 10 years after regular measles; 25% with the highest hemagglutinating-inhibiting (HI) antibody titers] contained detectable antibodies to M antigen. Similarly, M antigen antibodies were only seen in 2 of 6 sera from patients with definite multiple sclerosis (supplied by Dr. B. Vandvik, Department of Neurology, Rikshospitalet, Oslo). SSPE sera (supplied by Dr. B. Vandvik) contained high titers of HI antibodies and NP antigen antibodies, both determined by RIPA. However, confirming observations by others (3, 22) only one out of 6 samples contained M antigen antibodies (Fig. 2A). As a consequence the ratios of antibodies to NP and M antigens were high. A similar finding was somewhat unexpectedly made in tests with selected high titer sera from patients with chronic active hepatitis (clinically and liver biopsy verified; 25% with the highest HI antibody titers) (Fig. 2B). Only 1 of 6 samples contained demonstrable antibodies to M antigen, whereas antibodies to NP antigen occurred in high titers.

Sera from cases of atypical measles (supplied by Dr. J. D. Cherry, Department of Pediatrics, University of California, Los Angeles, California) contained high titers of HI antibodies, corresponding to titers found in the sera selected from patients with chronic active hepatitis. As a further similarity, sera of both categories contained high titers of NP antigen antibodies, as determined by RIPA tests. However, whereas M antigen antibodies were rarely seen in sera from patients with SSPE or chronic active hepatitis they occurred in readily measurable titers in sera from all patients with atypical measles (Fig. 2C). In the latter cases ratios of antibodies

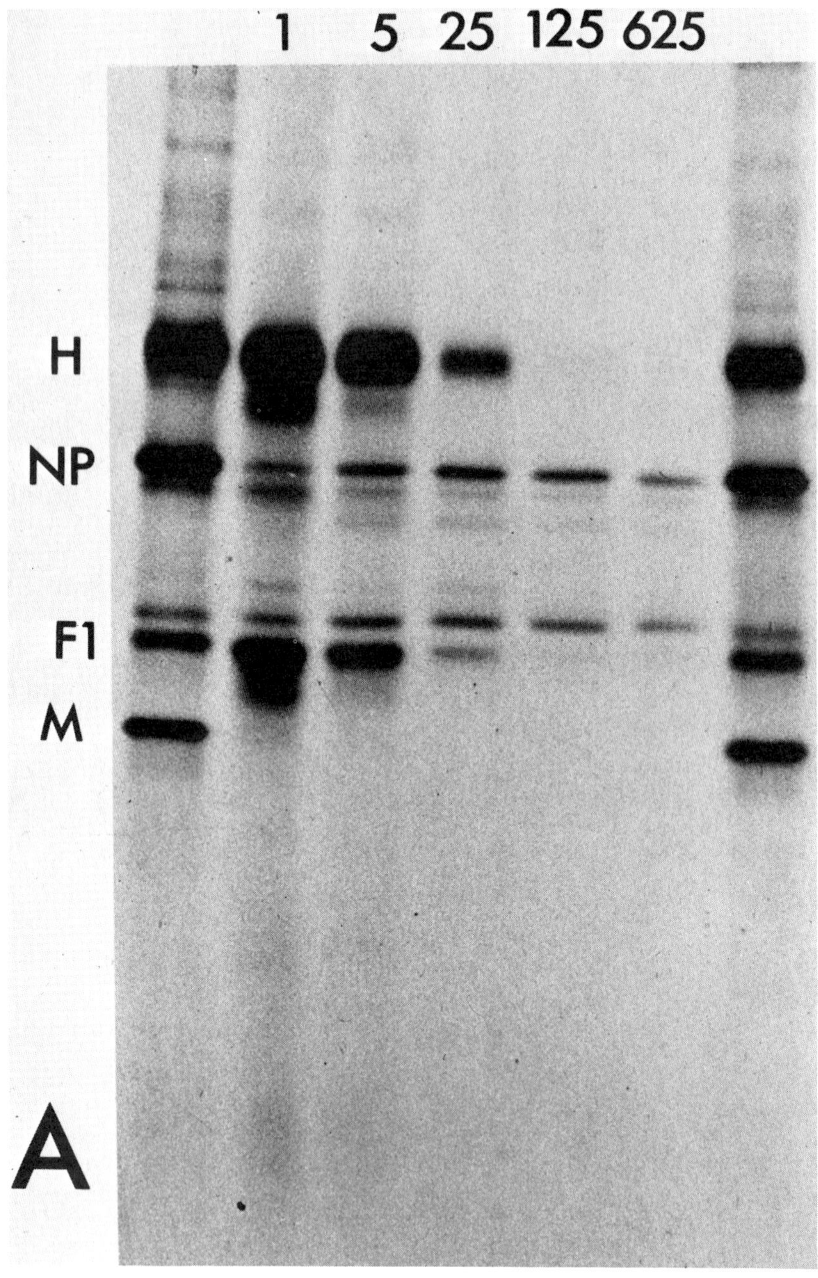

FIGURE 2. Radioimmune precipitation of measles virus polypeptides by sera collected from patients with (A) SSPE, (B) chronic active hepatitis, and (C) atypical measles. For explanation of markings see Fig. 1.

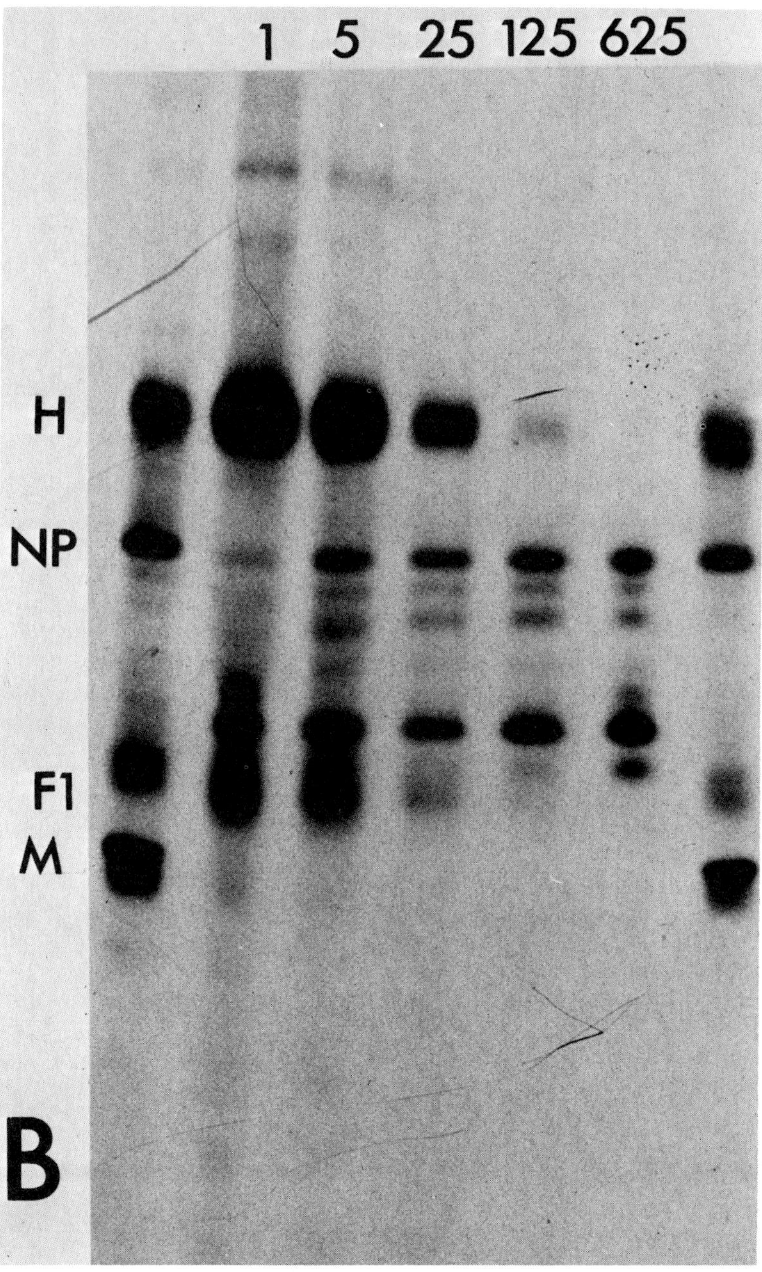

FIGURE 2 (*Continued*)

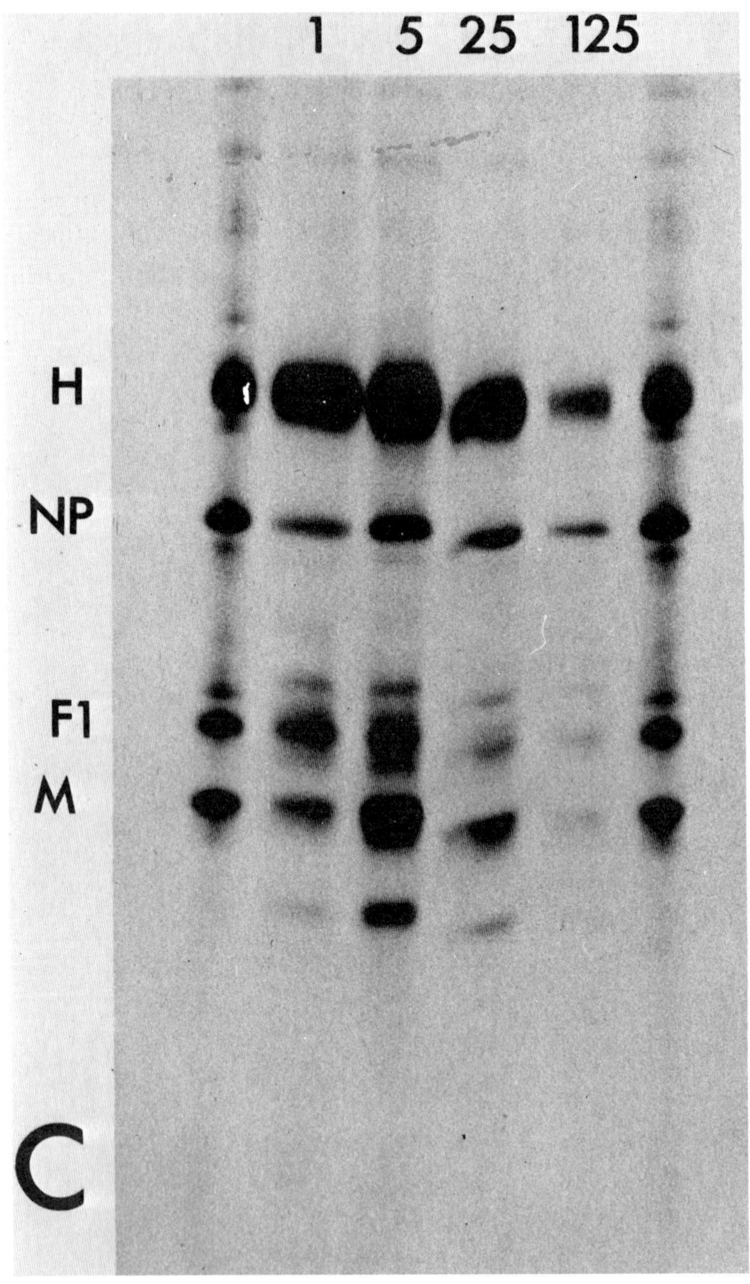

FIGURE 2 (*Continued*)

against NP and M antigens corresponded to, or in many cases were even lower than, those found in tests of early measles convalescent sera.

III. CHARACTERIZATION BY CF TESTS WITH PURIFIED VIRUS COMPONENTS OF THE OCCURRENCE OF ANTIBODIES TO NP AND M ANTIGENS IN DIFFERENT GROUPS OF PATIENTS AND IN HEALTHY INDIVIDUALS

There was good agreement between occurrence of NP and M antigen antibodies as determined by RIPA tests and by CF tests with purified antigens. However, antibodies to M antigen were more readily identified by the CF test than by the RIPA test, and in a few cases where no antibodies to M antigen were detected by the RIPA test, a moderate titer of M antigen-specific antibodies was found. This was interpreted to mean that the CF test allowed detection of antibodies to a larger spectrum of antigenic sites than the RIPA test (see Discussion). Table II gives a summary of data obtained in NP and M antigen CF tests.

After regular measles the antibody response to M antigen was weak, and in about half the cases no antibodies were detectable in late convalescent sera or in sera from patients with multiple sclerosis. Sera from five of six SSPE patients contained detectable M antigen antibodies but the titer was 10 times lower than the matching titer of CF antibody titer against NP antigen. Only two out of six sera from patients with chronic active hepatitis contained detectable CF antibodies against M antigen and the titers were 20 and 160. Relatively high titers of CF antibodies against M antigen were found in patients with atypical measles. The ratio of NP to M antigen CF antibody titers, as in the case of measles early convalescent sera, was about 4.

TABLE II. The Antibody Response to Measles Virus NP and M Antigen in Different Sets of Sera as Determined by CF Tests with Purified Antigens*

Set of serum samples	No. of sera	CF antibody titer in test with: NP antigen** range (mean value)	CF antibody titer in test with: M antigen** range (No. of positive samples; mean value)	Range of ratios of NP/M CF antibody titers
Measles early convalescent	10	40- 640 (260)	<10- 160 (9;68)	1 - >32
Measles late convalescent	14	<10- 640 (160)***	<10- 320 (8;-)****	1 - >32
Multiple sclerosis	6	20- 320 (110)	<10- 320 (1;-)	1 - >32
SSPE	6	80- 5,120 (450)	<10- 640 (5;46)	8 - >32
Chronic active hepatitis	6	1,280-20,480 (3800)	<10- 160 (2;-)	128 - >2,048
Atypical measles	5	640- 2,560 (2100)	80-2,560 (5;550)	2 - 32

* *Range and mean of antibody titers and range of ratios of CF antibody titers with the two antigens are given.*

** *The technique used for preparation of antigens is described in Tyrrell* et al. *(19).*

*** *12 of 16 sera contained detectable antibodies.*

**** *Mean value not calculated.*

IV. DISCUSSION

The two methods used for determination of antibodies against NP and M antigens gave results that were in good agreement, but the CF test appeared relatively more efficient for demonstration of the M antigen antibodies. Since the CF test in general has a low sensitivity compared to the RIPA test, this difference in efficacy for demonstration of M antigen antibodies is probably due to inherent limitations of the RIPA test. Several factors can be of importance in this context.

1. The relative labeling of different polypeptides with [^{35}S]methionine may vary due both to the relative amount of individual components produced and to the relative content of methionine. The degree of labeling influences their detectability after autoradiography of the electrophoretically separated polypeptides. In the present experiments antigen preparations labeled for a relatively long time (3 days) were used to allow maximal labeling of individual polypeptides. The effective labeling of M antigen was shown by the precipitation of this component by antibodies in sera from cases from acute and atypical measles.

2. The sensitivity to proteolytic breakdown varies for different structural polypeptides. The P component shows the highest sensitivity to proteolytic breakdown (4), and because of the long time used for labeling of antigens no P antigen antibodies were detected in this study. Also, the NP antigen is degraded to a certain extent by proteolytic enzymes, but antibodies to this component are readily detected by identification of uncleaved polypeptides and degradation products in the autoradiogram. The M component appears relatively resistent to proteolytic cleavage.

3. The overall number of antigenic sites in different components varies, and furthermore there may be a variation in sensitivity of different components to the denaturing effects of the treatment used to dissociate virus products in the cell lysate.

It seems likely that phenomena discussed under 3 may be of major importance in explaining differences in the capacity of RIPA and CF tests to detect antibodies against M antigen. Thus, M antigen may have both a relatively low number of antigenic sites, which could partly explain the limited and transient response to M antigen after a regular infection, and also a relatively higher susceptibility to denaturing effects of the lysis buffer than, for example, the NP antigen.

Whereas the RIPA test, in confirmation of results obtained by others (3, 9, 22), in most cases of SSPE did not detect M antigen antibodies, the CF test detected M antigen antibodies in five of six patients. However, the relative titer of antibodies to M antigen in relationship to antibodies to NP antigen is low compared with the relative occurrence of these antibodies in sera from patients with acute or atypical measles, emphasizing that there may be some defect in the production of M antigen in SSPE patients. This defect may be both quantitative, although a complete absence of M antigen production appears uncommon, and qualitative, with a change of certain antigenic sites on which reactivity in the RIPA test is dependent. Defective SSPE measles virus strains propagated *in vitro* have been shown to lack the capacity to produce M antigen (2, 7, 9).

A very limited antibody response to M antigen was found not only in serum samples from patients with SSPE but also in sera from patients with chronic active hepatitis. This was somewhat unexpected since increased titers of antibodies against measles virus as well as certain other viruses, for example, rubella, has been interpreted to signify that there is a general activation of Ig production in these patients. One would therefore anticipate that there should be a certain parallel between the rise in titers of antibodies against NP and M antigens. The fact that this is not the case could have either of two explanations. One possibility is that, similar to what has been proposed for SSPE, a defective measles virus infection is involved in chronic active hepatitis. This explanation appears less likely in view of the fact that the accentuated production of Ig does not concern only antibodies to measles virus. However, there are examples of a nonspecific activation of antibody production to one virus in connection with an intense immune response to another virus in the central nervous sytem (20), and further a transient production of autoantibodies is observed in connection with a regular measles infection [see Fagraeus *et al.* (1)]. The other possibility is that the primary antibody response to the M antigen is weak and poorly memorized and that therefore a polyclonal activation of B cells a long time after the primary infection might be less disposed to include an antibody response to M antigen.

The high titer antibody response to M antigen in patients with atypical measles is of interest. It shows that the M antigen produced during the acute infection in these patients can give an intense immunization. This immunization probably implies that the preceding immunization with inactivated measles vaccine also included a sensitization with M antigen, but it can also be true that the conditions of immune pathological reactions in patients with atypical measles enhances the immune response, including antibodies to the M antigen.

ACKNOWLEDGMENT

The technical assistance of Miss Anna Aleman and Miss Mariethe Ehnlund is gratefully acknowledged. This investigation was supported by a grant from the Swedish Medical Research Council (project No. B81-16X-00116-17A).

REFERENCES

1. Fagraeus, A., Tyrrell, D. L. J., Norberg, R., and Norrby, E. Actin filaments in paramyxovirus-infected human fibroblasts studied by indirect immunofluorescence. *Arch. Virol. (Engl. Ed.) 57*, 291-296 (1978).

2. Hall, W. W. and Choppin, P. W. Evidence for lack of synthesis of the M polypeptide of measles virus in brain cells in subacute sclerosing panencephalitis. *Virology 99*, 443-447 (1979).

3. Hall, W. W., Lamb, R. A., and Choppin, P. W. Measles and subacute sclerosing panencephalitis virus proteins: Lack of antibodies to the M protein in patients with subacute sclerosing panencephalitis. *Proc. Natl. Acad. Sci. U.S.A. 76*, 2047-2051 (1979).

4. Hall, W. W., Lamb, R. A., and Choppin, P. W. The polypeptides of canine distemper virus: Synthesis in infected cells and relatedness to the polypeptides of other morbilliviruses. *Virology 100*, 433-449 (1980).

5. Hayes, C. E., Gollobin, D. S., Machamer, E. C., Westfall, K. L., and Zweerink, J. H. Measles specific antibodies in sera and cerebrospinal fluids of patients with multiple sclerosis. *Infect. Immunol. 27*, 1033-1037 (1980).

6. Laitinen, O. and Vaheri, A. Very high measles and rubella virus antibody titers associated with hepatitis, systemic lupus erythematosus and infectious mononucleosis. *Lancet 1*, 194-198 (1974).

7. Lin, F. H. and Thomar, H. Absence of M protein in a cell-associated subacute sclerosing panencephalitis virus. *Nature (London) 285*, 490-492 (1980).

8. Machamer, C. E., Hayes, E. C., Gollobin, D. S., Westfall, K. L., and Zweerink, J. H. Antibodies against the measles matrix polypeptide after clinical infection and vaccination. *Infect. Immunol. 27*, 817-825 (1980).

9. Machamer, C. E., Hayes, E. C., and Zweering, J. H. Cells infected with a cell-associated subacute sclerosing panencephalitis virus do not express M protein. *Virology 108*, 515-520 (1981).

10. Mountcastle, W. E. and Choppin, P. W. A comparison of the polypeptides of four measles virus strains. *Virology 78*, 463-474 (1977).

11. Norrby, E. Viral antibodies in multiple sclerosis. *Prog. Med. Virol. 24*, 1-39 (1978).

12. Norrby, E. and Gollmar, Y. Appearance and persistence of antibodies against different virus components after regular measles infections. *Infect. Immunol. 6*, 240-247 (1972).

13. Norrby, E., Enders-Ruckle, G., and ter Meulen, V. Differences in the appearance of antibodies to structural components of measles virus after immunization with inactivated and live virus. *J. Infect. Dis. 132*, 262-269 (1975).

14. Örvell, C. and Norrby, E. Immunological and molecular relationships between homologous structural polypeptides of measles and canine distemper virus. *J. Gen. Virol. 50*, 231-245 (1980).

15. Stephenson, J. R. and ter Meulen, V. Antigenic relationships between measles and canine distemper virus: Comparison of immune response in animals and humans to individual virus-specific polypeptides. *Proc. Natl. Acad. Sci. U.S.A. 76*, 6601-6605 (1979).

16. ter Meulen, V., Katz, M., and Müller, D. Subacute sclerosing panencephalitis. *Curr. Top. Microbiol. Immunol. 57*, 1-38 (1972).

17. Togashi, T., Örvell, C., Vartdal, F., and Norrby, E. Production of antibodies against measles virions by use of the mouse hybridoma technique. *Arch. Virol. (Engl. Ed.) 67*, 149-157 (1981).

18. Tyrrell, D. L. J. and Norrby, E. Structural polypeptides of measles virus. *J. Gen. Virol. 29*, 219-229 (1978).

19. Tyrrell, D. L. J., Rafter, D. J., Örvell, C., and Norrby, E. Isolation and immunological characterization of the nucleocapsid and membrane proteins of measles virus. *J. Gen. Virol. 51*, 307-315 (1981).

20. Vandvik, B., Nilsen, R. E., Vartdal, F., and Norrby, E. Mumps meningitis: Specific and nonspecific antibody responses in the central nervous system. *Acta Neurol. Scand.* In press.

21. Vartdal, F., Vandvik, B., and Norrby, E. Viral and bacterial antibody response in multiple sclerosis. *Ann. Neurol. 8*, 248-255 (1980).

22. Wechsler, S. L., Weiner, H. L., and Fields, B. N. Immune response in subacute sclerosing panencephalitis: Reduced antibody response to the matrix protein of measles virus. *J. Immunol. 123*, 884-889 (1979).

Immunopathology: VIIIth International Symposium, 1980

MECHANISMS OF COMPLEMENT-DEPENDENT VIRAL NEUTRALIZATION[1]

Neil R. Cooper
Deborah P. Beebe
Glen R. Nemerow

Department of Molecular Immunology,
Research Institute of Scripps Clinic,
La Jolla, California

I. INTRODUCTION

The complex, well-integrated immunologic network has evolved to cope with the great diversity of potential pathogens. Viruses represent a major category of such infectious agents and are probably largely responsible for driving the components of the immune system to ever greater diversity through evolution. On first exposure, defense against virus infection is largely nonimmunologic and includes phagocytic cells, natural killer cells, and possibly also, as indicated below, the complement system, and natural or cross-reacting

[1]*This is publication number 2401 from the Research Institute of Scripps Clinic. This work was supported by Grants AI-07007, CA-14692, and 1-S07-RR05514 from the National Institutes of Health.*

ISBN 0-12-218320-7

antibody, originally stimulated by other agents. Since viruses are potent immunogens, on subsequent exposure viruses and virus-infected cells encounter a formidable array of humoral and cellular defense mechanisms. These include antibodies, the complement system, phagocytic cells, and various effector lymphocytes which act individually and collaboratively to neutralize or destroy viruses and virus-infected cells. Nevertheless, viruses frequently elude these formidable defenses, become established, and directly or indirectly cause a number of acute and chronic diseases. As replicating agents, they have the potential to amplify their pathogenic effects. Furthermore, a number of types of viruses may become latent in cells by any of several mechanisms and reappear at a later time with resulting disease. One important goal of contemporary immunopathology is the elucidation on a molecular basis of the interactions of viruses and virus-infected cells with the various humoral and cellular defense mechanisms. Such basic knowledge is essential to the understanding of the many facets of virus infection and is necessary for devising rational approaches to effective therapy for chronic virus diseases.

This contribution focuses exclusively on interactions of free viruses with the primary constituents of the humoral immune system, antibody (Ab) and the complement system (C). The various mechanisms by which these reactants inactivate viruses are discussed. Also considered in several model systems is the evidence that these humoral factors may function to inactivate viruses on first exposure.

II. ASPECTS OF VIRUS STRUCTURE

Certain aspects of virus structure as related to interactions with humoral elements will be briefly considered. Viruses contain nucleic acid and proteins which perform various functions in viral replication. The nucleic acid and protein core, or nucleocapsid, are surrounded by a protein coat, termed the capsid, which is made up of multiple copies of protein molecules. Many viruses also contain an outer envelope composed of lipid and glycolipid molecules arranged in bilayer configuration which is acquired in the process of budding through the host cell membrane. Accordingly, the lipid and carbohydrate composition of the external membrane of enveloped viruses largely reflects that of the cell of origin of the virus. In addition however, projecting through or situated on the surface of the lipid bilayer of enveloped viruses are multiple copies of one or more proteins which are encoded by the viral genome. Most host cell proteins are excluded from areas of cellular membranes where viruses bud, although reduced concentrations of certain host cell proteins are often also found. The external, exposed proteins are frequently glycosylated, which renders enveloped viruses hydrophilic.

It is obvious that humoral elements as well as cellular defense mechanisms are only effective if directed against external structural features of the virus. Thus, the recognition structure and also the target for such effector mechanisms are the surface viral proteins since these are the only exposed viral encoded structures.

III. FEATURES OF ANTIBODY AND COMPLEMENT REACTION SEQUENCES IMPORTANT FOR VIRUS NEUTRALIZATION

A. *Antibody*

Specific Ab directed against surface viral structures essential for attachment and/or penetration of susceptible cells obviously effectively neutralizes infectivity and prevents spread of viral infection even though the virions in such complexes are not irreversibly inactivated. Ab attached to surface viral structures that are not essential for viral attachment to cells may also neutralize if sufficient numbers of molecules bind to alter the surface characteristics of the virus so as to prevent attachment. The multivalent nature of immunoglobulin molecules and the repeating array of antigens on the viral surfaces facilitates the formation of Ab-virus aggregates.

Most antibodies in complex with antigen have the ability to fix C, i.e., to activate the complement system. The effects of the activated complement system on viral neutralization are considered in detail in Section IV.

B. *Complement*

The complement system, which consists of more than 20 distinct plasma proteins, is a major mediator of inflammatory processes *in vivo*. Activation of the C system triggers an orderly, carefully regulated series of interactions between the C proteins. The reactions of the C factors or components with one another and with membranes generate the mediators and biological activities of the C system. The system is generally entered by triggering one of the two activation pathways. Each of the activation pathways, which are termed the classical and the alternative or properdin pathways,

COMPLEMENT REACTION UNITS

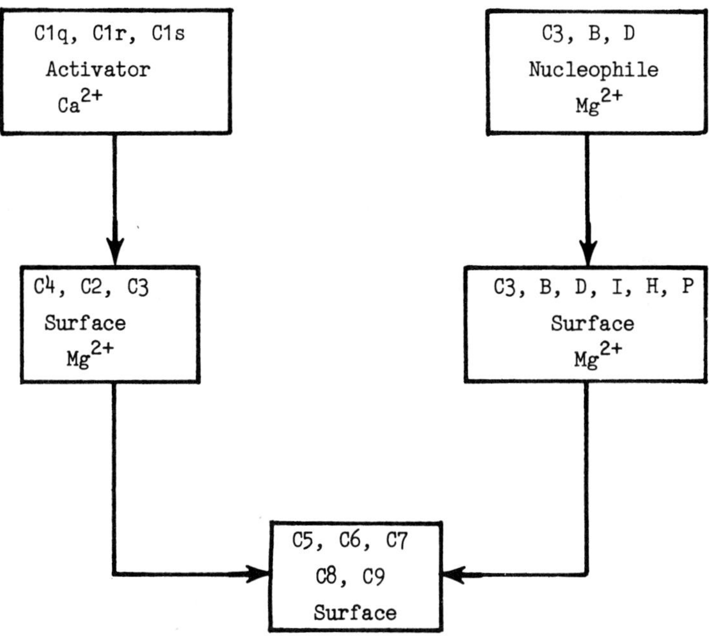

FIGURE 1. Schematic representation of the complement pathways.

consists of a series of enzyme-substrate interactions which lead to the generation of a complex multicomponent enzyme which cleaves C3 and subsequently C5 (Fig. 1). The terminal portion of the complement reaction sequence, which is common to both pathways, involves the assembly of a large multimolecular complex termed the membrane attack complex. After cleavage of C5 by the enzymes of the classical or alternative pathway, this complex self-assembles. The membrane attack complex in nascent form has the ability to insert into and damage cellular membranes.

There are three phases of the C reaction sequence that are particularly relevant for interactions with viruses. These are (a) the activation step, during which the classical or alternative pathways are activated by viruses or virus-antibody complexes; (b) the step involving C3; and (c) the membrane attack phase.

IgG or IgM antibodies in complex with viruses activate the first component of the classical pathway in the same manner as do other immune complexes. The repeating array of viral external proteins probably facilitates the formation of the clusters of IgG molecules in close proximity required for C1 activation. The activation process is initiated by the binding of the first complement component C1 through its C1q subunit to a site(s) located in the Fc region of immunoglobulin molecules. This is followed by several steps within the C1 molecule which lead to the conversion of two zymogens into proteolytic enzymes. One of these, termed C1s, then hydrolyzes the next two reacting factors, C4 and C2, and mediates their assembly into a proteolytic enzyme which cleaves C3 and, subsequently, C5. Recently, it has become apparent that the classical pathway can be activated in the complete absence of Ab by a number of substances of different chemical and physical structures. These include lipid A-rich lipopolysaccharides (8, 17), monosodium urate crystals (11), C-reactive protein (7, 14), polyanions and polycations (27), certain membranes and lipid vesicles (2, 23), and type-C RNA tumor viruses or retroviruses (4, 9). In these instances the first C component interacts directly with the activator. In such reactions the C1 molecule fulfills the recognition function normally associated with the Ab molecule. In the case of retroviruses, the activator is a 15,000-dalton surface protein, p15E (4). It is not yet clear whether activation proceeds by exactly the same process in this case. Nevertheless, once initiated on the retroviral surface, the C sequence may proceed to completion and result in lysis and therefore irreversible inactivation of the virus (4, 9, 32).

The alternative pathway is activated in a different manner. It is initiated following cleavage of C3 in the fluid phase by any of several enzymes. The responsible enzyme is probably composed of factor B, factor D, and C3 modified by interaction with a nucleophile to assume a C3b-like structure. A proportion of C3b molecules generated by this cleavage reaction deposits on surfaces in the vicinity of the cleaving enzyme. On most such surfaces this C3b is rapidly degraded by the control protein C3b inactivator (I) and β1H (H). On surfaces termed activators, the C3b is protected from degradation. The chemical structures involved in this protection phenomenon and the molecular nature of the process involved are not yet completely understood. Structures that present such surfaces are widespread in nature and include certain kinds of membranes, complex carbohydrates, and glycolipids. C3b on such protected surfaces interacts with factors B and D to form an enzyme that cleaves additional C3, thus generating more C3b, some of which also deposits on the surface. This enzyme is stabilized by attachment of a protein termed properdin (P). This process efficiently amplifies the reaction sequence and triggers the membrane attack complex in close proximity to the target cell membrane. A role for the alternative or properdin pathway in virus neutralization was first suggested in reports of studies by Wedgwood *et al.* (30). These workers found that the properdin system, now known as the alternative pathway, was responsible for neutralization of Newcastle disease virus (NDV). There have been few recent studies employing contemporary technology of possible direct viral neutralization, although Welsh (31) confirmed that NDV could be neutralized by human serum through the alternative pathway. Similarly, Hirsh *et al.* (13) have found that Sindbis virus can also directly activate the alternative C pathway. These studies suggest that some viruses are able to bind C3b and provide the protective surface required for alternative pathway activation.

Thus, viruses in conjunction with specific Ab can activate the classical pathway; and, in addition, certain viruses can directly activate the classical or the alternative pathway without the participation of Ab. After activation the C reaction sequence proceeds on the viral capsid or envelope.

The second phase of the C reaction sequence particularly important for virus neutralization is the C3 activation step. C3 is activated by cleavage of the molecule into a minor fragment C3a, a potent mediator that will not be considered here, and a major fragment C3b. This cleavage is normally accomplished by C enzymes. As noted earlier, a proportion of the C3b molecules thus generated arrives on the surface of nearby membranes and particles. Since many molecules of C3 may be cleaved by the C3 activating enzymes and C3 is also the complement protein present in highest concentration in the serum, large numbers of C3b molecules may become bound. This reaction sequence is particularly efficient when the activating enzyme is surface bound, as for example, on viral envelopes. In Berry and Almeida's electron micrographic studies of avian infectious bronchitis virus, the thick additional enveloping layer of protein following complement addition to antibody-sensitized virus undoubtedly represents deposited C3b (6). It is not difficult to visualize how such a blanket of protein would interfere with the ability of the virus to attach to potentially susceptible cells.

The third phase of the reaction sequence particularly relevant for viral neutralization is the action of the membrane attack complex. As noted earlier, this complex can only bind to lipid-containing membranes and only such membranes are susceptible to C-mediated lytic damage. Lysis of enveloped viruses by the membrane attack complex differs little from lysis of other cells except that viruses generally do not contain free protein and so there is not a contribution of colloid osmotic lysis to the lytic process. Nevertheless C very effectively disassembles the lipid bilayer membrane of many kinds of enveloped viruses leading to exposure of the nucleocapsid, which may be digested by various serum enzymes. Regardless of whether or not they are degraded, such exposed nucleocapsids are usually not infectious. Various workers have analyzed the events occurring during lysis of enveloped viruses. Welsh *et al.* (33) examined sections of lymphocytic choriomeningitis virus incubated with Ab and C and showed thickening and separation of the envelope from the nucleocapsid, loss of bilayer structure, and decreased density of the nucleocapsid, suggesting degradation. Numerous other electron microscopic studies of negatively stained enveloped viruses incubated with Ab and C (1, 3, 12, 28) also reveal thickening and the presence of membrane lesions now known to represent the membrane attack complex. Studies employing other approaches have shown that C-dependent lysis of enveloped viruses leads to release of the nucleocapsid, internal enzymes, or other proteins (22, 24, 26, 28, 29, 32, 33).

IV. HUMORAL MECHANISMS OF VIRUS NEUTRALIZATION

There are three basic mechanisms by which Ab, Ab and C, or C alone can neutralize viruses. First, these reactants may induce viral aggregation which reduces the net number of infectious particles and thus diminishes infectivity. Second, Ab and/or C binding may envelope viruses in a blanket of protein which interferes with attachment, adsorption, or penetration. Third, complement may alter viral structure. The first two of these mechanisms can occur with either Ab, C, or the two reactants together, whereas the latter process is restricted to C. Also, in the first two mechanisms, the virus is not irreversibly destroyed.

A. Aggregation

The ability of antibody to aggregate viruses has been observed and studied by many workers. Many, although not all types of virions can be aggregated by antibody *in vitro*. An example comes from studies of a nonenveloped virus, polyoma (21). Increasing amounts of IgG antibody increase the sedimentation rate of the virus in sucrose density in distinct increments. With binding of approximately 2 antibody molecules per virus the sedimentation rate increased from 242 to 260 S (Fig. 2). An Ab:virus ratio of 10:1 increased the sedimentation rate to 350 S whereas an Ab:virus ratio of 20:1 was characterized by a 410 S sedimentation rate (Fig. 2). Electron microscopic examination of the reaction mixtures showed viral aggregates. Polyoma virus was directly neutralized by the larger doses of antibody (10:1 and 20:1) but not by the lower dose (2:1).

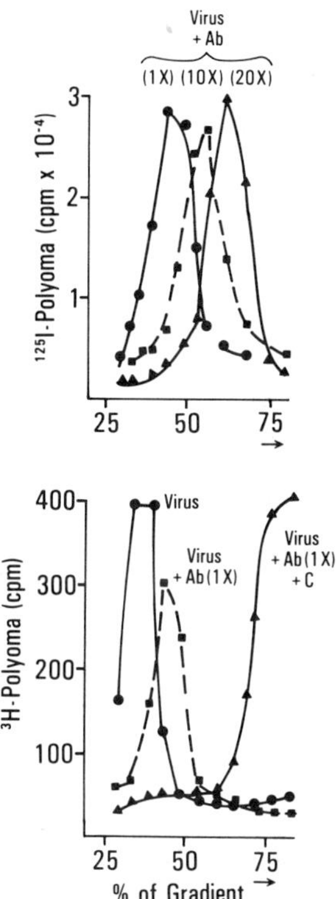

FIGURE 2. Sucrose density gradient ultracentrifugal analysis of interactions of IgG antipolyoma Ab and C with polyoma virus. In the upper panel the sedimentation characteristics of ^{125}I-labeled polyoma virus bearing 2 (1X), 10 (10X), or 20 (20X) molecules of bound IgG-Ab per virion incubated with C (Ab1x + C) are shown.

Polyoma virus sensitized with the lower dose of Ab was not neutralized. Complete neutralization, however, occurred on addition of C to the virus-Ab complex (21). As anticipated from the fact that polyoma is not an enveloped virus, complement did not potentiate neutralization by inducing lysis (21). Rate zonal ultracentrifugal studies with labeled virus revealed that C greatly increased the sedimentation rate of the virus sensitized with the lowest dose of Ab (Fig. 2). This phenomenon of C-induced aggregation was further investigated to determine the C components involved. It was found that either Clq or C3b produced C-mediated aggregation of the Ab-coated polyoma virus particles (21). The ability of Clq to aggregate was not unexpected since Clq is a multivalent molecule able to bind at least six IgG molecules. Although C3b has multiple functional sites related to its various activities, there is no evidence that either the labile binding site utilized in binding to membranes or the site involved in C3b receptor functions is multivalent; thus, C3b-dependent aggregation remains unexplained. No other virus has been demonstrated to be aggregated by C.

Antibody-dependent aggregation can be readily demonstrated *in vitro* when appropriate concentrations of reactants are mixed. Aggregation is not, however, an invariable consequence of the incubation of Ab with virus. The occurrence of aggregation depends on the class, affinity, and concentration of Ab, on the concentration of virus, and on the exposure, concentration, and spatial distribution of antigen subunits on the viral surface. Ab-dependent aggregation is probably an infrequent occurrence *in vivo* because of the restricted combinations of Ab and virus which lead to aggregation, and in particular, the simultaneous requirements for relatively high virus concentrations and for relatively low concentrations of avid Ab.

B. *Envelopment*

A second process leading to viral neutralization is envelopment by Ab and/or C protein. Numerous viruses are probably neutralized in this manner. Among the viruses studied is avian infectious bronchitis virus which can be significantly neutralized by certain antibodies alone (6). Electron microscopic studies of such mixtures showed a halo of protein up to 30 nm surrounding the virus. As studied by Berry and Almeida, the addition of C, particularly nonlytic avian C, to Ab-sensitized virus increased the visualized halo of protein from 30 to 70 nm (6). C also potentiated neutralization in these studies. Herpes simplex virus (HSV), studied by Daniels *et al.* (10), was found to be neutralized by IgM Ab together with only the first two reacting (Cl and C4) or first four reacting (Cl, C2, C3, and C4) components of the C system. Such combinations are nonlytic. Since Notkins *et al.* found that C does not aggregate HSV (20), C apparently neutralizes the virus by envelopment by protein, particularly C3b and C4b. Newcastle disease virus (16), equine arteritis virus (25), and vesicular stomatitis virus (15) are all neutralized by immune Ab and C by nonlytic mechanisms involving Cl, C2, C3, and C4. In further studies we found VSV (5) to be neutralized by a normal human serum reagent containing a naturally occurring IgM antibody present in all normal human sera thus far tested and Cl, C2, C3, and C4 (Table I). Neutralization did not occur if the IgM Ab or any of the C components were omitted.

TABLE I. Neutralization of VSV by Normal Human IgM, Cl, C2, C3, and C4

VSV treatment*	$-\log_{10}$ pfu/ml change in titer
IgM	0
IgM + Cl	0
IgM + Cl + C4	0
IgM + Cl + C2 + C4	0
IgM + Cl + C2 + C3 + C4	2.0
Buffer + Cl + C2 + C3 + C4	0

**Cl was at one tenth, IgM at one fifth, and C2, C3, and C4 were at normal serum concentrations.*

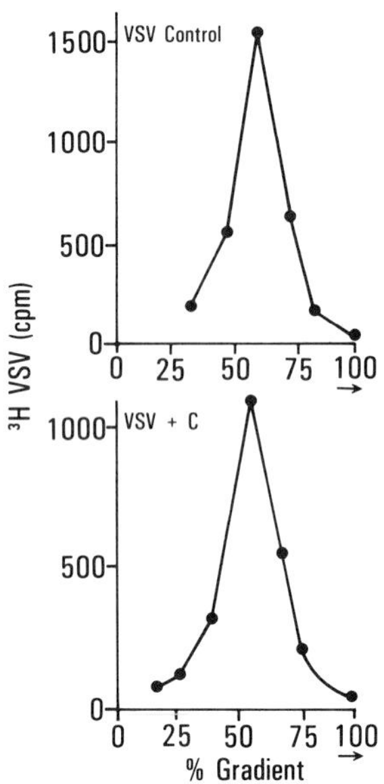

FIGURE 3. Sucrose density gradient ultracentrifugal analysis of [^{3}H]VSV (upper panel) and [^{3}H]VSV incubated with a human serum reagent lacking C5 (lower panel).

Neutralization thus required completion of the C sequence through the C3 step. Since no evidence for IgM- or C-dependent aggregation of VSV was obtained in these studies (Fig. 3), it is highly probable that neutralization was secondary to envelopment by C protein. Consistent with this interpretation was the direct demonstration of presence of C3b on the viral envelope (5). It is likely that each of these viruses is neutralized by a blanket of protein.

C. *Lysis*

C-dependent viral lysis leads to loss of viral structure and irreversible inactivation. Two principal approaches have been employed to show viral lysis. The first of these, electron microscopy, has revealed numerous changes in C-lysed viruses. These include characteristic, roughly circular lesions with a diameter of approximately 100 nm, now known to represent the bound C5b-9 membrane attack complex. Other changes indicative of lysis are envelope destruction, stripping of the envelope from the nucleocapsid, and various changes in the staining characteristics of the nucleocapsid, probably indicating nucleic acid degradation. An example of this approach is found in our studies of Ab- and C-dependent lysis of purified Epstein-Barr virus (19) as shown in Fig. 4. With Ab addition (a high titered Ab from a patient with nasopharyngeal carcinoma) the virus became coated with an amorphous electron dense material approximately 25 nm in thickness. With the addition of C, thickening of the envelope, dramatic separation of the envelope from the nucleocapsid and varying stages of disintegration of the viral nucleoid were seen (Fig. 4).

The second general approach has been to demonstrate that viral nucleic acid or internal proteins, enzymes or other constitutents are released after Ab and/or C action. Most commonly used has been release of radiolabeled nucleic acid. Release has most frequently been demonstrated by density gradient ultracentrifugation. An example of this approach, also from our recent studies (19) with Epstein-Barr virus (EBV), is found in Fig. 5. Purified EBV, internally labeled with tritium, sedimented as a discrete peak in the middle of the dextran gradient. After addition of high titered Ab from a patient with nasopharyngeal carcinoma, the virus was found on the bottom of dextran density gradients (not shown). After addition of DNase and fresh serum as a C source, viral nucleic acid was released from the virus and found on the top of the gradient (Fig. 5). DNase was necessary to demonstrate lysis of EBV in this manner, for in its absence, the viral DNA was found on the bottom of the gradients, exactly as was observed on addition of Ab alone (19). DNase had no effect on the EBV and Ab samples unless C was also added.

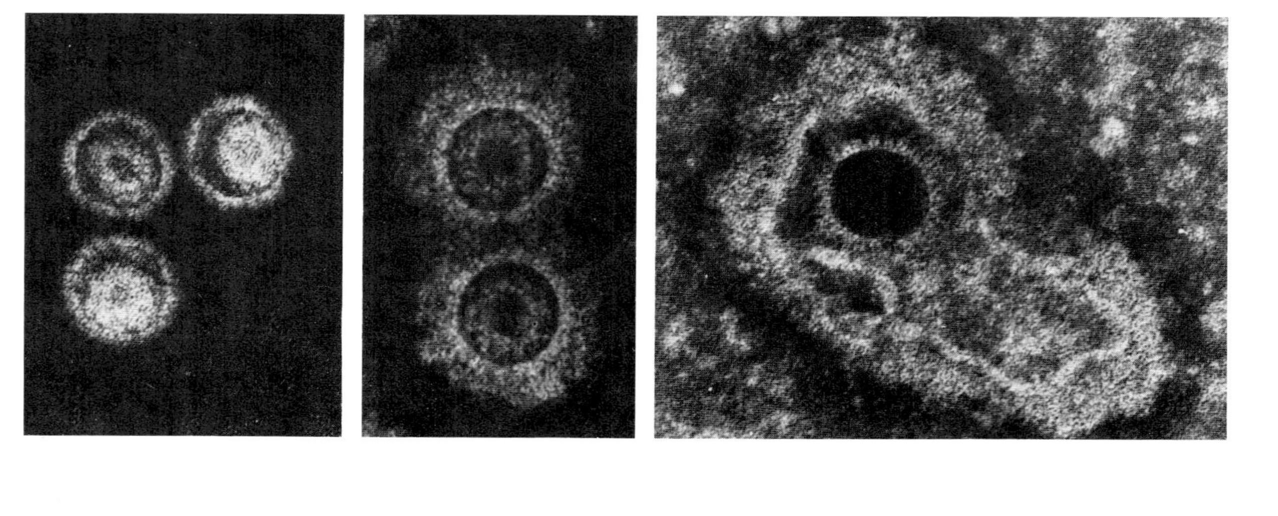

FIGURE 4. Electron microscopic examination of interactions of EBV with Ab and C. EBV was examined alone (left panel), and after interaction with immune IgG Ab (center panel) or with immune IgG Ab and C (right panel).

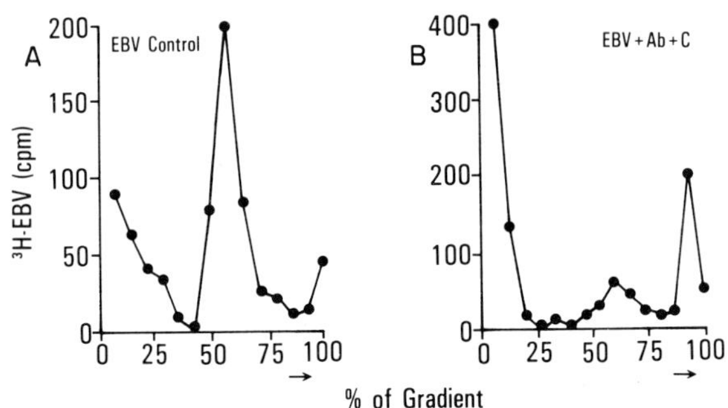

FIGURE 5. A: Dextran density gradient ultracentrifugal analysis of ^{3}H-labeled EBV. B: ^{3}H-labeled EBV incubated with immune IgG-Ab, C, and DNase.

The above techniques have been used to show that numerous enveloped viruses are lysed by specific antiviral Ab in conjunction with C. These include EBV (19), retroviruses (22), avian infectious bronchitis virus (1, 6), equine arteritis virus (24, 26), influenza virus (1), Newcastle disease virus (3), rubella virus (28), sendai virus (12), sindbis virus (29), and vesicular stomatitis virus (15, 18).

Some viruses are lysed by C without the participation of Ab. Welsh *et al.* (32) first noted that multiple retroviruses were lysed by normal human serum not containing Ab. Multiple techniques including electron microscopy and the release of labeled nucleic acid, reverse transcriptase, and the internal core protein have been used to demonstrate lysis (32). A number of approaches have definitively ruled out the presence of Ab, including ultimately, experiments in which purified virus was shown to interact with and activate highly purified immunoglobulin-free components of the C system (9). The viral surface protein has been isolated and demonstrated to be a 15,000-dalton protein (4). In isolated form it possesses the ability to bind and activate C1 and thus trigger the C system.

In this system the first complement component C1, fulfills the recognition role normally associated with the Ab molecule.

V. SUMMARY

This chapter has focused exclusively on serum-dependent mechanisms of viral neutralization. Such mechanisms are likely to play a major role in preventing reinfection and in limiting dissemination of viral infections through the blood stream and lymphatic system. The ability of naturally occurring or cross-reacting Ab together with the C system and with the C system alone to directly neutralize certain viruses suggests a role for humoral immunity on first encounter with a virus. Three processes resulting in neutralization have been considered. Viral aggregation leads to neutralization as a result of a reduction in the net number of infectious particles, although individual virions in such aggregates are not irreversibly inactivated. Antibody alone, or in rare instances C alone, can mediate neutralization; however, the requirements for high virus concentrations together with low concentrations of avid Ab make aggregation an unlikely mechanism of viral neutralization to be important *in vivo*.

A second process leading to neutralization is envelopment with protein. Either Ab or C may, under appropriate circumstances, contribute a blanket of protein which prevents viruses from attaching to and/or entering a potentially susceptible cell. A number of viruses have been found to be neutralized by Ab or by Ab and only a portion of the C reaction sequence. Since aggregation has not been observed in these instances and since such combinations of C components are nonlytic, neutralization presumably results from an enveloping coat of Ab or of Ab and C4b and C3b protein.

The third mechanism is C-dependent lysis. Only enveloped viruses are susceptible to lytic attack by C, which results in irreversible inactivation. Most enveloped viruses thus far examined can be lysed by the C system. Viral lysis by the membrane attack complex is quite similar to that observed with many cells except for the lack of an osmotic gradient. Various stages of thickening of the lipid bilayer, probably due to insertion of the membrane attack complex, stripping of the envelope from the nucleocapsid, and degradation of nucleic acid have been visualized. Studies have also revealed release of internal enzymes and nucleic acid, often in a degraded state after C action.

The focus of this chapter has thus been on humoral mechanisms of virus neutralization which are important in preventing infection and reinfection. Indications that these systems may operate in some instances prior to development of acquired immunity have been noted. However, it is important to appreciate that the humoral mechanisms described here are only one facet of a very complex and balanced interrelationship between humoral and cellular antiviral defense systems. The ultimate understanding of the interplay between these systems with each type of virus infection requires a detailed appreciation of each constituent system. The emphasis on humoral mechanisms in this chapter must be considered in this context.

REFERENCES

1. Almeida, J. D. and Waterson, A. P. The morphology of virus-antibody interaction. *Adv. Virus Res. 15*, 307 (1969).

2. Alving, C. R. and Guirguis, A. A. Cholesterol-dependent human complement activation resulting in damage to liposomal model membranes. *J. Immunol. 118*, 342 (1977).

3. Apostolov, K. and Sawa, M. I. Enhancement of haemolysis of Newcastle disease virus (NDV) after pretreatment with heterophile antibody and complement. *J. Gen. Virol. 33*, 459 (1976).

4. Bartholomew, R. M., Esser, A. F., and Müller-Eberhard, H. J. Lysis of oncornaviruses by human serum: Isolation of the viral complement (C1) receptor and identification as p15E. *J. Exp. Med. 147*, 844 (1977).

5. Beebe, D. P. and Cooper, N. R. Neutralization of vesicular stomatitis virus (VSV) by human complement requires a natural IgM antibody present in human serum. *J. Immunol. 126*, 1562 (1981).

6. Berry, D. M. and Almeida, J. D. The morphological and biological effects of various antisera on avian infectious bronchitis virus. *J. Gen. Virol. 3*, 97 (1968).

7. Claus, D. R., Siegel, J., Petras, K., Osmand, A. P. and Gewurz, H. Interactions of C-reactive protein with the first component of human complement. *J. Immunol. 119*, 187 (1977).

8. Cooper, N. R. and Morrison, D. C. Binding and activation of the first component of human complement by the lipid A region of lipopolysaccharides. *J. Immunol. 120*, 1862 (1978).

9. Cooper, N. R., Jensen, F. C., Welsh, R. M., Jr., and Oldstone, M. B. A. Lysis of RNA tumor viruses by human serum: Direct antibody independent triggering of the classical complement pathway. *J. Exp. Med. 144*, 970 (1976).

10. Daniels, C. A., Borsos, T., Snyderman, R., and Notkins, A. L. Neutralization of sensitized virus by the fourth component of complement. *Science 165*, 508 (1969).

11. Giclas, P. C., Ginsberg, M. H., and Cooper, N. R. Immunoglobulin G independent activation of the classical complement pathway by monosodium urate crystals. *J. Clin. Invest. 63*, 759 (1979).

12. Haukenes, G. Demonstration of host antigens in the myxovirus membrane: Lysis of virus by antibody and complement. *Acta Pathol. Microbiol. Scand., Sect. B 85*, 125 (1977).

13. Hirsch, R. L., Winkelstein, J. A., and Griffin, D. E. The role of complement in viral infections. III. Activation of the classical and alternative complement pathways by Sindbis virus. *J. Immunol. 124*, 2507 (1980).

14. Kaplan, M. H. and Volanakis, J. E. Interaction of C-reactive protein complexes with the complement system. I. Consumption of human complement associated with the reaction of C-reactive protein with pneumococcal C-polysaccharide and with the choline phosphatides, lecithin and sphingomyelin. *J. Immunol. 112*, 2135 (1974).

15. Leddy, J. P., Simons, R. L., and Douglas, R. G. Effect of selective complement deficiency on the rate of neutralization of enveloped viruses by human sera. *J. Immunol. 118*, 28 (1977).

16. Linscott, W. D. and Levinson, W. E. Complement components required for virus neutralization by early immunoglobulin antibody. *Proc. Natl. Acad. Sci. U.S.A. 64*, 520 (1969).

17. Loos, M., Bitter-Suerman, D., and Dierich, M. Interaction of the first (C1) and second (C2) and fourth (C4) components of complement with different preparations of bacterial lipopolysaccharides and with lipid A. *J. Immunol. 112*, 935 (1974).

18. Mills, B. J., Beebe, D. P., and Cooper, N. R. Antibody-independent neutralization of vesicular stomatitis virus by human complement. II. Formation of VSV-lipoprotein complexes in human serum and complement-dependent viral lysis. *J. Immunol. 123*, 2518 (1979).

19. Nemerow, G. R. and Cooper, N. R. Isolation of Epstein-Barr virus and studies of its neutralization by human IgG and complement. *J. Immunol. 127*, 272 (1981).

20. Notkins, A. L., Rosenthal, J., and Johnson, B. Rate-zonal centrifugation of herpes simplex virus-antibody complexes. *Virology 43*, 321 (1971).

21. Oldstone, M. B. A., Cooper, N. R., and Larson, D. L. Formation and biologic role of polyoma-antibody complexes: A critical role for complement. *J. Exp. Med. 140*, 549 (1974).

22. Orozlan, S. and Gilden, R. V. Immune virolysis: Effect of antibody and complement on C-type RNA virus. *Science 168*, 1478 (1970).

23. Pinckard, R. N., Olson, M. S., Kelley, R. E., DeHeer, D. H., Palmer, J. D., O'Rourke, R. A., and Goldfein, S. Antibody-independent activation of human Cl after interaction with heart subcellular membranes. *J. Immunol. 110*, 1376 (1973).

24. Radwan, A. I., Burger, D., and Davis, W. C. The fate of sensitized equine arteritis virus following neutralization by complement or anti-IgG serum. *Virology 53*, 372 (1973).

25. Radwan, A. I. and Burger, D. The complement-requiring neutralization of equine arteritis virus by late antisera. *Virology 51*, 71 (1973).

26. Radwan, A. I. and Crawford, T. B. The mechanisms of neutralization of sensitized equine arteritis virus by complement components. *J. Gen. Virol. 25*, 229 (1974).

27. Rent, R., Ertel, N., Eisenstein, R., and Gewurz, H. Complement activation by interaction of polyanions and polycations. I. Heparin-protamine induced consumption of complement. *J. Immunol. 114*, 120 (1975).

28. Schluederberg, A., Ajello, C., and Evans, B. Fate of rubella genome ribonucleic acid after immune and nonimmune virolysis in the presence of ribonuclease. *Infect. Immunol. 14*, 1097 (1976).

29. Stollar, V. Immune lysis of Sindbis virus. *Virology 66*, 620 (1975).

30. Wedgwood, R. J., Ginsberg, H. S., and Pillemer, L. The properdin system and immunity. VI. The inactivation of Newcastle disease virus by the properdin system. *J. Exp. Med. 104*, 107 (1956).

31. Welsh, R. M., Jr. Host cell modification of lymphocytic choriomeningitis virus and Newcastle disease virus altering viral inactivation by human complement. *J. Immunol. 118*, 348 (1977).

32. Welsh, R. M., Jr., Cooper, N. R., Jensen, F. C., and Oldstone, M. B. A. Human serum lyses RNA tumor viruses. *Nature (London) 257*, 612 (1975).

33. Welsh, R. M., Jr., Lampert, P. W., Burner, P. A., and Oldstone, M. B. A. Antibody complement interactions with purified lymphocytic choriomeningitis virus. *Virology 73*, 59 (1976).

Index

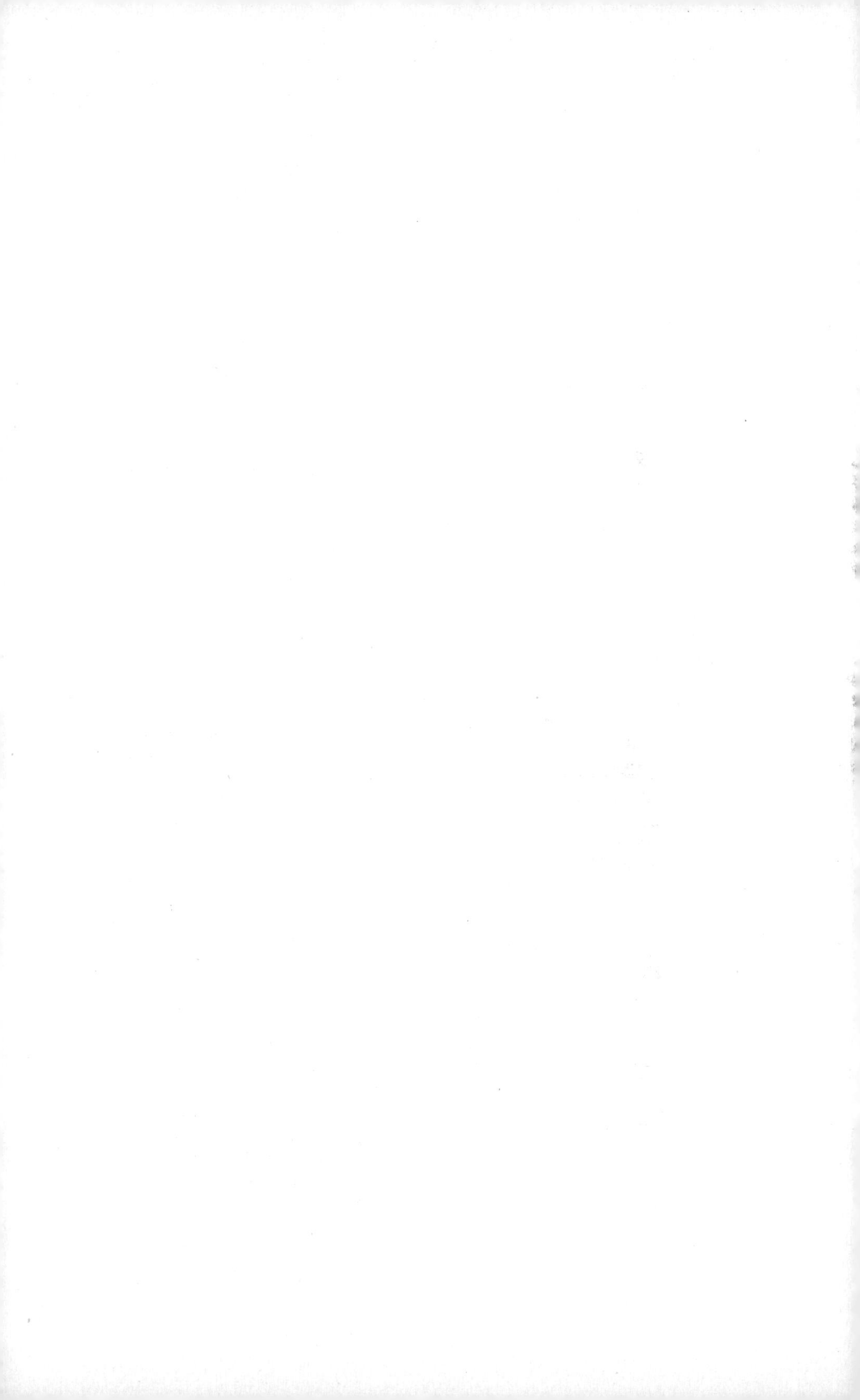